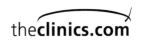
theclinics.com

EMERGENCY MEDICINE CLINICS OF NORTH AMERICA

Geriatric Emergency Medicine

GUEST EDITORS
Brendan Magauran, MD, MBA,
Joseph H. Kahn, MD, and
Jonathan S. Olshaker, MD, FACEP

CONSULTING EDITOR
Amal Mattu, MD, FAAEM, FACEP

May 2006 • Volume 24 • Number 2

SAUNDERS
An Imprint of Elsevier, Inc.
PHILADELPHIA   LONDON   TORONTO   MONTREAL   SYDNEY   TOKYO

W.B. SAUNDERS COMPANY
A Division of Elsevier Inc.

1600 John F. Kennedy Boulevard, Suite 1800 • Philadelphia, Pennsylvania 19103-2899

http://www.theclinics.com

EMERGENCY MEDICINE CLINICS
OF NORTH AMERICA
May 2006
Editor: Karen Sorensen

Volume 24, Number 2
ISSN 0733-8627
ISBN 1-4160-3614-8

Reprints. For copies of 100 or more, of articles in this publication, please contact the Commercial Reprints Department, Elsevier Inc., 360 Park Avenue South, New York, New York 10010-1710. Tel. (212) 633-3813; Fax: (212) 462-1935; e-mail: reprints@elsevier.com.

The ideas and opinions expressed in *Emergency Medicine Clinics of North America* do not necessarily reflect those of the Publisher. The Publisher does not assume any responsibility for any injury and/or damage to persons or property arising out of or related to any use of the material contained in this periodical. The reader is advised to check the appropriate medical literature and the product information currently provided by the manufacturer of each drug to be administered to verify the dosage, the method and duration of administration, or contraindications. It is the responsibility of the treating physician or other health care professional, relying on independent experience and knowledge of the patient, to determine drug dosages and the best treatment for the patient. Mention of any product in this issue should not be construed as endorsement by the contributors, editors, or the Publisher of the product or manufacturers' claims.

Emergency Medicine Clinics of North America (ISSN 0733-8627) is published quarterly by W.B. Saunders, 360 Park Avenue, South, New York, NY, 10010-1710. Months of Publication are February, May, August, and November. Business and Editorial Offices: 1600 John F. Kennedy Boulevard, Suite 1800, Philadelphia, PA 19103-2899. Accounting and Circulation Offices: 6277 Sea Harbor Drive, Orlando, FL 32887-4800. Periodicals postage paid at New York, NY, and additional mailing offices. Subscription prices are $175.00 per year (US individuals), $275.00 per year (US institutions), $235.00 per year (international individuals), $325.00 per year (international institutions), $215.00 per year (Canadian individuals), and $325.00 per year (Canadian institutions). International air speed delivery is included in all *Clinics'* subscription prices. All prices are subject to change without notice. POSTMASTER: Send address changes to *Emergency Medicine Clinics of North America*, Elsevier Periodicals Customer Service, 6277 Sea Harbor Drive, Orlando, FL 32887-4800. **Customer Service: 1-800-654-2452 (US). From outside of the US, call 1-407-345-4000. E-mail: hhspcs@harcourt.com.**

Emergency Medicine Clinics of North America is covered in *Index Medicus, Current Contents/Clinical Medicine, EMBASE/Excerpta Medica, BIOSIS, SciSearch, CINAHL, ISI/BIOMED,* and *Research Alert.*

Printed in the United States of America.

CONSULTING EDITOR

AMAL MATTU, MD, FAAEM, FACEP, Associate Professor and Program Director, Division of Emergency Medicine, University of Maryland School of Medicine, Baltimore, Maryland

GUEST EDITORS

BRENDAN MAGAURAN, MD, MBA, Assistant Professor of Emergency Medicine, Boston University School of Medicine, Boston, Massachusetts

JOSEPH H. KAHN, MD, Clinical Associate Professor of Emergency Medicine, Boston University School of Medicine, Boston, Massachusetts

JONATHAN S. OLSHAKER, MD, FACEP, Professor and Chairman, Department of Emergency Medicine, Boston University School of Medicine, Boston, Massachusetts; Chief, Emergency Services, Boston Medical Center, Boston, Massachusetts

CONTRIBUTORS

ADEYINKA ADEDIPE, MD, Attending Physician, Department of Emergency Medicine, Boston Medical Center, Boston, Massachusetts

MIRIAM T. ASCHKENASY, MD, MPH, Assistant Professor of Emergency Medicine; Associate Director, Section on Public Health and International Health; Director of Medical Informatics, Department of Emergency Medicine, Boston University School of Medicine, Boston, Massachusetts

MICHELLE P. BLANDA, MD, FACEP, Professor and Chairman, Department of Emergency Medicine, Northeastern Ohio, University Summa Health System, Akron, Ohio

JONATHAN A. EDLOW, MD, Department of Emergency Medicine, Beth Israel Deaconess Medical Center, Boston, Massachusetts

ADAM J. GEROFF, MD, Assistant Professor, Division of Emergency Medicine, Department of Surgery, University of Maryland School of Medicine

ROHIT GUPTA, MD, Staff Emergency Physician, Advocate Christ Medical Center, Oak Lawn, Illinois

LORI HARRINGTON, MD, Resident Physician, Department of Emergency Medicine, Boston Medical Center, Boston, Massachusetts

JASON IMPERATO, MD, MBA, Clinical Instructor, Harvard Medical School, Department of Emergency Medicine, Mount Auburn Hospital, Cambridge, Massachusetts

JOSEPH H. KAHN, MD, Clinical Associate Professor of Emergency Medicine, Boston University School of Medicine, Boston, Massachusetts

SETH KAUFMAN, MD, Resident, Emergency Medicine; Chief Resident EMS, University of Chicago, Chicago, Illinois

LARA K. KULCHYCKI, MD, Department of Emergency Medicine, Beth Israel Deaconess Medical Center, Boston, Massachusetts

ROBERT LOWENSTEIN, MD, Assistant Professor, Boston University School of Medicine, Department of Emergency Medicine, Boston Medical Center, Boston, Massachusetts

ANEESH T. NARANG, MD, Clinical Instructor, Department of Emergency Medicine, Boston Medical Center, Boston, Massachusetts

BRENDAN MAGAURAN, MD, MBA, Assistant Professor of Emergency Medicine, Boston University School of Medicine, Boston, Massachusetts

JOSEPH P. MARTINEZ, MD, Assistant Professor and Assistant Medical Director, Division of Emergency Medicine, University of Maryland School of Medicine, Baltimore, Maryland

AMAL MATTU, MD, FAAEM, FACEP, Associate Professor and Program Director, Division of Emergency Medicine, University of Maryland School of Medicine, Baltimore, Maryland

JONATHAN S. OLSHAKER, MD, FACEP, Professor and Chairman, Department of Emergency Medicine, Boston University School of Medicine, Boston, Massachusetts; Chief, Emergency Services, Boston Medical Center, Boston, Massachusetts

JOANNA PIECHNICZEK-BUCZEK, MD, Division of Psychiatry, Boston University School of Medicine, Boston, Massachusetts

TODD C. ROTHENHAUS, MD, FACEP, Assistant Professor of Emergency Medicine, Department of Emergency Medicine; Director of Medical Informatics, Boston University School of Medicine, Boston, Massachusetts

LEON D. SANCHEZ, MD, MPH, Clinical Instructor, Harvard Medical School, Department of Emergency Medicine, Beth Israel Deaconess Medical Center, Boston, Massachusetts

JEFFREY I. SCHNEIDER, MD, Assistant Professor of Emergency Medicine; Assistant Residency Director, Department of Emergency Medicine, Boston Medical Center, Boston, Massachusetts

RISHI SIKKA, MD, Assistant Professor, Department of Emergency Medicine, Boston Medical Center, Boston, Massachusetts

SCOTT T. WILBER, MD, Associate Professor of Emergency Medicine, Northeastern Ohio Universities College of Medicine, Akron, Ohio; Director, Emergency Medicine Research Center, Summa Health System, Akron, Ohio

CONTENTS

vulnerability of elderly patients to neurologic disease and injury and the comparative subtlety of clinical presentation mean that physicians should have a lower threshold for laboratory studies, radiologic imaging, consultation, and admission. Transferring appropriate patients to tertiary centers that offer specialized trauma and neurologic and neurosurgical care greatly enhances survival and functional outcomes.

This article reviews the significance of altered mental status in older emergency department patients. Specific diagnoses are discussed, including delirium, stupor and coma, and dementia, with a focus on delirium. Finally, an approach to all older patients is suggested that should result in increased clinician comfort with older patients, improved ability to communicate with other physicians, increased quality of care, and improved patient and family satisfaction.

The aging process results in changes in pulmonary physiology that make the elderly population more susceptible to pulmonary disease. These physiologic changes also alter the clinical presentation of such diseases, making the diagnosis and treatment of pulmonary disorders particularly challenging for the clinician. It is important for the clinician to have a high index of suspicion for pulmonary disorders to make the proper diagnosis. It is essential to keep in mind the subtle differences between pulmonary diseases in the elderly compared with younger patients.

Already the major cause of mortality in the United States, cardiovascular emergencies will become increasingly prevalent in the future as the geriatric population doubles. This article discusses five cardiovascular emergencies: acute coronary syndrome, congestive heart failure, dysrythmias, aortic dissection, and ruptured abdominal aortic aneurysm. The discussion focuses on the differences in presentation, management, and outcomes that characterize each disease amongst the elderly. As a rule, the elderly have significantly worse outcomes than younger patients.

FORTHCOMING ISSUES

RECENT ISSUES

GOAL STATEMENT

The goal of *Emergency Medicine Clinics of North America* is to keep practicing physicians up to date with current clinical practice in emergency medicine by providing timely articles reviewing the state of the art in patient care.

ACCREDITATION

The *Emergency Medical Clinics of North America* is planned and implemented in accordance with the Essential Areas and Policies of the Accreditation Council for Continuing Medical Education (ACCME) through the joint sponsorship of the University of Virginia School of Medicine and Elsevier. The University of Virginia School of Medicine is accredited by the ACCME to provide continuing medical education for physicians.

The University of Virginia School of Medicine designates this educational activity for a maximum of 15 AMA PRA Category 1 Credits™. Physicians should only claim credit commensurate with the extent of their participation in the activity.

The American Medical Association has determined that physicians not licensed in the US who participate in this CME activity are eligible for 15 AMA PRA Category 1 Credits™.

Category 1 credit can be earned by reading the text material, taking the CME examination online at http://www.theclinics.com/home/cme, and completing the evaluation. After taking the test, you will be required to review any and all incorrect answers. Following completion of the test and evaluation, your credit will be awarded and you may print your certificate.

FACULTY DISCLOSURE/CONFLICT OF INTEREST

The University of Virginia School of Medicine, as an ACCME accredited provider, endorses and strives to comply with the Accreditation Council for Continuing Medical Education (ACCME) Standards of Commercial Support, Commonwealth of Virginia statutes, University of Virginia policies and procedures, and associated federal and private regulations and guidelines on the need for disclosure and monitoring of proprietary and financial interests that may affect the scientific integrity and balance of content delivered in continuing medical education activities under our auspices.

The University of Virginia School of Medicine requires that all CME activities accredited through this institution be developed independently and be scientifically rigorous, balanced and objective in the presentation/discussion of its content, theories and practices.

All authors/editors participating in an accredited CME activity are expected to disclose to the readers relevant financial relationships with commercial entities occurring within the past 12 months (such as grants or research support, employee, consultant, stock holder, member of speakers bureau, etc.). The University of Virginia School of Medicine will employ appropriate mechanisms to resolve potential conflicts of interest to maintain the standards of fair and balanced education to the reader. Questions about specific strategies can be directed to the Office of Continuing Medical Education, University of Virginia School of Medicine, Charlottesville, Virginia.

The authors/editors listed below have identified no professional or financial affiliations for themselves or their spouse/partner:
Adeyinka Adedipe, MD; Miriam T. Aschkenasy, MD, MPH; Michelle P. Blanda, MD, FACEP; Jonathan A. Edlow, MD; Adam J. Geroff, MD; Rohit Gupta, MD; Carla Holloway, Acquisitions Editor; Lori Harrington, MD; Jason Imperato, MD, MBA; Joseph H. Kahn, MD; Seth Kaufman, MD; Lara K. Kulchycki, MD; Robert Lowenstein, MD; Brendan Magauran, MD, MBA; Joseph Martinez, MD; Amal Mattu, MD; Aneesh T. Narang, MD; Jonathan S. Olshaker, MD, AAEM, FACEP; Joanna Pierchniczek-Buczek, MD; Todd C. Rothenhaus, MD, FACEP; Leon D. Sanchez, MD, MPH; Jeffrey I. Schneider, MD; and, Rishi Sikka, MD.

The author listed below has identified the following professional or financial affiliation for himself or spouse/partner:
Scott T. Wilber, MD is an independent contractor for Merck and Novartis.

Disclosure of Discussion of non-FDA approved uses for pharmaceutical products and/or medical devices:
The University of Virginia School of Medicine, as an ACCME provider, requires that all faculty presenters identify and disclose any "off label" uses for pharmaceutical and medical device products. The University of Virginia School of Medicine recommends that each physician fully review all the available data on new products or procedures prior to instituting them with patients.

TO ENROLL

To enroll in the Emergency Medicine Clinics of North America Continuing Medical Education program, call customer service at 1-800-654-2452 or visit us online at www.theclinics.com/home/cme. The CME program is available to subscribers for an additional fee of $195.00

EMERGENCY
MEDICINE
CLINICS OF
NORTH AMERICA

ELSEVIER
SAUNDERS

Emerg Med Clin N Am
24 (2006) xiii–xiv

Foreword

Geriatric Emergency Medicine

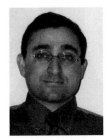

Amal Mattu, MD, FAAEM, FACEP
Consulting Editor

Anybody who has worked in emergency medicine for more than a few years has undoubtedly noticed a changing patient population: emergency department (ED) patients are getting older. The elderly represent the fastest growing segment of the U.S. population, and it is clearly reflected in the patients presenting to the nation's EDs and hospitals. The elderly currently constitute >15% of all ED patients, 40% of all ambulance arrivals to the ED, and almost 50% of all intensive care unit admissions. These patients tend to have greater comorbidities, they have more complicated workups, they utilize more laboratory and radiologic services, and they have longer lengths of stay in the ED and in the hospital than younger patients. Despite these more extensive workups, the rate of misdiagnoses, delayed diagnoses, and ED "bouncebacks" among discharged elderly patients is higher. The resulting morbidity and mortality in this patient group is also much higher than in younger patients with similar chief complaints. So why the problem?

The medical community is now starting to understand the significant changes that occur with aging that produce altered disease conditions and presentations in elderly patients. Alterations in physiologic processes, for example, predispose elderly patients to infection, drug toxicity, dehydration, and fractures. The elderly are also well known to present with atypical presentations of common disease, including myocardial infarction, pneumonia, urinary tract infection, appendicitis, and shock. There are also certain diseases that are almost exclusive to elderly patients, including temporal arteritis, aortic dissection, and dementia. Much like pediatric patients,

doi:10.1016/j.emc.2006.01.015   *emed.theclinics.com*

elderly patients should be thought of as a completely separate patient population with "their own" physiology, "their own" diseases, and "their own" presentations.

In this issue of *Emergency Medicine Clinics*, Guest Editors Drs. Kahn, Magauran, and Olshaker have assembled an outstanding group of physicians to educate and update us on the challenging topic of geriatric emergency medicine. The editors and authors have addressed physiologic changes, high-risk conditions, and atypical presentations associated with elderly patients in the ED. This issue represents an important contribution to education, and is certain to improve the care of our patients in the ED.

Amal Mattu, MD, FAAEM, FACEP
Emergency Medicine Residency
University of Maryland School of Medicine
110S Paca Street, 6th Floor, Suite 200, Baltimore, MD 21201, USA

E-mail address: amattu@smail.unmaryland.edu

ELSEVIER
SAUNDERS

Emerg Med Clin N Am
24 (2006) xv–xvi

EMERGENCY
MEDICINE
CLINICS OF
NORTH AMERICA

Preface

Geriatric Emergency Medicine

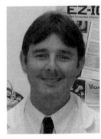 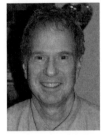 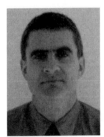

Brendan Magauran,   Joseph H. Kahn, MD   Jonathan S. Olshaker,
MD, MBA   MD, FACEP

Guest Editors

The percentage of the United States population that is 65 years and over will rise from the current 12% to 21% by 2050. Currently the elderly comprise 15% of all emergency department visits in the United States, so we can expect there will be an even greater increase in the proportion of emergency department patients who are elderly. Elderly emergency department patients have a high acuity level, often without the typical presentation of serious illness. In this edition, we attempt to provide the emergency physician with a framework for the resuscitation, evaluation, management, and disposition of the elderly patient in the emergency department. We focus on the unique pathophysiology of geriatric patients that makes them susceptible to serious disease without the usual outward manifestations we expect to see. We have tried to present the special needs of this vulnerable patient population so that as practitioners of Emergency Medicine we can care for the elderly patient as effectively, efficiently, and humanely as possible.

We wish to thank all of the authors who so meticulously researched and wrote the various articles in this edition of *Emergency Medicine Clinics of North America*. We also wish to thank our families for their support in the hours needed to revise and assemble this issue. We would like to thank Karen Sorensen and the staff at Elsevier for their support and patience.

doi:10.1016/j.emc.2006.01.014   *emed.theclinics.com*

Most of all, we wish to thank those of you who read this edition; we sincerely hope you find it useful in your practice.

Brendan Magauran, MD, MBA
Boston Medical Center
Department of Emergency Medicine
1 Boston Medical Center Place
Boston, MA 02118, USA

E-mail address: magauran@bu.edu

Joseph H. Kahn, MD
Boston Medical Center
Department of Emergency Medicine
1 Boston Medical Center Place
Boston, MA 02118, USA

E-mail address: jkahn@bu.edu

Jonathan S. Olshaker, MD, FACEP
Boston Medical Center
Department of Emergency Medicine
1 Boston Medical Center Place
Boston, MA 02118, USA

E-mail address: jonathan.olshaker@bmc.org

ELSEVIER
SAUNDERS

Emerg Med Clin N Am
24 (2006) 243–260

EMERGENCY
MEDICINE
CLINICS OF
NORTH AMERICA

Trends in Geriatric Emergency Medicine

Joseph H. Kahn, MD*, Brendan Magauran, MD, MBA

Department of Emergency Medicine, Boston Medical Center,
1 Boston Medical Center Place, Boston, MA 02118-2393, USA

In the 2002 National Hospital Ambulatory Medical Care Survey (NHACMS) [1], emergency department (ED) use by patients over the age of 64 years accounted for 15% of the 110.2 million patient visits. Patients over the age of 64 years presently account for 12% of the population. The demographics of the United States are changing, and projections show a substantial increase in the number and percentage of the population that is older than 64 years of age by the year 2050. This will have tremendous impact on the use of all healthcare resources by this population. People over 64 years of age presenting to the ED are at high risk for having significant medical and surgical illnesses. To better understand future ED use, it is valuable to analyze the current ED use rates of this population. This article reviews ED use by demographics, causes of death, principal reason for ED visits, number of ED visits per person per year, prescription drugs used, and recent trends in ED visits.

Demographics

According to the U.S. Census Bureau, the number of people 65 years of age and older in the United States on July 1, 2004 totaled 36.3 million. This age group accounts for 12% of the total population. This is an increase of 1% over 2003, when 351,000 people moved into this age group. The number of people 85 years of age and older in the United States on July 1, 2004 totaled 4.9 million. By the year 2050, the projected population of people over 65 years of age will be 86.7 million, comprising 21% of the total population. This represents a 147% increase in the population 65 years of age and older between 2000 and 2050, whereas in comparison the under 65 years of age population is projected to increase between 2000 and 2050 by only 49%.

* Corresponding author.
E-mail address: jkahn@bu.edu (J.H. Kahn).

0733-8627/06/$ - see front matter © 2006 Elsevier Inc. All rights reserved.
doi:10.1016/j.emc.2006.01.012
emed.theclinics.com

The oldest old, those 85 years of age and older, will increase by 388%, and the population aged 65 to 84 years of age will increase by 114% [2]. As of August 1, 2004, there were an estimated 64,658 centenarians in the United States [3].

With regard to race and sex within the population over 64 years of age, women predominate over men and live longer, to represent an increasing percentage in each age subgroup (Table 1) [4]. The racial disparity is striking in this population. Caucasians far outnumber all other racial groups almost 10:1 (Table 2) [5]. Broken down by gender, Caucasian men represent 94% of all men over 64 years of age, whereas African American and Hispanic men represent the remaining 6% with a slight predominance for African American men. Caucasian women represent 91% of all women over 64 years of age. African American women, however, outnumber Hispanic women by a 2:1 ratio or 6% to 3%. Life expectancy projections at birth and at ages over 64 years of age indicate that Caucasian men and women live slightly longer than African American men and women (Table 3) [6,7].

Cause of death

Based on death certificates and ICD-10 codes, the five leading causes of death for all persons are (1) diseases of the heart, (2) malignant neoplasms, (3) cerebrovascular disease, (4) chronic lower respiratory diseases, and (5) unintentional injuries. These five categories account for 67% of all deaths. In the population over 64 years of age, four disease categories account for two thirds of death in the following order: (1) diseases of the heart, (2) malignant neoplasms, (3) cerebrovascular disease, and (4) chronic lower respiratory diseases (Table 4) [8]. The death rate per 100,000 population for heart disease is higher in African American men and women than either Caucasian or Hispanic men and women (Table 5) [9]. The death rate per 100,000 population from malignant neoplasms is slightly higher for African American women than Caucasian women, but it is much higher for African American women than for Hispanic women. In men, African Americans have a much higher death rate from neoplasms than either Caucasian or Hispanic men (Table 6) [10].

Across the major racial groups there is an interesting variation among the top five causes of death for the population over 64 years of age. Interesting to

Table 1
Percentage of population by sex and age subgroup

Age	65–74	75–84	>85
Total	18.3 million	12.6 million	4.4 million
Male	45%	40%	30%
Female	55%	60%	70%

National Center for Health Statistics. Health, United States, 2004. Table 1. Hyattsville, MD: National Center for Health Statistics; 2004. p. 39–40.

Table 2
Percentage of population by sex, race, and age subgroup

	65–74 years	%	75–84 years	%	85+ years	%
Caucasian male	7.3 million	86	4.5 million	94	1.2 million	95
African American male	0.7 million	8	0.1 million	4	0.01 million	1
Hispanic male	0.5 million	6	0.2 million	2	0.05 million	4
Caucasian female	8.7 million	84	6.8 million	88	2.8 million	91
African American female	1.0 million	10	0.6 million	8	0.2 million	6
Hispanic female	0.6 million	6	0.3 million	4	0.1 million	3

National Center for Health Statistics. Health, United States, 2004. Table 1. Hyattsville, MD: National Center for Health Statistics; 2004. p. 39–40.

note is that cardiovascular disease, malignant neoplasm, and cerebrovascular disease are commonly the first three diagnoses in order, but after that there are racial differences. Chronic lower respiratory disease is fourth for Caucasians and Hispanics; for African Americans diabetes mellitus is fourth; diabetes is third and cerebrovascular disease is fourth for American Indians; and pneumonia/influenza is fourth for Asian/Pacific Islanders (Table 7) [11].

Principal reason for emergency department visit

Contained within the National Ambulatory Care Hospital survey, data were collected on the patient's principal reason for the ED visit. These visits were coded according to "A Reason for Visit Classification for Ambulatory Care" (RVC) [12]. The data are not broken down by age, but injuries, general symptoms such as pain or fever, abdominal symptoms, and respiratory symptoms were the major reasons for ED visits overall (Table 8) [13]. Patients over 64 years of age seen in the ED had a higher percentage of visits classified as emergent (within 15 minutes) and urgent (15–60 minutes) when compared with their younger counterparts (Table 9) [14].

Prescription drugs

The population over 64 years of age comprises 12% of the population but accounts for 41% of all prescription drug expenses [15]. The expenditures

Table 3
Life expectancy in years by age, sex, and race

AGE				
Race	Caucasian	Caucasian	African American	African American
Sex	Male	Female	Male	Female
65	16.6	19.5	14.6	18.0
75	10.3	12.3	9.5	11.7

National Center for Health Statistics. Health, United States, 2004. Table 27. Hyattsville, MD: National Center for Health Statistics; 2004. p. 77.

Table 4
Leading causes of death, age over 64 years in 2002

Cause of death	Deaths	Percentage
All causes	1,811,720	100
Diseases of the heart	576,301	32
Malignant neoplasms	391,001	22
Cerebrovascular diseases	143,293	8
Chronic lower respiratory diseases	108,313	6
Influenza and pneumonia	58,826	3
Alzheimer disease	58,289	3
Diabetes mellitus	54,715	3
Nephritis, nephritic syndrome, nephrosis	34,316	2
Unintentional injuries	33,641	2
Septicemia	26,670	1.5
Other	326,355	18

National Center for Health Statistics. Health, United States, 2004. Table 32. Hyattsville, MD: National Center for Health Statistics; 2004. p. 92–93.

SOURCES: Centers for Disease Control and Prevention, National Center for Health Statistics, National Vital Statistics System: *Vital Statistics of the United States, vol II, mortality, part A*, 1980. Washington: Public Health Service 1985: Anderson RN, Smith BL. Deaths: Leading causes for 2002. National vital statistics reports. Vol 53. Hyattsville. Maryland: National Center for Health Statistics. 2004.

associated with prescription medicine increased from $13.9 billion in 1992 to $35.6 billion in 2000 [16]. Seniors are three times as likely to use prescription drugs as compared with persons under 64 years of age [17]. Adverse reactions to medications can occur for multiple reasons: altered physiology in

Table 5
Death rate per 100,000 persons for heart disease by sex, race, and age

Age	65–74	75–84	85+
Male overall	827	2,110	5,823
Female overall	440	1390	5,283
Caucasian male	808	2,112	5,940
African American male	1,193	2,450	5,126
Hispanic male	658	1,600	4,302
Caucasian female	415	1,368	5,351
African American female	734	1,822	5,111
Hispanic female	346	1,091	4,033

National Center for Health Statistics. Health, United States, 2004. Table 36. Hyattsville, MD: National Center for Health Statistics; 2004. p. 103–5.

SOURCES: Centers for Disease Control and Prevention, National Center for Health Statistics, National Vital Statistics System; numerator data from annual mortality files; denominator data from national population estimates for race groups from table 1 and unpublished Hispanic population estimates for 1985–96 prepared by the Housing and Household Economic Statistics Division. U.S. Bureau of the Census, additional mortality tables are available at www.cdc.gov/nchs/datawh/statab/unpubd/mortabs.htm: Kochanek KD, Murphy SL, Anderson RN, Scott C. Deaths: Final data for 2002. National vital statistics reports. Vol 53 no 5. Hyattsville. Maryland: National Center for Health Statistics. 2004.

Table 6
Death rate per 100,000 persons for malignant neoplasm by sex, race, and age

Age	65–74	75–84	85+
Male overall	965	1,711	2,491
Female overall	649	1,047	1,391
Caucasian male	955	1,695	2,487
African American male	1,275	2,223	2,976
Hispanic male	622	1,191	1,869
Caucasian female	650	1,053	1,395
African American female	741	1,123	1,468
Hispanic female	396	692	1,031

National Center for Health Statistics. Health, United States, 2004. Table 38. Hyattsville, MD: National Center for Health Statistics; 2004. p. 109–12.

SOURCES: Centers for Disease Control and Prevention, National Center for Health Statistics, National Vital Statistics System: Grove RD, Hetzel AM. Vital statistics rates in the United States. 1940–1960. Washington: U.S. Government Printing Office, 1968: numerator data from National Vital Statistics System, annual mortality files; denominator data from national population estimates of race groups from table 1 and unpublished Hispanic population estimates for 1985–96 prepared by the Housing and Household Economic Statistics Division. U.S. Bureau of the Census; additional mortality tables are available at www.cdc.gov/nchs/datawh/statab/unpubd/mortabs.htm; Kochanek KD, Murphy SL, Anderson RN, Scott C. Deaths: Final data for 2002. National vital statistics reports. Vol 53 no 5. Hyattsville. Maryland: National Center for Health Statistics. 2004.

absorbing, metabolizing, and eliminating medications, and memory impairment or vision problems complicating adherence to complex medical regimens [18]. The prescription drugs used by patients in the outpatient setting (ED and physician offices) are characterized in the attached table by age (Table 10) [19].

Table 7
Top five death rates by race

	Caucasian	African American	American Indian	Asian/Pacific Islander	Hispanic
1	Heart disease	Heart disease	Heart disease	Heart disease	Heart disease
2	Cancer	Cancer	Cancer	Cancer	Cancer
3	Stroke	Stroke	Diabetes	Stroke	Stroke
4	COPD	Diabetes	Stroke	Pneumonia/influenza	COPD
5	Pneumonia Influenza	Pneumonia Influenza	COPD	COPD	Pneumonia Influenza

National Center for Health Statistics. Health, United States, 2004. Table 31. Hyattsville, MD: National Center for Health Statistics; 2004. p. 154–7.

SOURCES: Centers for Disease Control and Prevention, National Center for Health Statistics, National Vital Statistics System; Vital statistics of the United States, vol II, mortality, part A. 1980. Washington: Public Health Service. 1985: Anderson RN, Smith BL. Deaths: Leading causes for 2002. National vital statistics reports. Vol 53. Hyattsville. Maryland: National Center for Health Statistics. 2004.

Table 8

Number and percent distribution of ED visits with corresponding standard errors, by patient's principal reason for visit: United States, 2002

Principal reason for visit and RVC code[a]		Number of visits in thousands	Standard error in thousands	Percent distribution	Standard error of percent
All visits		110,155	4,416	100.0	—
Symptom module	S001–S999	79,192	3,446	71.9	0.6
General symptoms	S001–S099	17,510	851	15.9	0.3
Symptoms referable to psychologic/ mental disorders	S100–S199	2,049	123	1.9	0.1
Symptoms referable to the nervous system (excluding sense organs)	S200–S259	6,653	314	6.0	0.2
Symptoms referable to the cardiovascular/ lymphatic system	S260–S299	914	85	0.8	0.1
Symptoms referable to the eyes and ears	S300–S399	3,694	240	3.4	0.1
Symptoms referable to the respiratory system	S400–S499	13,247	825	12.0	0.4
Symptoms referable to the digestive system	S500–S639	14,429	602	13.1	0.3
Symptoms referable to the genitourinary system	S640–S829	3,785	199	3.4	0.1
Symptoms referable to the skin, hair, and nails	S830–S899	2,724	171	2.5	0.1
Symptoms referable to the musculoskeletal system	S900–S999	14,185	709	12.9	0.4
Disease module	D001–D999	4,543	267	4.1	0.2
Diagnostic/screening and preventive module	X100–X599	946	123	0.9	0.1
Treatment module	T100–T899	2,449	150	2.2	0.1
Injuries and adverse effects module	J001–J999	21,847	907	19.8	0.5
Test results module	R100–R700	333	51	0.3	0.0
Administrative module	A100–A140	156	31	0.1	0.0
Other	U990–U999	690	134	0.6	0.1

Quantity more than zero but less than 0.05

Numbers may not add to totals because of rounding.

[a] Includes problems and complaints not elsewhere classified entries of "none" blanks, and illegible entries.

McCaig LF, Burt CW. National Ambulatory Hospital Medical Care Survey: 2002 Emergency Department Summary. Advance data from vital and health statistics; No. 340. Table 5. Hyattsville, MD: National Center for Health Statistics; 2004. p. 15.

Emergency department use

Overall ED visits over the time period from 1992 to 2002 increased 23% from 89.8 million annual visits to 110.2 million annual visits. Trends in ED visit rates over the same time period increased from 35.7 visits per 100 persons to 38.9 visits per 100 persons. In persons over 64 years of age, the visit rate per 100 persons was 49, the highest rate for any age group. The visit rate ranged from 37 visits per 100 persons for the 65 to 74 years of age group to 61 visits per 100 persons in the 75 years and older group. The most significant increases for types of visits by the population over age 64 years was 87% increase for arthropathies, 84% for diabetes mellitus, 45% for stroke, and by 29% for spinal disorders (Table 10) [20]. ED visits by race measured by number of visits per 1,000 persons stayed constant over the period 1992 to 2002 (Fig. 1) [21].

Special needs of elderly patients

Elderly patients presenting to the ED have a higher likelihood of significant pathology than their younger counterparts. Furthermore, the presentation of myocardial infarction, surgical abdomen, and sepsis may be subtle and easily missed in elderly patients. Resuscitation of elderly patients and management of acute medical and surgical illnesses in the elderly population are covered elsewhere in this issue. Elderly patients presenting to the ED often have special needs in addition to the medical complaints for which they are presenting. People over 65 years of age frequently have multiple medical problems that may affect their chief complaint. The presentation of serious medical or surgical illness is often atypical and subtle. Elderly patients may not be able to express themselves clearly as a result of various causes, including cognitive impairment, confusion, and dysarthria [22,23]. In fact, the acute medical condition leading to the ED visit may worsen the patient's existing cognitive impairment, making communication even more difficult [24]. It is not unusual for elderly people to not remember why they were sent to the ED, making reading of ambulance trip sheets, nursing triage notes, and documents from sending facilities essential. In fact, the routine use of transfer forms from extended care facilities to the ED has been shown to improve the care of elderly patients [25].

ED evaluations are usually brief and goal-directed; a more thorough history and physical is required when evaluating the geriatric patient [24]. More liberal use of laboratory evaluation and imaging modalities also is required to avoid missing subtle presentations of serious disease.

Admission to the hospital sometimes is required for observation of elderly patients with nonspecific complaints. There has been research on the development of ED observation units for elderly patients [26].

Managing agitated elderly patients in the ED and as inpatients can be challenging. Delirium may complicate the hospitalization of elderly patients and is

Table 9
Urgency of ED visit by category and age

Patient and visit characteristics	Number of visits in thousands	Total	Immediacy with which patient should be seen									
			Percent distribution					Standard error of percent				
			Emergent[a]	Urgent[b]	Semiurgent[c]	Nonurgent[d]	Unknown/ no triage[e]	Emergent[a]	Urgent[b]	Semiurgent[c]	Nonurgent[d]	Unknown/ no triage[e]
All visits	110,156	100.0	22.3	34.2	18.5	10.2	14.5	1.7	1.5	1.3	1.4	1.7
Age												
Under 15 years	24,077	100.0	16.3	33.5	19.7	15.6	14.9	1.6	2.1	1.4	3.4	2.0
15–24 years	17,215	100.0	16.6	33.9	20.8	11.6	15.1	2.0	1.9	1.8	1.6	2.0
25–44 years	32,432	100.0	20.7	34.3	20.1	10.1	14.9	1.8	1.6	1.6	1.4	1.6
45–64 years	19,943	100.0	24.8	34.4	17.5	8.1	15.2	1.7	1.5	1.3	1.1	1.9
65–75 years	6,759	100.0	32.4	35.1	19.6	4.1	14.8	2.2	1.9	1.5	0.8	2.0
75 years and over	9,726	100.0	36.9	34.6	12.1	3.1	13.3	2.2	1.6	1.2	0.6	1.9
Sex												
Female	59,594	100.0	22.0	34.9	18.7	9.6	14.7	1.7	1.5	1.4	1.3	1.7
Male	50,561	100.0	22.6	33.3	18.4	10.8	15.0	1.7	1.4	1.2	1.5	1.7
Race[f]												
White	81,704	100.0	23.6	34.0	18.3	9.1	15.1	1.8	1.5	1.4	1.3	1.7
Black or African American	24,861	100.0	17.8	34.5	19.7	14.4	13.6	1.8	2.1	1.4	2.8	2.3
Other	3,590	100.0	23.2	36.6	16.5	6.1	17.6	2.7	3.8	2.5	1.1	5.6

Expected source of payment

Private insurance	42,802	100.0	21.6	35.1	18.5	9.7	15.1	1.7	1.6	1.4	1.3	2.0
Medicaid/SCHIP[g]	21,751	100.0	18.1	34.8	19.6	13.5	14.0	1.8	2.1	1.7	2.5	2.1
Medicare	16,964	100.0	34.1	34.3	13.9	3.9	13.9	2.2	1.5	1.5	0.6	2.2
Self-pay	15,935	100.0	20.8	34.9	21.0	11.5	11.7	2.3	2.1	1.6	1.7	1.7
Worker's Compensation	2,148	100.0	20.6	33.6	21.4	9.5	14.9	2.9	2.9	2.9	2.0	2.9
No change	*1,155	100.0	8.5	17.7	*20.1	*36.5	17.0	2.2	4.5	6.9	14.0	6.5
Other	2,551	100.0	22.2	37.6	17.0	10.2	13.0	4.4	3.4	2.3	2.2	2.4
Unknown blank	6,848	100.0	16.9	26.3	20.4	10.9	25.5	2.4	2.2	3.1	2.0	4.0

Numbers may not add to totals because of rounding.

* Figure does not meet standard of reliability or precision.

[a] A visit in which the patient should be seen in less than 15 minutes.

[b] A visit in which the patient should be seen within 15–60 minutes.

[c] A visit in which the patient should be seen within 61–120 minutes.

[d] A visit in which the patient should be seen within 121 minutes–24 hours.

[e] A visit in which there is no mention of an immediacy rating or triage level in the medical record or the hospital did not perform triage or the patient was dead on arrival.

[f] Other race includes visits by Asians, Native Hawaiians or other Pacific Islanders. American Indians or Alaska Natives, and multiple races. All race categories include visits by persons of Hispanic origin. Persons of Hispanic origin may be of any race. Staying with data year 1999, race-specific estimates have been tabulated according to 1997 Standards for Federal Data on Race and Ethnicity and are not strictly comparable with estimates for earlier years. However, the percent of visit records with multiple races indicated is small and lower than what is typically found for self-reported race. See "Technical Notes" for more details.

[g] SCHIP is State Children's Health Insurance Program.

McCaig LF, Burt CW. National Ambulatory Hospital Medical Care Survey: 2002 Emergency Department Summary. Advance data from vital and health statistics; No. 340. Table 3. Hyattsville, MD: National Center for Health Statistics; 2004. p. 14.

Table 10

Selected prescription and nonprescription drugs recorded during MD office visits and hospital outpatient visits by age and sex: United States, 1995–1996 and 2001–2002

Age group and National Drug Code (NDC) therapeutic class[a] (common reasons for use)	Total		Male		Female	
	1995–96	2001–02	1995–96	2001–02	1995–96	2001–02
Age 65 years and over		Visits with at least one drug per 100 population[b]				
Drug visits[c]	399.4	470.8	378.1	439.2	414.7	493.8
		Number of drugs per 100 population[d]				
Total number of drugs[e]	1,047.4	1,422.9	956.9	1,309.5	1,112.5	1,505.4
Hyperlipidemia (high cholesterol)	24.7	71.3	25.1	79.5	24.5	65.3
Hypertension control drugs, not otherwise specified (high blood pressure)	29.1	69.8	22.7	62.3	33.8	75.2
Nonnarcotic analgesics (pain relief)	44.9	66.7	49.0	69.4	42.0	64.7
Diuretics (high blood pressure, heart disease)	55.2	65.6	48.5	61.7	60.0	68.4
ACE inhibitors (high blood pressure, heart disease)	42.6	64.7	41.2	66.5	43.6	63.4
NSAID[f] (pain relief)	41.8	62.2	31.9	47.5	49.0	72.9
Blood glucose/sugar regulators (diabetes)	37.5	62.0	38.0	69.9	37.1	56.3
Calcium channel blockers (high blood pressure, heart disease)	57.3	59.6	52.2	52.3	60.9	64.9
Beta blockers (high blood pressure, heart disease)	25.5	54.2	23.6	54.0	26.8	54.4
Acid/peptic disorders (gastrointestinal reflux, ulcers)	42.2	53.3	36.0	48.2	46.6	56.9
Antiasthmatics/bronchodilators (asthma, breathing)	31.3	45.9	37.1	52.1	27.0	41.5
Thyroid/antithyroid (hyper- and hypothyroidism)	22.2	30.4	10.0	12.1	31.0	43.7
Antidepressants (depression and related disorders)	23.5	39.0	16.7	26.2	28.5	48.3
Estrogen/progestins (menopause, hot flashes)					37.1	47.4
65–74 years		Visits with at least one drug per 100 population[b]				
Drug visits[c]	362.8	432.5	323.0	398.3	394.9	460.8

	Number of drugs per 100 population[d]					
Total number of drugs[e]	930.5	1,273.1	804.7	1,175.2	1,032.1	1,354.4
Blood glucose/sugar regulators (diabetes)	35.7	66.7	32.4	77.9	38.4	57.5
Hyperlipidemia (high cholesterol)	27.3	77.2	27.1	86.5	27.4	69.4
Nonnarcotic analgesics (pain relief)	38.0	56.0	40.5	63.2	35.9	50.1
NSAID[f] (pain relief)	42.0	59.1	31.2	50.3	50.8	66.4
ACE inhibitors (high blood pressure, heart disease)	37.1	62.0	35.6	63.8	38.3	60.4
Diuretics (high blood pressure, heart disease)	40.0	44.1	32.3	43.0	46.3	45.1
Calcium channel blockers (high blood pressure, heart disease)	48.9	53.5	46.2	49.3	51.2	57.0
Acid/peptic disorders (gastrointestinal reflux, ulcers)	38.7	51.1	30.6	44.2	45.2	56.9
Hypertension control drugs, not otherwise specified (high blood pressure)	24.8	65.3	19.2	58.6	29.3	70.9
Beta blockers (high blood pressure, heart disease)	23.7	50.8	20.7	54.2	26.1	48.0
Antiasthmatics/bronchodilators (asthma, breathing)	31.1	42.7	33.0	42.9	29.5	42.5
Antidepressants (depression and related disorders)	22.7	36.9	14.2	25.4	29.6	46.5
Vitamins/minerals (dietary supplements)	14.5	33.3	10.8	31.0	17.5	35.3
Estrogens/progestins (menopause, hot flashes)					47.5	59.1
Age 75 years and over						
	Visit with at least one drug per 100 population[b]					
Drug visits[c]	449.2	514.6	466.3	494.3	438.7	527.3
	Number of drugs per 100 population[d]					
Total number of drugs[e]	1,206.8	1,594.2	1,200.9	1,490.8	1,210.4	1,658.7
Diuretics (high blood pressure, heart disease)	75.8	90.1	74.5	87.1	76.6	92.0
Nonnarcotic analgesics (pain relief)	54.4	79.0	62.6	77.9	49.4	79.6
Hypertension control drugs, not otherwise specified (high blood pressure)	35.1	74.9	28.4	67.4	39.2	79.6
ACE inhibitors (high blood pressure, heart disease)	50.2	67.9	50.2	70.2	50.1	66.4
Calcium channel blockers (high blood pressure, heart disease)	68.6	66.5	61.8	56.3	72.7	72.8
NSAID[f] (pain relief)	41.5	65.7	33.1	43.6	46.7	79.5

(continued on next page)

Table 10 (*continued*)

Age group and National Drug Code (NDC) therapeutic class[a] (common reasons for use)	Total		Male		Female	
	1995–96	2001–02	1995–96	2001–02	1995–96	2001–02
Hyperlipidemia (high cholesterol)	21.3	64.5	21.8	70.1	21.0	61.0
Beta blockers (high blood pressure, heart disease)	27.9	58.1	28.3	53.8	27.6	60.9
Blood glucose/sugar regulators (diabetes)	39.8	56.6	46.9	59.1	35.5	55.1
Acid/peptic disorders (gastrointestinal reflux, ulcers)	47.0	55.7	44.7	53.7	48.3	56.9
Antiasthmatics/bronchodilators (asthma, breathing)	31.5	49.7	43.7	64.5	24.0	40.4
Anticoagulants/thrombolytics (blood thinning, reduce or prevent blood clots)	27.6	46.2	33.8	59.1	23.7	38.1
Antidepressants (depression and related disorders)	24.6	41.4	20.7	27.2	27.0	50.2
Glaucoma (elevated eye pressure)	32.6	40.1	32.6	42.8	32.6	38.4

Category not applicable.

NOTE: Drugs recorded on the patient record form are those prescribed, continued, administered, or provided during a physician office visit or hospital outpatient department visit.

SOURCE: Centers for Disease Control and Prevention, National Center for Health Statistics. National Ambulatory Medical Care Survey and National Hospital Ambulatory Medical Care Survey.

[a] The National Drug Code (NDC) therapeutic class is a general therapeutic or pharmacological classification scheme for drug products reported to the Food and Drug Administration (FDA) under the provisions of the Drug Listing Act. See Appendix II. National Drug Code (NDC) Directory therapeutic class and table XI.

[b] Estimated number of drug visits during the 2-year period divided by the sum of population estimates for both years times 100.

[c] Drug visits are physician office and hospital outpatient department visits in which at least one prescription or nonprescription drug was recorded on the patient record form.

[d] Estimated number of drugs recorded during visits during the 2-year period divided by the sum of population estimates for both years times 100.

[e] Up to six prescription and nonprescription drugs may be recorded per visit. See Appendix II, Drugs.

[f] NSAID is nonsteroidal anti-inflammatory drug. Aspirin was not included as an NSAID in this analysis. See Appendix II. National Drug Classification (NDC) system.

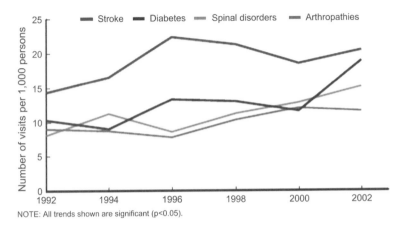

Fig. 1. Annual rate of emergency department visits for persons 65 years of age and older by selected diagnosis groups: United States, 1992 to 2002. Used with permission from McCaig LF, Burt CW. National Ambulatory Hospital Medical Care Survey: 2002 Emergency Department Summary. Advance data from vital and health statistics; No. 340. Hyattsville, MD: National Center for Health Statistics; 2004. Fig. 11, p . 8.

difficult to prevent and more difficult to treat [27]. Restraint-free care is highly desirable, because restraints not only deprive elders of their dignity but also may be associated with injuries [28–30]. In addition, medications used to control agitation in elderly patients actually may make them worse [31].

The long list of medications that many geriatric patients are receiving requires the clinician to screen for interactions before adding a medication for their chief complaint [32,33].

Elderly patients may be nonambulatory for various reasons, including musculoskeletal and neurologic disorders. They may be confused and frightened of the ED environment. They may have poor bowel and bladder control. Elderly ED patients require more attention and nursing care and overall use of ED resources than their younger counterparts [24].

Separate space for elderly patients

The very ED environment may work against the evaluation of the geriatric patient. Geriatric patients may decompensate further when exposed to the noisy, fast-paced, stressful ED setting, making them less amenable to thorough, efficient evaluations [34]. Geriatric patients frequently also have trouble focusing on the acute event (even if they can recall it) that brought them to the ED and often do not respond well to the rapid, pressured assessments that emergency physicians and nurses in a crowded ED impose on them. Geriatric patients may have more trouble lying on a hard stretcher without a pillow for hours than younger patients, and in fact may be more comfortable in reclining chairs [35]. Increasing elderly patient comfort in the ED is not only humane, it may aid in assessment, decrease decompensation, and reduce falls.

Many screening tools have been introduced in recent years to determine the elder ED patient's level of functioning, risk for falling, risk for repeat ED visits, use of alcohol and drugs, mental illness, exposure to elder abuse, and risk for medication interactions [36–42]. Unfortunately the pressures of emergency medicine in the twenty-first century make it difficult to obtain accurate, timely assessment of elder patients, much less screen for at-risk behaviors. For this reason, some investigators have advocated the development of geriatric EDs, with a quieter setting and better resources aimed at the special needs of the geriatric ED patient [43]. Although this idea may seem unlikely to succeed, other special units have been implemented successfully, including trauma teams for multiple trauma patients, urgent care centers and fast tracks for people with minor illnesses and injuries, and pediatric EDs [43]. Because of the population shift with ever-increasing numbers of geriatric patients in EDs anticipated over the next 20 years, the concept of geriatric EDs or a designated space within an ED for elderly patients is worth considering. Emergency physicians with a special interest in geriatrics or advanced training in geriatrics could staff these units. In fact, the first fellowship program in Geriatric Emergency Medicine was launched recently [44]. This may pave the way for the development of a board-certified subspecialty in Geriatric Emergency Medicine.

Geriatric assessment

To maximize an older person's chance for independent living, an assessment can be undertaken by a team consisting of the patient's primary care physician, a geriatric specialist, a visiting nurse, and a social worker. This interdisciplinary approach can attempt to identify all medical problems and formulate a comprehensive plan to improve the person's quality of life and level of functioning. This approach uses existing elder services and optimizes the living environment to enhance the person's independence [45,46].

There is a multitude of assessment instruments for elder patients. In determining the person's level of functioning, there is the Activities of Daily Living scale (ADLs), which assesses use of toilet, feeding, dressing, grooming, and ambulation [47]. Another way of assessing level of functioning is with the Instrumental Activities of Daily Living scale (IADLs), which assesses use of phone, shopping, food preparation, housekeeping, laundry, transportation, responsibility for medications, and ability to handle finances [47]. There are screens for hearing loss [48,49], vision [49], and memory impairment [49], gait disturbance [50], fall-risk, depression [51], substance abuse, dementia [52], balance [53], and elder abuse and global geriatric screens [54,55]. Geriatric screening using these instruments is not a practical task for the emergency physician, and some ED geriatric screen tools have been developed [39,56]. ED screening helps the emergency physician determine who may be suitable for discharge from the ED after treatment of an acute medical problem. Communication with the primary caregiver and expedited follow-up are certainly the keys to avoiding admission after treatment of minor medical conditions in the elderly population. If the emergency physician is not convinced that the elderly patient is returning to a safe environment and there is no family member present to accept responsibility, then it is reasonable to admit the patient until a more thorough assessment can be performed.

Comprehensive care

Primary care for the geriatric patient can serve as a bridge between the ED and return to home. Geriatric services, including home visits by nurses and physicians, can reduce loss of functioning in the geriatric patient and can reduce ED visits. Such services have not yet been shown to demonstrate clearly a decrease in hospitalizations [57]. Comprehensive primary care for geriatric patients also can facilitate movement between the ED, the inpatient service, rehabilitation services, home care, and the various levels of long-term care. The key role of emergency physicians in these services is communication with primary caregivers when geriatric patients are in the ED, so that appropriate disposition and follow-up can be achieved. The emergency physician should be aware of the services available for geriatric patients in their community.

Summary

Geriatrics is becoming an increasing portion of the practice of emergency medicine. Knowledge of the resuscitation, diagnosis, treatment, and disposition of this challenging group of patients is essential for the emergency physician of the twenty-first century.

References

[1] McCaig LF, Burt CW. National Ambulatory Hospital Medical Care Survey: 2002 Emergency Department Summary. Advance data from vital and health statistics; no 340. Hyattsville, MD: National Center for Health Statistics; 2004. Available at: http://www.cdc.gov/nchs/data/ad/ad340.pdf. Accessed March 18, 2004.
[2] U.S. Census Bureau, 2004. U.S. interim projections by age, sex, race, and Hispanic origin. Available at: http://www.census.gov/ipc/www/usinterimproj/natprojtab02a.pdf. Accessed April 25, 2005.
[3] U.S. Census Bureau. Releases, facts for features & special editions. CB05-FF.07–2. Available at: http://www.census.gov/PressRelease/www/releases/archives/facts_for_features_special_editions/004210.html. Accessed on April 25, 2005.
[4] National Center for Health Statistics. Health, United States, 2004. With chartbook on trends in the health of Americans. Table 1. Hyattsville, MD: National Center for Health Statistics; 2004. p. 39–40. Available at: http://www.cdc.gov/nchs/data/hus/hus04trend.pdf.

[5] National Center for Health Statistics. Health, United States, 2004. With chartbook on trends in the health of Americans. Table 35. Hyattsville, MD: National Center for Health Statistics; 2004. p. 99–102. Available at: http://www.cdc.gov/nchs/data/hus/hus04trend.pdf. Accessed April 25, 2005.

[6] National Center for Health Statistics. Health, United States, 2004. With chartbook on trends in the health of Americans. Table 27. Hyattsville, MD: National Center for Health Statistics; 2004. p. 77. Available at: http://www.cdc.gov/nchs/data/hus/hus04trend.pdf. Accessed April 25, 2005.

[7] National Vital Statistics Reports. Table 12. 2004;53(6):1. Available at: http://www.cdc.gov/nchs/date/dvs/nvsr53_06t12.pdf. Accessed November 10, 2004.

[8] National Center for Health Statistics. Health, United States, 2004. With chartbook on trends in the health of Americans. Table 35. Hyattsville, MD: National Center for Health Statistics; 2004. p. 99–102. Available at: http://www.cdc.gov/nchs/data/hus/hus04trend.pdf. Accessed April 25, 2005.

[9] National Center for Health Statistics. Health, United States, 2004. With chartbook on trends in the health of Americans. Table 36. Hyattsville, MD: National Center for Health Statistics; 2004. p. 103–5. Available at: http://www.cdc.gov/nchs/data/hus/hus04trend.pdf. Accessed April 25, 2005.

[10] National Center for Health Statistics. Health, United States, 2004. With chartbook on trends in the health of Americans. Table 38. Hyattsville, MD: National Center for Health Statistics; 2004. p. 109–12. Available at: http://www.cdc.gov/nchs/data/hus/hus04trend.pdf. Accessed April 25, 2005.

[11] National Center for Health Statistics. Health, United States, 2004. With chartbook on trends in the health of Americans. Table 31. Hyattsville, MD: National Center for Health Statistics; 2004. p. 154–7. Available at: http://www.cdc.gov/nchs/data/hus/hus04trend.pdf. Accessed April 25, 2005.

[12] Schneider D, Appleton L, McLemore T. A reason for visit classification for ambulatory care. National Center for Health Statistics. Vital and Health Statistics 1979;2(78):1–63.

[13] McCaig LF, Burt CW. National Ambulatory Hospital Medical Care Survey: 2002 Emergency Department Summary. Advance data from vital and health statistics; no 340. Table 5. Hyattsville, MD: National Center for Health Statistics; 2004. p. 15. Available at: http://www.cdc.gov/nchs/data/ad/ad340.pdf. Accessed April 25, 2005.

[14] McCaig LF, Burt CW. National Ambulatory Hospital Medical Care Survey: 2002 Emergency Department Summary. Advance data from vital and health statistics; no 340. Table 3. Hyattsville, MD: National Center for Health Statistics; 2004. p. 14. Available at: http://www.cdc.gov/nchs/data/ad/ad340.pdf. Accessed April 25, 2005.

[15] Goulding MR. Trends in prescribed medicine use and spending by older Americans 1992–2001. Aging Trends. No. 5. Hyattsville, MD: National Center for Health Statistics; 2005.

[16] National Center for Health Statistics. Health, United States, 2004. Agency for Healthcare Research and Quality, Center for Financing, Access, and Cost Trends (CFACT). August 2004 e-mail to MR Goulding, from M. Stagniti of AHRQ/CFACT with estimates from the household component of the 2001 Medical Expenditure Panel Survey. Available at: http://www.cdc.gov/nchs/data/hus/hus04trend.pdf. Accessed April 25, 2005.

[17] Cunningham PJ. Prescription drug access: not just a medicare problem. Washington, DC: Center for Studying Health System Change; 2002. Available at: http://www.hschange.org/CONTENT/429/429.pdf. Accessed April 25, 2005.

[18] American Society on Aging. Live well, live long. Health promotion and disease prevention for older adults. Optimal medications use module. Available at: http://www.americansocietyonaging.org/cdc/module3/phase1. Accessed April 25, 2005.

[19] National Center for Health Statistics. Health, United States, 2004. With chartbook on trends in the health of Americans. Table 87. Hyattsville, MD: National Center for Health Statistics; 2004. p. 215–7. Available at: http://www.cdc.gov/nchs/data/hus/hus04trend.pdf.

[20] U.S. Census Bureau. Releases, facts for features & special editions. CB05-FF.07–2. April 25, 2005. p. 7. Available at: http://www.census.gov/PressRelease/www/releases/archives/facts_for_features_special_editions/004210.html. Accessed April 25, 2005.

[21] McCaig LF, Burt CW. National Ambulatory Hospital Medical Care Survey: 2002 Emergency Department Summary. Advance data from vital and health statistics; no 340. Figure 11. Hyattsville, MD: National Center for Health Statistics; 2004. p. 8. Available at: http://www.cdc.gov/nchs/data/ad/ad340.pdf. Accessed April 25, 2005.

[22] Hustey FW, Meldon SW. The prevalence and documentation of impaired mental status in elderly emergency department patients. Ann Emerg Med 2002;39:248–53.

[23] Sanders AB. Missed delirium in older emergency department patients: a quality-of-care problem. Ann Emerg Med 2002;39:338–41.

[24] Wilber ST. Geriatric emergency medicine. New frontiers in geriatrics research: an agenda for surgical and related medical specialties. American Geriatrics Society; 2004.

[25] Terrell KM, Brizendine EJ, Bean WF, et al. An extended care facility-to-emergency department form improves communication. Acad Emerg Med 2005;12:114–8.

[26] Ross MA, Compton S, Richardson D, et al. The use and effectiveness of an emergency department observation unit for elderly patients. Ann Emerg Med 2003;41:668–77.

[27] Inouye SK, Bogardus ST, Charpentier PA, et al. A multicomponent intervention to prevent delirium in hospitalized older patients. N Engl J Med 1999;340:669–76.

[28] Rafter RH, Strumpf NE, Robinson J, Wagner J, et al. Caring for the person who interferes with treatment. In: Restraint-free care, individualized approaches for frail elders. New York: Springer Publishing; 1998. p. 85–123.

[29] Evans LK, Strumpf NE, Allen-Taylor SE, et al. A clinical trial to reduce restraints in nursing homes. J Am Geriatr Soc 1997;45:675–81.

[30] Tinetti ME, Liu WL, Gunter SF. Mechanical restraint use and fall-related injuries among residents of skilled nursing facilities. Ann Int Med 1992;116:369–74.

[31] Breier A. Safety data on Zyprexa (olanzapine) and Symbyax (olanzapine and fluoxetine HCl): elderly patients with dementia-related psychosis [letter]. Indianapolis, IN: Eli Lilly and Company; January 15, 2004.

[32] Goulding MR. Inappropriate medication prescribing for elderly ambulatory care patients. Arch Intern Med 2004;164:305–12.

[33] Gurwitz JH, Field TS, Harrold LR, et al. Incidence and preventability of adverse drug events among older persons in the ambulatory setting. JAMA 2003;289:1107–16.

[34] Wilber ST, Gerson LW. A research agenda for geriatric emergency medicine. Acad Emerg Med 2003;10:251–60.

[35] Wilber ST, Burger B, Gerson LW, et al. Reclining chairs reduce pain from gurneys in older emergency department patients: a randomized controlled trial. Acad Emerg Med 2005;12:119–23.

[36] Meldon SW, Mion LC, Palmer RM, et al. A brief risk-stratification tool to predict repeat emergency department visits and hospitalizations in older patients discharged from the emergency department. Acad Emerg Med 2003;10:224–32.

[37] McCusker J, Dendukuri N, Tousignant P, et al. Rapid two-stage emergency department intervention for seniors: impact on continuity of care. Acad Emerg Med 2003;10:233–43.

[38] Baraff LJ, Lee TJ, Kader S. Effect of a practice guideline for emergency department care of falls in elder patients on subsequent falls and hospitalizations for injuries. Acad Emerg Med 1999;6:1224–31.

[39] McCusker J, Jacobs P, Dendukuri N, et al. Cost-effectiveness of a brief two-stage emergency department intervention for high-risk elders: results of a quasi-randomized controlled trial. Ann Emerg Med 2003;41:45–56.

[40] Hohl CM, Robitaille C, Lord V, et al. Emergency physician recognition of adverse drug-related events in elder patients presenting to an emergency department. Acad Emerg Med 2005;12:197–205.

[41] Diggs BS, Lenfesty B, Arthur M, et al. The incidence and burden of ladder, structure, and scaffolding falls. Acad Emerg Med 2005;12:267–70.

[42] Hustey FM, Meldon SW, Smith MD, et al. The effect of mental status screening on the care of elderly emergency department patients. Ann Emerg Med 2003;41:678–84.

[43] Adams JG, Gerson LW. A new model for emergency care of geriatric patients. Acad Emerg Med 2003;10:271–4.

[44] Elder ER: first geriatric emergency medicine fellowship launched. Available at: http://www.modernheathcare.com/storyPreview.cms?articleID=350868archive=y. Accessed March 8, 2006.

[45] Reuben DB, Frank JC, Hirsch SH, et al. A randomized clinical trial of outpatient comprehensive geriatric assessment coupled with an intervention to increase adherence to recommendations. J Am Geriatr Soc 1999;47:269–76.

[46] Silliman RA, Barry PP. Outpatient comprehensive geriatric assessment: an intervention whose time has come, or has it. J Am Geriatr Soc 1999;47:371–2.

[47] Geriatrics at your fingertips. American Geriatrics Society. Available at: http://www.geriatricsatyourfingertips.org/ebook/Gayf_36.asp.

[48] Baloh RW. Evaluation of hearing. In: Dizziness, hearing loss and tinnitus. Philadelphia: FA Davis Company; 1988. p. 89–105; Table 6, p. 90.

[49] Moore AA, Siu A, Partridge JM, et al. A randomized trial of office-based screening for common problems in older persons. Am J Med 1997;102:371–8.

[50] Tinnetti M. Performance-oriented assessment of mobility problems in elderly patients. J Am Geriatr Soc 1986;34:119–26.

[51] Sheikh JI, Yesavage J. Yesavage Geriatric Depression Scale (GDS): Short Form. Clin Gerontol 1986;5:165.

[52] Cockrell JR, Fohlstein MF. Mini-Mental Status Examination (MMSE). Psychopharm Bull 1988;24:689–92.

[53] Lewis C. Balance, gait test proves simple yet useful. Psychopharm Bull 1993;2:9–40.

[54] Lachs MS, Feinstein AR, Cooney LM, et al. A simple procedure for screening for functional disability in elderly patients. Ann Int Med 1990;112:699–706.

[55] Moore AA, Siu AL. Screening for common problems in ambulatory elderly: clinical confirmation of a screening instrument. Am J Med 1996;100:438–43.

[56] Mion LC, Palmer RM, Meldon SW, et al. Case finding and referral model for emergency department elders: a randomized clinical trial. Ann Emerg Med 2003;41:57–68.

[57] Boult C, Boult L, Morishita L, et al. A randomized clinical trial of outpatient geriatric evaluation and management. J Am Geriatr Soc 2001;49:351–9.

ELSEVIER
SAUNDERS

Emerg Med Clin N Am
24 (2006) 261–272

EMERGENCY
MEDICINE
CLINICS OF
NORTH AMERICA

Resuscitation of the Elderly

Aneesh T. Narang, MD, Rishi Sikka, MD*

*Department of Emergency Medicine, Boston Medical Center, Dowling 1 South,
818 Harrison Avenue, Boston, MA 02118, USA*

The increasing proportion of elderly within the population has altered America's socioeconomic landscape and gradually transformed the practice of health care. Compared with the general population, the elderly are more acutely ill on presentation, consume more emergency department (ED) resources, are admitted more frequently to the hospital, and account for a greater proportion of intensive care unit admissions [1].

Given the current trends, EDs can anticipate an increase in the presentation of critically ill, elderly patients. Unfortunately, these patients remain a challenge to diagnose and to resuscitate. The normal physiologic changes associated with aging may masquerade a critical illness, and may impact the effectiveness of resuscitation. In many instances, physicians also must take into account issues of advance directives and medical futility when formulating their clinical decisions.

This article outlines the basic science and practical decision making involved in the resuscitation of the elderly patient. It is intended as a guide to assist in evidence-based, compassionate ED care for the critically ill, geriatric patient.

Epidemiology and outcomes

Elderly individuals who are ill are at high risk for hospitalization and death. On average, an elderly person has three to four chronic illnesses and nearly a 20% annual risk of hospitalization [2]. Once admitted, up to two thirds of elderly patients may be readmitted to the hospital within 6 months [3]. Unfortunately, the majority of elderly die in the hospital setting [4].

* Corresponding author.
E-mail address: sikka@att.net (R. Sikka).

0733-8627/06/$ - see front matter © 2006 Elsevier Inc. All rights reserved.
doi:10.1016/j.emc.2006.01.001   *emed.theclinics.com*

The first step in improving the resuscitation of the elderly in the ED is to better understand the outcomes and prognosis of resuscitation in this age group. The literature on the success of in-hospital and out-of-hospital cardiopulmonary resuscitation (CPR) provides some valuable guidance. The success of CPR in hospitalized patients has been well studied. Some earlier studies have demonstrated poor survival rates among hospitalized elderly patients after CPR, prompting some to question its utility in the geriatric population [5,6]. Contrary to older studies, more recent studies have reported more favorable results. Most studies have shown a hospital discharge survival rate ranging from 10% to 29%, and shown age not to be a significant determinant of survival [7–16]. The presence of ventricular tachycardia/ventricular fibrillation (VT/VF) substantially improves these rates, while relatively few patients who demonstrate asystole survive. Duration of CPR as well as the patient's prearrest comorbidities also significantly affect survival to hospital discharge [14]. Follow-up data in many of these studies have shown that more than half of the patients were alive, and most were living independently at home without any compromise in daily activities [12,16]. In general, patients who are highly functional with fewer chronic illnesses, hospitalized for a cardiac etiology, and closely monitored before the arrest are more likely to benefit from CPR. In these circumstances, CPR can be very successful, and elderly patients will benefit as much as younger patients [17].

The results of studies examining the effectiveness of out-of-hospital resuscitation have been conflicting. Survival rates following an out-of-hospital arrest for elderly patients with VF as a presenting rhythm is between 14% and 24% in most studies [18–23]. It is much lower in patients presenting with asystole or electromechanical dissociation. The wide range can be partially attributed to differences in study methodologies, down time before CPR, the availability of advanced cardiac life support in the field, and the training level of the paramedics. In general, the majority of analyses indicate favorable resuscitation outcomes in the elderly, particularly if the inciting event is a ventricular arrhythmia [17]. In contrast to studies of in-hospital and out-of-hospital cardiac arrests, there is little data regarding the effectiveness of resuscitation in nursing home residents. CPR is rarely, if ever, performed in this setting. Most analyses report poor rates of survival in the majority of patients who receive CPR [24–26]. However, there is some data to suggest that CPR can be effective if an arrest is witnessed and the initial rhythm is VT or VF [27,28].

The conclusions of these various studies have shown that age alone does not appear to be a significant determinant of survival in patients who receive CPR following cardiac arrest. Instead, those elderly patients with acute cardiac illnesses with fewer diseases and better baseline functional status have better resuscitation outcomes. Therefore, determining the potential success of resuscitation on the basis of age is shortsighted and not evidence-based. The potential response to CPR in an elderly patient with chronic, debilitating illnesses is not equivalent to that of an active, vigorous elderly patient with few comorbidities.

Pathophysiology

The difficulty in resuscitating elderly patients often can be attributed to significant pathophysiologic changes associated with aging, particularly within the cardiovascular system. Over time, there is a progressive decrease in the number of myocytes as well as an increase in collagen content, connective tissue, and fat. This results in a decline in ventricular compliance and in an increase in the incidence of sick sinus syndrome, atrial arrhythmias, and bundle branch blocks. There is also a substantial hardening of the major vessels, resulting in elevated systolic blood pressure, increased resistance to ventricular emptying, and ventricular hypertrophy. These physiologic changes lead to decreases in maximal heart rate, maximal aerobic capacity, peak exercise cardiac output, and peak ejection fraction. The elderly often are unable to compensate for decreased cardiac output by increasing their heart rate. Instead, they rely on augmenting ventricular filling and stroke volume to increase cardiac output. As a consequence, minor hypovolemia may precipitate a significant deterioration in cardiac function [29].

Pulmonary function is also affected by aging. As individuals age, there is a substantial decrease in the strength of respiratory muscles, chest wall compliance, and rib mobility. This results in a decline in maximum inspiratory and expiratory force by as much as 50%. Ventilatory responses to hypoxia and hypercapnia also fall by 50% and 40%, respectively. The respiratory system's ability to guard against environmental injury and infection also declines. A decline in T-cell function, mucociliary clearance, swallowing function, and the cough reflex all predispose the elderly to aspiration, with an increase in the incidence of respiratory infections and failure. All of these changes within the respiratory system combine to increase the incidence and severity of pneumonia, other respiratory infections, and respiratory failure [29].

Renal function is also not spared from the effects of the aging process. Along with a decline in glomerular filtration rate (GFR) of approximately 45% by age 80 years, renal tubular function also declines. As a result, assessing renal function and calculating creatinine clearance becomes important when determining the type and dosage of drugs used in the elderly. In addition, regulation of volume status becomes more problematic in the elderly. The ability to conserve sodium and excrete hydrogen ions falls, and therefore, the aging kidney is not able to regulate fluid and acid-base balance as well. Dehydration may become exacerbated because the kidney does not compensate well for nonrenal losses of sodium and water, which is thought to be due to a decline in the renin–angiotensin system and decreased end-organ responsiveness to antidiuretic hormone. Volume overload also can be a problem due to the decline in GFR and functional impairment of the diluting segment of the nephron [29].

Other significant changes that occur with aging involve the central nervous system. Components of sensory perception such as visual acuity, proprioception, balance, and tactile sensation all decline with age and make it difficult for patients to adjust to new environments. When placed in this situation, they are more likely to become confused and depressed, and suffer a serious fall. Decline in hypothalamic function along with decreased basal metabolic rates and changes in threshold for peripheral vasoconstriction and shivering cause a decrease in the ability to generate and conserve heat. In the postoperative or postinjury period, fever responses may be blunted as well. Changes in acute pain perception with aging are also problematic, and can lead to misdiagnosis and undertreatment. Several clinical observations have confirmed this, such as in the incidence of silent myocardial infarction and asymptomatic duodenal ulcer disease in this population [29].

Management of resuscitation

The elderly undergo many changes that pose challenges for emergency medicine (EM) physicians in recognizing a critically ill patient and impact the efficacy of various interventions during all stages of CPR. The initial steps in basic life support are aimed at establishing an airway and providing adequate oxygenation and ventilation. Unfortunately, the aging process renders the management of the geriatric airway slightly different from typical airway management. In the elderly, mouth opening may be limited by temporomandibular joint disease. Because there is often poor dentition and teeth can be dislodged into the oropharynx, special care must be taken during direct laryngoscopy. Dentures and bridges should be removed, although ventilation can be more difficult in an edentulous airway because the seal may be hard to establish in mouth-to-mouth or mouth-to-mask procedures. There may also a decrease in the range of motion of the cervical spine, especially at the atlanto-occipital joint, sometimes making positioning of the head and visualization of the glottis difficult. Forced extension of the neck can result in atlanto-occipital subluxation and spinal cord injury [30].

Due to these numerous anatomic changes, the emergency physician often must use alternative strategies and techniques in securing an airway. Intubation and mechanical ventilation of the elderly often become necessary, due to respiratory insufficiency and depressed mental status, and should not be withheld because of the patient's age. However, intubation should not be undertaken lightly. The risk of barotrauma and nosocomial pneumonia increase substantially, and weaning an elderly patient from the ventilator often becomes very difficult. In patients with respiratory insufficiency from easily reversible causes, it is reasonable to attempt noninvasive ventilatory support such as continuous positive airway pressure or bilevel positive airway pressure in efforts to avoid intubation. If intubation is necessary, avoid the small priming dose of nondepolarizing neuromuscular blocker, which is often administered before succinylcholine in younger patients. In the elderly, even a small priming dose of nondepolarizing neuromuscular blockers can abolish ventilation and airway reflexes completely. Furthermore, doses of induction agents, including barbiturates, benzodiazepines, and etomidate, should be reduced between 20% to 40% to minimize cardiac depression and hypotension in this population. On the other hand, doses of neuromuscular blocking agents should not be reduced. A Miller blade can be useful because it has a smaller flange than a Macintosh and allows easier visualization of landmarks and passage of the endotracheal tube [1]. It is also important to consider adjunctive airway devices, such as laryngeal mask airways and lighted stylets, in elderly patients with difficult airways [30].

The assessment of breathing in the elderly also becomes problematic, as there are wide arrays of changes in respiratory physiology that occur in this group. Decreasing baseline arterial oxygen tension with advancing age is due to an age-related decrease in diffusion capacity and an age-related ventilation–perfusion mismatch. The increased work of breathing along with frequent underlying nutritional deficiency puts the elderly at increased risk of respiratory failure. Because both ventilatory and heart rate responses to both hypoxia and hypercapnia are reduced, diagnosing occult respiratory insufficiency is very difficult and requires careful and frequent monitoring. A chest radiograph is important to perform in assessing respiratory distress. An EKG in the elderly is also critical, as silent myocardial ischemia is common among acute illnesses. If concern for carbon dioxide retention exists, a venturi mask is favorable over a nasal cannula because it provides a more precise method of oxygen delivery and does not vary depending on whether the patient is primarily mouth or nose breathing. For chronic obstructive pulmonary disease patients requiring intubation, ventilatory therapy should avoid respiratory alkalosis, which is a significant hurdle in attempts at subsequent weaning and extubation. It is generally agreed that using higher respiratory rates in conjunction with tidal volumes from 6 to 8 mL/kg is more physiologic and reduces the patient's work of breathing, as well as minimizing peak pressures and chances of barotrauma. Pulmonary oxygen toxicity is minimized by using the lowest amount of oxygen necessary to keep the PO_2 at least 60 mmHg [1].

After ventilation, the next step is the assessment of the circulation. Although the usual recommendation is to palpate a carotid pulse, this is often difficult in the elderly, secondary to carotid artery lesions and severe vascular narrowing. Potential complications include carotid flow occlusion or disruption of a plaque with subsequent distal embolization. Using the femoral pulse is a reasonable alternative in this population [30]. It is important to note that the elderly often do not have enough cardiac reserve to mount a significant response to stresses such as hypovolemia, sepsis, trauma, acute coronary ischemia, or respiratory failure. The initial approach to shock after addressing the airway begins with intravenous access and use of intravenous resuscitative fluids. Multiple small (250 cc) fluid boluses with repeated reassessment will often prevent significant volume overload and cardiogenic pulmonary edema. If time permits, using a central venous or pulmonary artery catheter will help improve outcome and guide therapy. By measuring filling pressures, it will be easy to assess whether the patient may need inotropic support to maintain an adequate blood pressure [1].

The predicament for the emergency physician lies in determining which patients with normal vital signs may still have significant tissue hypoperfusion. Capillary refill and extremity temperature are late signs of shock in the elderly. A venous lactate level can be helpful, and has shown to be a sensitive marker for intensive care unit admission and death. Unexplained metabolic acidosis on an arterial blood gas also suggests lactate production, although it is not as sensitive. Causes of shock in the elderly are numerous and include sepsis, dehydration, cardiac failure, and blood loss. A full laboratory workup is essential, as well as a chest radiograph. It is important to note that fever may be absent in elderly patients with focal infections, bacteremia, or sepsis, and hypothermia can occur in the setting of sepsis because of significant hypoperfusion. An EKG is mandatory to determine whether acute coronary ischemia or an arrhythmia is playing a role [1].

Managing shock in the elderly is also problematic for other reasons. Although chest compressions are to be instituted to maintain cardiac output when the patient does not have evidence of adequate circulation, it may be even less effective in the elderly who have higher incidence of underlying valvular dysfunction. It also produces significant injuries in the elderly, including those to the ribs, sternum, heart, lungs, great vessels, liver, and upper gastrointestinal tract. In patients with osteopenia and dorsal kyphosis, there have been case reports of chest compression induced thoracolumbar transvertebral fractures. Several studies have addressed the use of manual and mechanical compression devices to standardize the force and depth of compression and minimize injuries and complications [30].

The aging process also may impact the standard dosages of medications used during resuscitation. The changes in body composition during aging results in an increase in the volume of distribution of lipophilic drugs, and a decrease in the volume of distribution for hydrophilic drugs. The degree of drug binding to plasma proteins is also affected because of the decrease in albumin often seen in aging. In addition, there also is evidence of decreased beta-adrenergic responsiveness in the elderly. Despite all of these physiologic changes, the current recommended Advanced Cardiac Life Support (ACLS) guidelines on the use of drugs during resuscitation do not require modification in the elderly because there is no compelling evidence to suggest that they are not effective in this population. However, one ACLS medication of particular importance in the elderly may be magnesium. The elderly are susceptible to hypomagnesiumia due to poor daily intake, diuretic therapy, as well as malabsorption and diabetes mellitus. Magnesium deficiency is often associated with cardiac arrhythmias, cardiac insufficiency, and sudden cardiac death. There have been no reports regarding the use of magnesium or incidence of torsades de pointes in the elderly, but there have been studies showing decreased in-hospital mortality in patients 70 years or older who received magnesium versus placebo following an acute myocardial infarction [30].

Ethics of resuscitation and end-of-life care

In addition to facing complex dilemmas regarding resuscitating elderly patients, EM physicians increasingly will also confront a myriad of other issues associated with end-of-life care. Unfortunately, some aspects of the care of the dying may be at odds with the professional mission of EM physicians and the environment of the ED [4]. EM physicians possess a reflexive instinct toward saving the dying and averting death. Expertise in difficult resuscitation is a hallmark of the specialty. However, the impulse to save life at all costs must be relinquished by the EM physician when approaching the terminal patient. Although the rapid pace and lack of privacy of the ED may conspire against optimal end-of life care, EM physicians should attempt to embrace a more patient-centric, humane imperative. EM physicians should acknowledge and respect an individual patient's needs for end-of-life care. This requires a working knowledge of advance directives and the concepts underlying medical futility.

Advance directives

An advance directive (AD) is a document providing guidance for a patient's wishes when they are unable to do so themselves. ADs may take the form of either a living will or a durable power of attorney. A living will outlines the interventions that should or should not be performed under certain clinical scenarios, particularly when the patient is terminally ill [2]. Living wills may vary in substance from highly detailed documents to vague instructions with dubious interpretation [31]. In contrast, a power of attorney identifies a surrogate decision maker in the event that a patient no longer has the capacity to make decisions [2].

ADs secure the autonomy of an individual who currently lacks, but once possessed, an appropriate decision-making ability [32]. This extension of patient autonomy has been protected and encouraged through legislation. All 50 states recognize the patient autonomy embodied within an AD [33]. The federal Patient Self-Determination Act of 1991 requires that patients admitted to the hospital have the opportunity to complete and incorporate an AD within their medical record [34].

Although ADs have been embraced by professional organizations and the general patient community, their use remains sporadic, and their implementation is problematic [35–37]. In one study of approximately 700 nursing home residents, only 8% possessed an AD [38]. A second analysis of over 13,000 US deaths found that less than 10% of the deceased had an AD [39]. However, the mere creation of an AD far from guarantees its application. It is not uncommon for individuals at the end-of-life to arrive in the ED without their AD. The AD may have been lost, placed in an outpatient chart, or simply forgotten at the place of residence [31,32,40]. Patients also may fail to inform the treating physician of the presence of an AD [41].

Equally concerning is the reticence of EM physicians to engage their patients about ADs and resuscitation options [4]. EM physicians may feel inappropriate initiating this process, and may wish to defer to a primary care provider who has an ongoing, established relationship with the patient. EM physicians may also feel that the process is difficult and too time-consuming. However, neither of these concerns is supported by the available evidence. Most patients welcome the opportunity to discuss their end-of-life care with a physician, and a do not resuscitate order may be established in as little as 16 minutes in an ambulatory care setting [42–44].

EM physicians require a strategy to cope with the implementation problems associated with ADs and the moral ambiguities associated with end-of-life care. If an AD exists but cannot be produced in the ED, the EM physician must evaluate the reliability of the information available and attempt to make a series of clinical decisions adhering to the patient's previously stated wishes [45]. Physicians must resist the temptation to infer a patient's preferences for life-sustaining treatment. In general, physicians are unable to accurately predict an individual patient's preferences for resuscitation at the end of life [46].

If an AD can be produced in the ED, then the EM physician should not overrule it. Overriding an AD has been described as morally abhorrent and an act of profound disrespect toward patient autonomy [4]. Physicians should adhere to the instructions of an AD, although this may be difficult when the patient is comatose and the patient's next of kin or health care proxy wants the patient fully resuscitated [47]. If there is doubt about the validity of the AD, or the next of kin or health care proxy insist on resuscitation, it is reasonable to resuscitate the patient and then discuss these issues in more detail. Physicians may also override an AD if there is clear evidence that the patient's preferences have changed since the drafting of the original document [4].

If an AD does not exist and the timing and moment are appropriate, EM physicians should embrace the opportunity to discuss ADs with the appropriate patients. It is a component of the process to facilitate the follow-up of inpatient and outpatient care for the terminally ill. This is a proactive stance that promotes the cooperation and accountability of the entire health care team that serves patients at the end of their life [4].

Medical futility

Often, an unknown elderly patient may present to the ED on the verge of death. In such a situation, there may be neither the time nor the means to engage in meditative reflection regarding a patient's wishes. A delay in action may significantly hinder the effectiveness of a resuscitation. Although the impulse may be to resuscitate, a physician is not under an overriding legal or ethical obligation to treat if they believe an intervention may be futile.

A futile intervention may encompass a variety of potential outcomes. It may be used to refer to an intervention with a low likelihood of success, or an intervention with a low probability of survival, or an intervention with an unlikely restoration of an adequate quality of life [48]. Physicians lack a consensus definition of the meaning of futility [49,50]. As a result of these ambiguities, any discussion with families and other professionals requires an exact specification of the interpretation of a potentially futile intervention [48].

Both professional organizations and the judicial system have made meaningful contributions to the debate on withholding ineffective interventions. The American College of Emergency Physicians (ACEP) has issued a policy statement stating that EM physicians may withhold a treatment that has no realistic chance of medical benefit toward the patient [51]. Although this recommendation provides some guidance, the legal ramifications also need to be considered. In the majority of jurisdictions, there is no state or federal law addressing the withholding of nonbeneficial treatments. Instead, case law provides some guidance regarding the legal implications of withholding care. In general, courts and juries are reluctant to override a family's desire for continuing care [48]. Similarly, they are reticent about holding a physician liable for their judgment regarding the ineffectiveness of an intervention [48]. Nonetheless, EM physicians must bear in mind that their determination of a treatment's effectiveness may be subject to legal scrutiny [48]. Any decision regarding a treatment's effectiveness should have a solid grounding in the evidence for the outcomes of resuscitation.

Desptie the endorsement of ACEP and recent legal precedent, EM physicians still remain reluctant to withhold care [52]. Legal concerns and the fear of liability continue to dominate EM physicians' decisions regarding resuscitation [52]. The best strategy to deal with these concerns and to promote ethical, humane care relies on open communication and knowledge of scientific data. The key is to engage the patient, their family, and their surrogates as early as possible regarding their preferences [48]. These preferences should be weighed in the context of the available evidence regarding the benefits and risks of various alternative interventions [48].

Allowing the family to be present during a patient's resuscitation may be considered by the emergency physician and staff. Some family members may prefer to be present, rather than waiting to see their loved one after she/he has been pronounced dead. Factors relevant to this decision include the emotional state of the family member(s) and the age and number of family members present. If a family member is present during the resuscitation, a staff member should be assigned to provide support to this person [53].

Summary

In the future, EM physicians can anticipate increasing ED visits from critically ill, elderly patients. These individuals require prompt identification and early, aggressive intervention. Unfortunately, the effects of aging on normal physiology conspire to make the recognition of the critically ill geriatric patient a challenge. These same physiologic effects may also impact the effectiveness of standard life-saving interventions. EM physicians must redouble their efforts toward understanding the pathophysiology and effective treatment of these patients.

A more thorough knowledge of this information will also assist in the ethic treatment of critically ill elderly patients toward the end of their life. An evidence-based comprehension of patient prognosis is a key component of an elderly individual's treatment toward the end of life. This information assists in the interpretation of ADs and patient and family preferences.

Ultimately, improving the care of the critically ill geriatric patient hinges on improved communication. EM physicians should actively engage primary care providers, specialists, prehospital providers, patients, and families in this process. Hopefully, initiating this process will further the goal of more humane, patient-centric care of all geriatric patients.

References

[1] Milzman D, Rothenhaus T. Resuscitation of the geriatric patient. Emerg Med Clin North Am 1996;14:233–44.

[2] Mueller PS, Hook CC, Fleming KC. Ethical issues in geriatrics: a guide for clinicians. Mayo Clin Proc 2004;79:554–62.

[3] Callahan E, Thomas D, Goldhirsch S, et al. Geriatric hospital medicine. Med Clin North Am 2002;86:707–29.

[4] Schears RM. Emergency physicians' role in end-of-life care. Emerg Med Clin North Am 1999;17:539–59.

[5] Murphy DI, Murry AM, Robinson BE, et al. Outcomes of cardiopulmonary resuscitation in the elderly. Ann Intern Med 1989;111:199–205.

[6] Taffet GI, Teasdale TA, Luchi RJ. In-hospital cardiopulmonary resuscitation. JAMA 1988; 260:2069–72.

[7] Gulati RS, Bhan GL, Horan MA. Cardiopulmonary resuscitation of old people. Lancet 1983;2:267–9.

[8] Bedell SE, Delbanco TL, Cook EF, et al. Survival after cardiopulmonary resuscitation in the hospital. N Engl J Med 1983;309:569–75.

[9] Woog RH, Torzillo PJ. In-hospital cardiopulmonary resuscitation: prospective survey of management and outcome. Anaesth Intensive Care 1987;15:193–8.

[10] George AL Jr, Folk BP III, Crecelius PL, et al. Pre-arrest morbidity and other correlates of survival after in-hospital cardiopulmonary arrest. Am J Med 1989;97:28–34.

[11] Tortolani AJ, Risucci DA, Rosati RJ, et al. In-hospital cardiopulmonary resuscitation: patient arrest and resuscitation factors associated with survival. Resuscitation 1990;20:115–28.

[12] Robinson GR II, Hess D. Postdischarge survival and functional status following in-hospital cardiopulmonary resuscitation. Chest 1994;105:991–6.

[13] Roberts D, Landolfo K, Light RB, et al. Early predictors of mortality for hospitalized patients suffering cardiopulmonary arrest. Chest 1990;97:413–9.

[14] Rosenberg M, Wang C, Hoffman-Wilde S, et al. Results of cardiopulmonary resuscitation. Arch Intern Med 1993;153:1370–5.

[15] Berger R, Kelley M. Survival after in-hospital cardiopulmonary arrest of noncritically ill patients. Chest 1994;106:872–9.

[16] Tresch DD, Heudebert G, Kutty K, et al. Cardiopulmonary resuscitation in elderly patients hospitalized in the 1990s: a favorable outcome. J Am Geriatr Soc 1994;42:137–41.

[17] Tresch DD, Thakur RK. Cardiopulmonary resuscitation in the elderly. Beneficial or an exercise in futility? Emerg Med Clin North Am 1998;16:649–63.

[18] Tresch DD, Thakur RK, Hoffmann RG, et al. Comparison of outcome of paramedic-witnessed cardiac arrest in patients younger and older than 70 years. Am J Cardiol 1990;65:453–7.

[19] Tresch DD, Thakur RK, Hoffmann RG, et al. Should the elderly be resuscitated following out-of-hospital cardiac arrest? Am J Med 1989;86:145–50.

[20] Bonnin MJ, Pepe PE, Clark PS. Survival in the elderly after out-of-hospital cardiac arrest. Crit Care Med 1993;21:1645–51.

[21] Denes P, Long L, Madison C, et al. Resuscitation from out-of-hospital ventricular tachycardia/fibrillation (VT/VF): the effect of age on outcome. Circulation 1990;82(Suppl):III-81.

[22] Eisenberg MS, Horwood BT, Larson MP. Cardiopulmonary resuscitation in the elderly. Ann Intern Med 1990;113:408–9.

[23] Longstreth WT Jr, Cobb LA, Fahrenbruch CE, et al. Does age affect outcomes of out-of-hospital cardiopulmonary resuscitation? JAMA 1990;264:2109–10.

[24] Applebaum GE, King JE, Finucane TE. The outcome of CPR initiated in nursing homes. J Emerg Geriatr Soc 1990;38:197–200.

[25] Awoke S, Mouton CP, Parrott M. Outcomes of skilled cardiopulmonary resuscitation in a long-term care facility: futile therapy? J Am Geriatr Soc 1992;40:593–5.

[26] Gordon M, Cheung M. Poor outcome of on-site CPR in a multilevel geriatric facility: three and a half years experience at the Baycrest Center for Geriatric Care. J Am Geriatr Soc 1993;41:163–6.

[27] Tresch DD, Neahring JM, Duthie EH, et al. Outcomes of cardiopulmonary resuscitation in nursing homes: can we predict who will benefit? Am J Med 1993;95:123–30.

[28] Ghusn HF, Teasdale TA, Pepe PE, et al. Older nursing home residents have a cardiac arrest survival rate to that of older persons living in the community. J Am Geriat Soc 1995;43:520–7.

[29] Rosenthal R, Kavic S. Assessment and management of the geriatric patient. Crit Care Med 2004;32:S92–105.

[30] Liu L, Carlisle A. Geriatric anesthesia: management of cardiopulmonary resuscitation. Anesthiol Clin North Am 2000;18:143–58.

[31] Walker RM, Schonwetter RS, Kramer DR, et al. Living wills and resuscitation preferences in the elderly popuation. Arch Intern Med 1995;155:171–5.

[32] Danis M, Southerland LI, Garrett JM, et al. A prospective study of advance directives for life-sustaining care. N Engl J Med 1991;324:882–8.

[33] Prendergast TJ. Advance care planning: pitfalls, progress, promise. Crit Care Med 2001;29:N34–9.

[34] Wolf SM, Boyle P, Callahan D, et al. Sources of concern about the Patient Self-Determination Act. N Engl J Med 1991;325:1666–71.

[35] American College of Physicians. Ethics manual. 4th ed. Ann Intern Med 1998;128:576–94.

[36] Orentlicher D. Advanced medical directives. JAMA 1990;263:2365–7.

[37] Emmanuel LL, Barry MJ, Stoeckle JD, et al. Advance directives for medical care—a case for greater use. N Engl J Med 1991;324:889–95.

[38] Jones JS, Dwyer PR, White LJ, et al. Patient transfer from nursing home to emergency department: outcomes and policy implications. Acad Emerg Med 1997;4:908–15.

[39] Hanson LC, Rodgman E. The use of living wills at the end of life: a national study. Arch Intern Med 1996;156:1018–22.

[40] Miles SH, Koepp R, Weber EP. Advanced end-of-life treatment planning: a research review. Arch Intern Med 1996;156:1062–8.

[41] Teno JM, Licks S, Lynn J, et al. SUPPORT Investigators. Do advance directives provide instructions that direct care? J Am Geriatr Soc 1997;45:508–12.

[42] Hakim RB, Teno JM, Harrell FE, et al. Factors associated with do-not-resuscitate orders: patients' preferences, prognoses, and physicians' judgments. Ann Intern Med 1996;125: 284–93.

[43] Schonwetter RS, Walker RM, Solomon M, et al. Life values, resuscitation preferences and the applicability of living wills in an older population. J Am Geriatr Soc 1996;44:954–8.

[44] Smith TJ, Desch CE, Hackney MK, et al. How long does it take to get a "do not resuscitate" order? J Palliat Care 1997;13:5–8.

[45] Marco CA. Ethical issues of resuscitation. Emerg Med Clin North Am 1999;17:527–38.

[46] Hamel MB, Lynn J, Teno JM, et al. Age-related differences in care preferences, treatment decisions, and clinical outcomes of seriously ill hospitalized adults: lessons from SUPPORT. J Am Geriatr Soc 2000;48:S176–82.

[47] Ramos T, Reagan JE. "No" when the family says "go": resisting families' requests for futile CPR. Ann Emerg Med 1989;18:898–9.

[48] Marco CA, Larkin GL, Moskop JC, et al. Determination of "futility" in emergency medicine. Ann Emerg Med 2000;35:604–12.

[49] Solomon MZ. How physicians talk about futility: making words mean too many things. J Law Med Ethics 1993;21:231–7.

[50] McCrary SV, Swanson JW, Youngner SJ, et al. Physicians' quantitative assessments of medical futility. J Clin Ethics 1994;5:100–5.

[51] American College of Emergency Physicians. Nonbeneficial ("futile") emergency medical interventions [policy statement]. Approved March 1998. Dallas (TX): American College of Emergency Physicians; 1998. Access at: http://www.acep.org/policy/PO400198.HTM.

[52] Marco CA, Bessman ES, Schoenfeld CN, et al. Ethical issues of cardiopulmonary resuscitation: current practice among emergency physicians. Acad Emerg Med 1997;4:898–904.

[53] Wagner JM. Lived experience of critically ill patients' family members during cardiopulmonary resuscitation. Am J Crit Care 2004;13:416–20.

ELSEVIER
SAUNDERS

Emerg Med Clin N Am
24 (2006) 273–298

EMERGENCY
MEDICINE
CLINICS OF
NORTH AMERICA

Geriatric Neurologic Emergencies

Lara K. Kulchycki, MD, Jonathan A. Edlow, MD*

Beth Israel Deaconess Medical Center, West Clinical Center 2,
Department of Emergency Medicine, One Deaconess Road West CC-2,
Boston, MA 02215, USA

The aging of the United States population is well publicized. Projections indicate that by 2030, 55 to 65 million people over the age of 65 years will live in this country, approximately 20% of the total population [1]. Elderly patients are more likely to require emergency care and have different disease patterns with increased risk for morbidity and mortality. Familiarity with geriatrics is becoming an increasingly important component of emergency practice. Yet surveys suggest that many emergency physicians are uneasy assessing and managing geriatric patients [2].

Elderly patients are particularly prone to serious neurologic problems. Chronic diseases common in this group, such as hypertension, diabetes, atherosclerosis, and obstructive sleep apnea, increase the risk for stroke. Older patients have an increased incidence of same-level falls and pedestrian accidents, mechanisms more likely to cause head and neck injuries. Aging patients have decreased innate and specific immunity, increasing the likelihood of infectious disease.

Clinical assessment of geriatric patients can be difficult. Such patients often have complicated medical histories that they may not be able to relate secondary to dementia or acute illness. Mental status changes may be missed or underestimated in patients who have underlying cognitive dysfunction. In addition, vital signs and examination findings are less reliable in predicting the severity of illness, resulting in diagnostic delays and misdiagnoses.

Aneurysmal subarachnoid hemorrhage

The Framingham data indicate that the incidence of aneurysmal subarachnoid hemorrhage (SAH) increases from 15 per 100,000 among people from 30 to 59 years of age to approximately 78 per 100,000 among those

* Corresponding author.
E-mail address: jedlow@bidmc.harvard.edu (J.A. Edlow).

aged 70 to 88 years [3]. Data from the International Cooperative Study on
the Timing of Aneurysm Surgery, however, which enrolled 3,521 patients
who had SAH, indicate the average age at presentation is 50 years [4].

Advanced age is an independent risk factor for death and severe disability
after aneurysmal SAH. Lanzino and colleagues examined data on 906 patients from 21 neurosurgical centers to define the relationship between
age, presentation, clinical course, and prognosis in SAH. Five age groups
were compared: younger than 40 years, 41 to 50 years, 51 to 60 years, 61
to 70 years, and older than 70 years. Mortality rates increased from only
12% in the youngest patients to 35% in the oldest. Good outcomes defined
by Glasgow Outcome Scores (GOS) [5] at 3 months were significantly less
likely in aged patients, decreasing steadily from 73% in patients younger
than 40 years to 25% in those older than 70 years (Fig. 1) [6]. This relationship
between age and morbidity and mortality persisted even when outcomes were
controlled for the severity of bleed and presence of pre-existing comorbidities.
Although there is no correlation between aneurysm size or location with age,
it is clear that elderly patients who have large aneurysms (>9 mm) are more
likely to be disabled and dependent [7].

Clear differences in presentation and hospital course appear in geriatric
patients who have SAH. Elderly patients more often present with thick subarachnoid clot and a profoundly depressed level of consciousness. The percentage of obtunded or comatose patients steadily increased from 12% in
those younger than 40 years to 27% in those older than age 70 years. Elderly
patients were more likely to re-bleed; rates of recurrent hemorrhage ranged

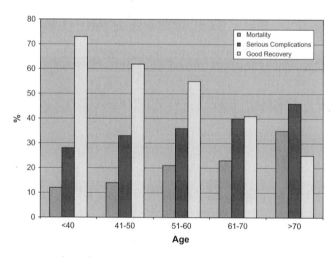

Fig. 1. Poor outcomes in patients who have aneurysmal subarachnoid hemorrhage (SAH) are
related to advanced age. The rates of mortality and life-threatening complications and the likelihood of a good functional recovery by Glasgow Outcome Scale (GOS) are depicted for each age
group [6].

from 4.5% in the youngest age group to 16.4% in patients older than age 70 years. The oldest patients were also more likely to develop intraventricular hemorrhage, hydrocephalus, and symptomatic vasospasm. Rates of life-threatening complications steadily increased with each decade [6].

Cardiac abnormalities, including electrocardiogram (ECG) changes, cardiac enzyme elevations, and regional wall motion abnormalities, are common in SAH. ECG abnormalities may include sinus tachycardia, ST segment elevation or depression, inverted T waves, or prolongation of the QT interval. Transient arrhythmias are common after acute bleeds, appearing in up to 9 out of 10 patients [8]. Approximately 20% to 30% of patients who have nontraumatic SAH display CK-MB and troponin spikes, usually within the first 24 hours [9]. Those patients often have some degree of left ventricular (LV) dysfunction, as evidenced by wall motion abnormalities on echocardiography.

Interpreting the clinical significance of new cardiac abnormalities in the setting of acute neurologic disease can be challenging in elderly patients who already may have underlying cardiac pathology. Ventricular dysfunction associated with SAH, although incompletely understood, does not arise from coronary occlusion. Pathology from animal models shows myofibrillar degeneration similar to that seen in states of catecholamine excess. The vast majority of patients exhibiting these deficits revert to their previous level of cardiac function within a few weeks [9]. Emergency physicians must be aware that ECG changes and cardiac enzyme elevations in such patients do not necessarily equate with ischemia; these patients are not de facto poor surgical candidates and still warrant aggressive treatment.

Advances in neurosurgical management continue to improve the overall outcome for these critically ill patients. Operative mortality has decreased drastically from more than 50% in the first Cooperative Study of Intracranial Aneurysms and Subarachnoid Hemorrhage in 1966 to only 20% in the Cooperative Study on the Timing of Aneurysm Surgery published in 1990 [10,11]. Inagawa studied 503 SAH patients and compared outcomes for those treated in the early versus the late 1980s. He showed a twofold increase in the number of elderly patients (from 17% to 34%) and in the percentage of good functional outcomes among this patient population (from 18% to 41%) [12].

Although no randomized controlled trial (RCT) specifically addresses the benefit of definitive management over medical therapy in elderly patients who have SAH, several lines of evidence argue that outcomes with surgical or endovascular treatment are superior. First, the prognosis in conservative management is bleak, with a 5-year survival of only 20% [13]. Also, geriatric patients are far more likely to re-bleed and suffer acute complications amenable to surgical correction, such as hydrocephalus. Also, some medical management strategies, such as Triple H therapy (hypertensive, hypervolemic, and hemodilution therapy), can be pursued more safely once the aneurysm has been obliterated.

The emergency physician's role is in the rapid detection and stabilization of patients who have ruptured aneurysms. Once computed tomography (CT) scans or cerebrospinal fluid (CSF) analysis reveal the presence of subarachnoid blood, the care pathways for elderly patients are similar to those for younger patients. All require careful monitoring, assessment of the airway, seizure prophylaxis, and control of pain and nausea. Coagulopathy, frequently present in elderly patients secondary to warfarin use, should be reversed. Although severe hypertension is associated with more dire outcomes, acute lowering of blood pressure has not proven to improve consistently the clinical course of aneurysmal bleeds [14].

Considerable uncertainty exists with regard to optimal blood pressure parameters in patients who have SAH; some surgeons advocate tolerance of mean arterial pressures (MAP) less than 130 mm Hg, whereas others insist on tight control of systolic blood pressures (SBP) to less than 140 mm Hg. When antihypertensive agents are needed, the use of a short-acting and titratable agent, such as nicardipine or labetalol is preferable. Nitroprusside, although effective in decreasing systolic pressures, has several disadvantages in neurologic emergencies; it dilates cerebral vasculature, placing the patient at risk for elevations in intracranial pressure (ICP), impairs autoregulation, and may induce excessive hypotension in elderly patients [15].

Patients who have known SAH must be monitored carefully in the emergency department (ED) for signs of decompensation. Patients who have a changing neurologic examination or alterations in mental status warrant a repeat CT scan to look for signs of progression. Nonspecific changes, such as increased confusion, also may be a postictal change or the presenting symptom of cerebral vasospasm [16].

Early involvement of a skilled neurosurgical consultant is a critical component of management. Emergency physicians should have a low threshold for transfer of surgical candidates to centers with experience in aneurysm repair, because increased surgical volume correlates with significantly lower in-hospital mortality [17]. Centers that offer the option of traditional open surgical clipping and endovascular coiling techniques are preferable. The International Subarachnoid Aneurysm Trial (ISAT), which randomized 2,143 patients eligible for both techniques to clipping versus coiling, showed a distinct advantage to endovascular repair; coiled patients had a 22.6% relative risk reduction for death and dependency without a significant increase in re-bleeding [18].

Emergency physicians also may be in the fortuitous position of diagnosing unruptured intracranial aneurysms. Such patients may present with symptoms such as headache, transient ischemic attack (TIA), seizure, third nerve palsy, or other evidence of mass effect. Patients who have unruptured aneurysms require neurosurgical evaluation, although management for asymptomatic lesions remains controversial [19,20]. Clinical data indicate that aneurysm repair can result in good functional outcomes even for elderly patients [21]. It is again critical to refer such patients to sites that offer open and endovascular techniques, because coiling may confer particular advantage to patients older than 65 years of age and those who have significant comorbidities [22].

Traumatic brain injury

Elderly patients are at particular risk for traumatic brain injury (TBI). The overall incidence of TBI cases seen in emergency departments in the United States is 444 cases per 100,000 persons. The incidence increases in the elderly population and peaks at 1,026 cases per 100,000 in patients older than 85 years of age. Younger patients are 1.6 times more likely to be male, but this sexual disparity reverses in the elderly population [23].

Elderly patients have higher morbidity and mortality from head injury. Worse outcomes do not seem to be the result of therapeutic nihilism. In most applicable studies, similar percentages of younger and elderly patients received ICP monitoring and neurosurgical intervention [24,25]. Even accounting for differences in the premorbid state, outcomes remain worse in old age; something innate to the aging brain lends a particular vulnerability to neurologic insult.

The relative frequency of different injuries and mechanisms of injury differ in geriatric patients. Subdural hematomas (SDH) are far more common, accounting for 46% of TBI cases in elderly patients versus only 28% in younger cohorts [24]. Epidural hematomas are less common among elderly trauma victims (Fig. 2). Although younger trauma patients are more likely to be injured in motor vehicle collisions (MVC), the elderly population has more pedestrian accidents and falls [25].

Falls represent an enormous cause of morbidity and mortality in older adults. Those older than 65 years of age have an annual fall incidence of

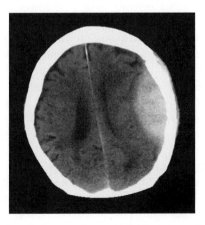

Fig. 2. Trauma is less likely to produce epidural hematomas in elderly patients.

30% and this rate increases to 50% in octogenarians [26]. This high predilection for falls is multifactorial. Normal aging adversely affects vision, joint function, and proprioception. Superimposed chronic diseases, such as diabetes, can result in autonomic dysfunction, peripheral neuropathy, and general deconditioning. Syncopal events may be associated with medication-related orthostasis or arrhythmias. Geriatric patients are not only more likely to fall, but they are also more likely to sustain serious injury when they do. Sterling noted that falls in elderly patients were seven times more likely to be the predominant etiology of injury (48% versus 7%) and seven times more likely to be the cause of death (55% versus 7.5%) than in younger patients [26].

Falls from a sitting or standing position can lead to surprisingly severe injuries in older people. Sterling and colleagues found that same-level falls resulted in serious injury in 30% of elderly persons compared with only 4% of a younger cohort. Head and neck injuries were particularly common, occurring more than twice as often (47% versus 22%) [26]. Mortality for these low falls in the elderly population approaches 15%, three times that seen in younger cohorts [27]. Paramedics and emergency physicians must be cautious with these patients and maintain a low threshold for cervical spine immobilization, imaging, and admission.

The increased number of pedestrian accidents seen in elderly patients has important implications for the nature and severity of injuries. Hui and colleagues studied elderly trauma patients admitted to the Surgical Intensive Care Unit (SICU) and compared patients injured in motor vehicle accidents with those injured in pedestrian traffic accidents. They found that pedestrian victims were significantly more likely to have subarachnoid (26% versus 9%) and subdural (29% versus 8%) bleeding. Pedestrians struck by motor vehicles had significantly greater Injury Severity Scores (ISS) [28] and higher mortality (19.6% versus 9.5%) [29].

Some researchers have argued that the threshold for scene triage and subsequent transfer to trauma centers should be lower for geriatric patients. Meldon and colleagues conducted a retrospective analysis of trauma outcomes in 455 patients older than age 80 years who were transported to a trauma center (level I or II) or an acute care hospital. Most of the deaths occurred in patients who had an ISS in the range of 21 to 45. Within that group, trauma center care conferred an enormous survival benefit (56% in trauma centers versus 8% in acute care hospitals). Using logistic regression to control for age, gender, ISS, and the presence of TBI, they demonstrated that very elderly patients are three times more likely to die at nontrauma centers [30].

Standard prehospital protocols may underestimate the severity of injury in older trauma patients. Traumatized elders are less likely to display clear hemodynamic distress. Changes in mental status may be under appreciated in patients who have underlying cognitive dysfunction. Changes in the aging brain may make standard clinical scoring mechanisms, such as the Glasgow

Coma Scale (GCS), less reliable. Low-energy mechanisms, such as same-level falls, do not commonly trigger transport to trauma centers.

Vital signs may not reveal the extent of injury in geriatric patients. In fact, up to 63% of elderly patients who have an ISS of greater than 15 and 25% who have an ISS greater than 30 did not display any of the standard hemo-dynamic criteria for trauma activation [31]. Tachycardia may be absent be-cause of inherent decline in the maximum output of the cardiovascular system or secondary to cardiac medications, such as beta blockers. Blood pressure that would be considered normal in a younger person may repre-sent significant relative hypotension in an elderly patient.

Use of GCS is a standard component of trauma evaluations but carries special import for patients who have TBI. Admission and postresuscitation GCS is correlated with survival and the ultimate degree of impairment after discharge [32], but physiologic data on the aging brain raise questions about the usefulness of GCS for elderly patients who have brain injury. Mosenthal and colleagues found significant mortality in aging adults whose sole de-tected injury was a minor TBI as defined by a GCS of 14 to 15 [24]. Normal age-related atrophy results in enlargement of the space between the brain and the inner table of the skull for hematoma accumulation. Significant brain injury may exist without midline shift on CT scans or clinical evidence of elevated ICP. Emergency physicians should not be falsely reassured by high GCS scores, especially in adults older than 70 years of age.

Even if prehospital protocols were optimized for geriatric trauma, several studies have shown a perplexing discrepancy in protocol compliance for el-derly patients. Scheetz examined a registry of 5,712 trauma victims with an ISS ≥ 16. In that analysis, young men were most likely to be brought to a trauma center (82%), whereas older women were least likely to be trans-ported to a trauma center (60%) [33]. Ma and colleagues conducted an anal-ysis of 32,950 EMS transports and similarly found that a disproportionate percentage of elderly trauma victims were transported to nontrauma centers [34]. More investigation is needed to elucidate the reason for this trend.

Age itself has been suggested as a potential criterion for trauma team ac-tivation and for the use of early intensive monitoring and resuscitation. De-metriades and colleagues prospectively evaluated outcomes once age greater than 70 years was used to trigger trauma team activation. Overall mortality in the elderly population was significantly lower, decreasing from 53.8% to 34.2%, without a concomitant increase in survivors who had permanent dis-ability (16.7% versus 12%) [35].

Most studies on TBI in the elderly population are muddied by the pres-ence of multisystem trauma. Mosenthal and colleagues gathered retrospec-tive data on elderly patients who had isolated TBI and found a persistent pattern of increasing mortality with each decade past 50 years. Overall in-hospital mortality for isolated TBI was twofold higher in elderly patients, 30% versus 14%, and remained significantly elevated even in mild to mod-erate brain injury. Even when pre-existing medical conditions and complications were removed from the equation by logistic regression, age remained an independent risk factor for death despite that similar percentages received invasive neurosurgical interventions [24].

Geriatric TBI patients who survive to discharge exhibit poorer cognitive and functional outcomes when compared with younger cohorts. As expected, more elderly patients are discharged to skilled nursing facilities, require longer periods of rehabilitation, and display less rapid clinical improvement [36].

Chronic subdural hematoma

Among types of traumatic brain injuries, chronic subdural hematoma (SDH) bears special mention, because it can be subtle and varied in presentation and hence frequently misdiagnosed. Epidemiologic data show the annual incidence of chronic SDH is approximately 1 to 2 cases per 100,000 population, but this number increases to more than 7 cases per 100,000 among patients older than 70 years of age [37]. Most studies show a clear male predominance in all age groups [38].

Although frequently attributed purely to cerebral atrophy and concomitant stretching of the bridging veins, the vulnerability of the elderly patient to chronic SDH likely has additional contributors. As previously mentioned, aging patients are prone to falls and have an increased incidence of head trauma. They also are more likely to be on antiplatelet or anticoagulant medicines that can exacerbate bleeding from minor injury. Certain structural brain lesions, such as meningiomas and metastatic tumors, increase the likelihood of hemorrhage into the subdural space. Intracranial hypotension, such as that caused by over shunting of CSF, represents another potential etiology of chronic SDH. In fact, up to 8% of adults shunted for normal pressure hydrocephalus (NPH) develop subdural bleeding [39].

Minor trauma, often long forgotten by the time of presentation, is postulated to be the initial insult in most cases of chronic SDH. Severe head injuries with brisk bleeding are likely to present as an acute SDH. More minor injuries with slow hematoma accumulation lead to the delayed presentation and more subtle spectrum of deficits seen in chronic SDH. The seemingly benign nature of many of these injuries, the time lag before symptom onset, and the frequent presence of cognitive deficits in these patients means that 25% to 50% of them are not able to relate any history of trauma [38].

The presence of cortical atrophy in aging adults directly affects clinical presentation. A comparatively large space between the brain and inner table exists for hematoma accumulation, meaning that significant blood collections with mass effect can occur over time without causing elevations in ICP. Older patients thus tend to have an insidious onset of symptoms and are less likely to present with the classic clinical picture of ICP elevation, including headache, visual changes, and vomiting [38,40]. Instead, aged adults are more likely to manifest seizures, focal neurologic signs, such as hemiparesis and aphasia, and subtle cognitive deficits, such as confusion, personality changes, memory loss, and impaired judgment. These changes can mimic many neurologic and psychiatric illnesses; common misdiagnoses include transient ischemic attack (TIA), stroke, vascular dementia, Alzheimer disease, and depression.

Emergency physicians must consider the diagnosis of chronic SDH when evaluating an elderly person who has mental status changes or sudden progression of known neurologic or psychiatric disease. It is diagnosed easily by CT scan (Fig. 3) and treatable by surgical intervention. Practitioners should seek a history of chronic SDH in such patients, because recurrence rates vary from 9% to 26% [41].

Spinal injury

Studies on cervical spine trauma show that elderly patients have different predominant mechanisms and patterns of injury. Older patients are more likely to be injured in falls and have increased likelihood of upper cervical injuries, particularly of the odontoid. Lomoschitz and colleagues conducted a retrospective analysis of 149 patients older than the age of 65 years with a total of 225 cervical spine injuries. C2 was the cervical bone injured most commonly, accounting for 40% of all fractures (Fig. 4). In the lower

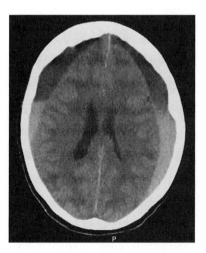

Fig. 3. The computed tomographic characteristics of subdural hematomas (SDH) change over time. Acute subdural blood usually appears hyperdense to brain parenchyma. After approximately 1 week, the hematoma becomes isodense. By 3 weeks, most SDHs appear hypodense to adjacent parenchyma [102]. Mixed density blood collections, as seen in this noncontrast CT, usually represent acute on chronic bleeding. This elderly woman was found down and had a recent history notable for 3 weeks of gait instability and confusion.

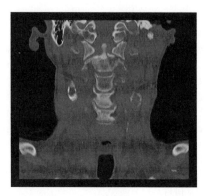

Fig. 4. Elderly patients are at particular risk for high cervical spine fractures, particularly of the dens. These injuries can be difficult to detect, because elderly patients are likely to present without signs of neurologic injury. This man suffered a comminuted C2 fracture during a fall from standing.

cervical spine, C5 and C6 were the most likely levels of injury, accounting for 12% each. Four in 10 elders sustained multilevel cervical injuries, most commonly at C1/2 or C5/6. The investigators specifically examined the differences in injury pattern, mechanism, and initial clinical presentation of those aged 65 to 75 years with those older than 75 years of age. The eldest patients (> 75 years) were significantly more likely to have upper cervical injuries regardless of mechanism [42].

Degenerative changes of the spine may result in increased risk for spinal fracture and specifically atlantoaxial injury in older persons. Osteopenia places bones at greater risk from what would otherwise be trivial trauma. In young patients, C4 to 7 is the most flexible portion of the cervical spine and the most likely to fracture. The presence of senile degenerative disease alters spinal mechanics, making the upper cervical levels comparatively more mobile and vulnerable to blunt trauma.

Cervical spine plain film interpretation in very elderly patients is complicated by relative osteopenia, the presence of degenerative changes, and unreliable markers of soft tissue injury. Cervical radiographs lack obvious prevertebral soft tissue swelling in 17% of upper cervical and 40% of lower cervical spine injuries [42]. Given the enhanced sensitivity of CT scans and the high incidence of pathology, some physicians have advocated bypassing plain films in this population.

It may be safe in certain clinical situations to forego spine imaging in elderly patients. Touger and colleagues conducted a subpopulation analysis of geriatric patients in the National Emergency X-radiography Use Study (NEXUS) database to determine if NEXUS criteria can identify safely low-risk patients who do not need cervical spine imaging. The database included information on 2,943 patients 65 years of age or older (8.6% of the total sample). Of these, 14% failed to meet the five criteria for imaging and qualified as low risk. Only two of these patients later proved to have cervical injury, specifically two cases of C2 lateral mass avulsion that the investigators classified as clinically insignificant. Based on this analysis, the sensitivity of NEXUS criteria for significant injury in patients older than 65 years of age was 100% (95% CI, 97.1%–100%) [43].

Many studies note the unnerving tendency for elders to suffer significant head and neck injuries from low-energy mechanisms, particularly same-level falls [26,27]. To further complicate clinical assessment, three in four elderly patients who have cervical spinal injury have normal neurologic examinations [42]. Aged patients are in fact less likely to exhibit paralysis at every level of spinal injury (Fig. 5) [44], despite their much higher risk for mortality [45]. Emergency physicians must be wary of such patients and have a low threshold for cervical immobilization and imaging.

It is not uncommon for geriatric patients to present to the ED with clinical evidence of vertebral or spinal cord injury in the absence of known trauma. The increased incidence of osteoporosis and cancer in this population substantially raises the risk for pathologic fracture. Degenerative spine disease may lead to canal or neural foraminal stenosis with subsequent motor and sensory findings. Unremitting back pain may be the herald of vertebral fracture, spinal metastasis, epidural hematoma, or abscess. The threshold for imaging the spine, whether by plain radiograph, CT, or magnetic resonance imaging (MRI) should be lower for geriatric patients. MRI is the modality of choice when there is clinical suspicion of spinal cord compression.

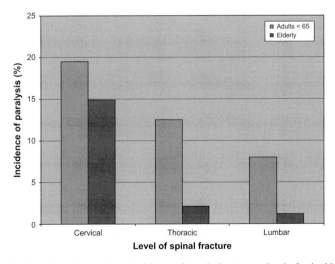

Fig. 5. Geriatric patients have a lower incidence of paralysis at every level of spinal injury [44].

Disparities exist in the rate of surgery in young and old patients who have spinal fractures. Elderly patients are significantly less likely to be selected for surgical intervention despite the clear mortality benefit in both groups [44].

Transient ischemic attacks

TIAs are common among older patients, occurring in as many as 1 in 15 adults older than the age of 65 years [46]. Up to 8.6% of patients have a stroke within 7 days of their index TIA, and more than half of these may occur within 48 hours of the initial ED visit [46,47]. Over 5 years, the stroke incidence exceeds 25% [48]. Correct diagnosis is paramount, because the institution of appropriate therapy can mitigate the risk for future stroke.

Diagnosing TIAs in the ED can be difficult. Such patients may present in a deceptively benign fashion; neurologic deficits have reversed often before physician evaluation, and brain CT is usually normal. A careful history is the key to diagnosis. Given these pitfalls, even experienced neurologists frequently disagree on the diagnosis [49].

Debate exists within the neurology community about the definition of a TIA. The classic definition of a sudden focal neurologic deficit caused by a vascular lesion that dissipates within 24 hours was framed before the availability of advanced brain imaging techniques, such as diffusion-weighted imaging (DWI) MRI. As a result, clinicians were unable to differentiate TIAs from strokes with reversible deficits. True TIAs usually resolve within 30 to 60 minutes. More than 98% of patients who do not reverse their deficit within 1 hour or rapidly improve within 3 hours are having a stroke, not a TIA [50]. These data have led some stroke experts to proffer a redefinition of TIA to include episodes that last typically less than 1 hour and are not associated with acute infarction [51]. This new proposed definition implies that an MRI has been performed.

TIA patients rarely require acute stabilization. All such patients warrant a finger stick blood glucose, a careful neurologic examination, and an ECG to look for arrhythmias. Any patient who has a persistent neurologic deficit must be treated as an acute stroke victim until proven otherwise. TIA patients whose deficits have resolved still should have some neuroimaging; at a minimum, a head CT without contrast should be performed to rule out other etiologies of neurologic dysfunction, such as hemorrhage or mass effect. No published guidelines argue for routine MRI for suspected TIA. MRI, however, detects small infarcts in up to 67% of patients who have traditionally-defined TIAs [52–54].

Further vascular assessment is indicated in patients diagnosed with TIA. Anterior circulation TIAs mandate urgent carotid evaluation, usually by ultrasonography, to look for high-grade stenosis. Two-year follow-up data from the North American Symptomatic Carotid Endarterectomy Trial (NASCET) revealed that patients who had high-grade stenosis defined as greater than 70% occlusion achieved a 17% absolute risk reduction for ipsilateral stroke from carotid endarterectomy (CEA) [55]. Benefits were more modest (6.5% absolute risk reduction) for patients who had moderate (50%–69%) stenosis and absent for those who had only low-grade (<50%) blockage [56]. Clinical trials are in progress to determine if angioplasty with stenting may be more advantageous than CEA [57,58]. To date no published data address the optimal timing for vascular intervention; the need for carotid evaluation has not been proven to be emergent. Posterior circulation TIAs require radiologic studies of the vertebrobasilar system, such as transcranial Doppler ultrasonography (TCD) or angiography. In patients who have a possible cardioembolic source, transthoracic or transesophageal echocardiography is indicated.

Most patients who have TIA should be placed on antiplatelet therapy, because aspirin alone confers a 20% relative risk reduction for subsequent stroke [49]. Considerable variation in clinical practice, however, exists among neurologists with regard to full anticoagulation for these patients. One of the few proven indications for emergent anticoagulation is a TIA in the setting of new onset atrial fibrillation. In the European Atrial Fibrillation Trial (EAFT) study, 1,007 patients who had atrial fibrillation and a history of recent TIA or minor stroke were randomized to anticoagulation, aspirin, or placebo treatment arms. The annual rate of stroke was 8%, 15%, and 19%, respectively [59]. TIA patients who had new atrial fibrillation or flutter should be admitted, anticoagulated, and assessed for intracardiac thrombus with echocardiography. Although controversial and not based on data from RCTs, up to one in two neurologists also recommend heparin for patients who have crescendo TIAs [60].

Given the high but unpredictable risk for further ischemic events, many clinicians routinely admit TIA patients to assure an expedited work-up and close monitoring. Certain patient subsets at particular risk and who may warrant admission and urgent neurologic consultation include: (1) patients who failed first-line therapy with antiplatelet agents, such as aspirin or clopidogrel, (2) patients on full anticoagulation, such as enoxaparin or warfarin, (3) patients who have crescendo TIAs, defined as three or more events over 72 hours with escalating severity or duration, and (4) patients who have suspected cardioembolic sources of TIA, such as new onset atrial fibrillation or valvular vegetations from endocarditis.

There are few data to guide admission decisions for TIA patients. Johnston and colleagues studied patients diagnosed with TIA in the ED to isolate risk factors associated with poor short-term prognosis. Using multivariate logistic regression, Johnston found five factors associated with higher short-term risk for ischemic stroke: age greater than 60 years, a history of diabetes, symptoms lasting more than 10 minutes, and the presence of motor weakness or speech difficulties with the event. The 3-month risk for stroke ranged from 0% in patients who had none of the five criteria to 34% in those who met all five [46]. The caveat to Johnston's data is that the average

length of symptoms in the study was 207 minutes; ergo by modern definition, this was a mixed population of TIAs and strokes.

Certain factors increase the likelihood of safe outpatient work-up and
management of a TIA. Benavente studied medically treated patients who
had amaurosis fugax versus those who had hemispheric TIA and discovered
that the 3-year risk for ipsilateral stroke was twice as great in the latter
group [61]. Patients who have this form of transient monocular blindness
thus may be discharged safely on aspirin if prompt carotid imaging and
close physician follow-up can be ensured. Greater caution is warranted in
patients who are male, older than 75 years of age, and have a past history
of hemispheric TIA or stroke, because their risk for subsequent ischemic
events is higher [61]. Elderly patients whose TIA occurred more than
1 week before arrival also may be safe for outpatient work-up, because the
period of greatest risk has passed.

A recent study showed that nearly 30% of patients discharged from the
ED with a preliminary diagnosis of TIA were not given antiplatelet agents
[62]. This inconsistency creates vulnerability of the patient to further ischemic events and of the physician to litigation. If considering outpatient TIA
management, it is essential for the emergency physician to discuss the risk
for future stroke with the patient, explicitly describe reasons to return for
emergent care, prescribe an antiplatelet agent or document its contraindication, and coordinate timely and appropriate follow-up.

Stroke

Stroke is the leading cause of disability and the third leading cause of
death in the United States. Detailed descriptions of stroke syndromes are
beyond the scope of this article but have been well described elsewhere [63].

One of the first steps in the evaluation of suspected stroke is to check
a blood glucose level, because hypoglycemia can mimic an infarct from
any vascular territory. Practitioners must keep in mind that such neurologic
deficits occasionally take several hours to reverse even after the restoration
of normal serum glucose levels. Although ongoing deficits persist, emergency physicians must continue to evaluate the patient for the possibility
of hemorrhagic or ischemic disease.

Many other clinical entities besides hypoglycemia can masquerade as
stroke. Other mimics include seizures with postictal Todd paralysis, CNS infections, toxic-metabolic defects, and intracranial mass lesions, such as
chronic SDH [64,65]. Libman and colleagues examined more than 400 patients diagnosed with acute stroke in the ED after the completion of a history
and physical examination and discovered that nearly 20% had an entirely
different source of CNS pathology [66]. The percentage of misdiagnosed
strokes decreases substantially to less than 5% once historical and physical
examination data are combined with brain imaging (Fig. 6) [64]. The potential for misdiagnosis bears special importance for patients who arrive shortly

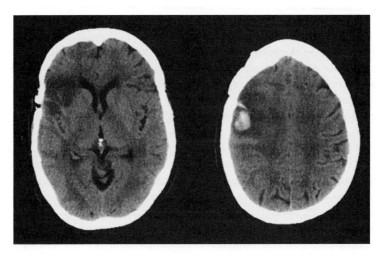

Fig. 6. These axial images from a noncontrast head CT scan reveal a wedge-shaped region of low attenuation in the right frontal lobe with a focal intraparenchymal hemorrhage at the superior margin. These images, consistent with a hemorrhagic transformation of a subacute infarct, were taken from a 65-year-old woman who had a history of TIAs and who presented with a right facial droop and slurred speech.

after the onset of symptoms. Although no clinician would intentionally treat a stroke mimic with thrombolytics, a recent small observational study showed no hemorrhagic complications in these patients [67].

The urgency of assessment and treatment implicit in the golden hour model of trauma care has been adapted successfully to stroke. Guidelines for optimal speed in treatment were established by the National Institute for Neurological Disorders and Stroke (NINDS) Study Group in 1997. The recommendations suggest an initial physician evaluation within 10 minutes of ED arrival, noncontrast CT scan within 25 minutes, radiologist interpretation within 45 minutes, and the administration of thrombolytics, if appropriate, within 1 hour [68]. Such a stringent timeline is only feasible with firm commitment from the departments of emergency medicine, radiology, and neurology within a given institution.

The incidence of spontaneous intracerebral hemorrhage (ICH) ranges from 10 to 20 cases per 100,000 population and is associated directly with advancing age [69]. Chronic hypertension and amyloid angiopathy, both more common in the elderly population, increase the likelihood of bleeding. Hemorrhagic strokes, although less frequent than ischemic events, are more deadly and have fewer effective therapeutic options. One-month mortality ranges from 35% to 52% [70].

Early progression of hemorrhage is common and linked with abrupt clinical decline. In a prospective study, Brott and colleagues found that 38% of ICH patients imaged within 3 hours of symptom onset developed significant hematoma expansion within 20 hours. Nearly 70% of these patients (26% of the ICH study population) progressed within 1 hour of the initial CT scan [71]. Because hematoma size has proven a powerful predictor of mortality and functional outcome in ICH, some researchers have focused on the therapeutic role of early hemostatic therapy. Activated factor VII is a candidate hemostatic agent that may have clinical benefit even for patients who do not have coagulopathy [72,73].

Acute medical management of geriatric patients who have ICH is the same as in younger patients and includes airway management, blood pressure and ICP monitoring, reversal of coagulopathy, and seizure prophylaxis. Patients who have evidence of elevated ICP may benefit from osmotherapy with mannitol and cautious hyperventilation. Because ICH patients are at risk for hematoma expansion and subsequent neurologic decline, they often benefit from admission to an intensive care unit.

The role for surgical drainage in ICH is still an area of active clinical investigation. Hankey and colleagues examined data on 249 ICH patients from three surgical trials and documented increased rates of death and dependency in the subset of patients randomized to craniotomy and hematoma evacuation (83% versus 70%) [74]. In 2005 the International Surgical Trial in Intracerebral Hemorrhage (STITCH) published data on 1,033 ICH patients from 83 medical centers and demonstrated that early surgery provided no clinical benefit for patients who had supratentorial ICH [75]. Craniotomy sometimes is recommended in cerebellar hematomas [69], but further study is needed to determine the clinical benefits of intervention for these patients.

Ischemia accounts for most strokes, with an incidence of 300 to 500 events per 100,000 population [76]. Acute medical management includes blood pressure monitoring, fever control, blood glucose regulation, and, if appropriate, thrombolysis. Hypotension is disastrous in patients who have stroke; given the loss of normal autoregulation and the marginal perfusion of the penumbra, mild to moderate hypertension should remain untreated. Antihypertensive medications should be administered only for specific indications, such as concurrent acute coronary syndrome (ACS), aortic dissection, malignant hypertension, or severe hypertension in a thrombolytic candidate.

Given the enormous potential for functional impairment and mortality in ischemic stroke, there is considerable interest in thrombolytic agents. The first published studies were not encouraging, leading to controversy within the medical community about continued clinical exploration. In 1995 the NINDS study was published [50]. In part one of the study, 291 ischemic stroke patients presenting within 180 minutes were randomized to treatment with intravenous tissue plasminogen activator (rt-PA) or to placebo. Researchers found no clinically significant improvement at 24 hours among patients in the treatment arm. In part two of NINDS, 333 patients were randomized to rt-PA versus placebo and patients in the rt-PA arm showed improved functional outcomes at 3 months. The data showed that eight to nine patients would require thrombolysis to have one patient recover with minimal or no deficit. The downside of thrombolysis was evident; patients treated with rt-PA were far more likely to have a symptomatic ICH (6.4% versus 0.6%). The subsequent FDA approval for thrombolytic agents later that year rested largely on the NINDS data.

Despite the volume of research published since NINDS, the use of thrombolytics remains a subject of academic discussion and dispute. The controversy surrounding rt-PA use culminated in the 2002 release of a position statement by the American Academy of Emergency Medicine (AAEM) stating that insufficient evidence existed on the efficacy of thrombolytics to support their inclusion in the standard of care for ischemic stroke [77]. In response to continued questions regarding the safety and usefulness of thrombolytics and methodologic concerns about the original study, the NINDS researchers commissioned an independent committee to reanalyze the data from the landmark 1995 article. This group confirmed the beneficial effect of rt-PA with an adjusted odds ratio (OR) for a favorable outcome of 2.1 (95% CI, 1.5–2.9) [78]. Meta-analysis has bolstered further the case for thrombolytics. In 2003 Wardlaw and colleagues compiled data from 14 RCTs investigating the use of thrombolytics within 6 hours of symptom onset for acute ischemic stroke. The data suggested that approximately 55 more patients would survive and live independently for every 1,000 treated. This number includes the approximately 20 deaths per 1,000 caused by ICH [79].

ICH is the immediate and often disastrous risk for thrombolytic treatment. Among the studies in Wardlaw's meta-analysis, symptomatic ICH occurred in 10% (153 of 1,496) of rt-PA patients and only 3% (46 of 1,459) of control subjects [79]. The risk for hemorrhage may be higher in geriatric patients; Heuschmann and colleagues found the rate of ICH was twice as high in patients older than 75 years of age as in those younger than 55 years of age (10.3% versus 4.9%) [80]. Attention to applicable contraindications is critical, because unacceptably high levels of ICH are associated with protocol violations. A study of Cleveland area hospitals reported a 15.7% incidence of symptomatic ICH, more than twice the 6.4% reported in NINDS [81]. Approximately 50% of those patients were treated outside of existing administration guidelines, leading some academicians to argue that thrombolytic agents could not be administered safely in the community setting. The rebuttal to this argument arrived 3 years later, when Katzan demonstrated that local quality improvement initiatives could increase overall use of rt-PA, decrease protocol violations, and result in a rate of hemorrhagic complications comparable to the original NINDS data [82]. Other investigators have confirmed that rt-PA can be administered successfully in community hospitals [83].

It is difficult to assess the safety of thrombolytics for ischemic stroke in very elderly patients given the paucity of data. Octogenarians are approximately 60% less likely and nonagenarians 85% less likely to be given the option of thrombolytic agents when compared with those younger than 60 years of age [79,84]. NINDS was perhaps the only published RCT that included patients older than age 80 years; data from only 42 such patients exists, making it impossible to form solid conclusions about the risk-to-benefit ratio of thrombolytics in the very elderly [79]. One recent observational study of 1,658 ischemic stroke patients treated with rt-PA showed that age increased in-hospital mortality with an adjusted OR of 1.6 for each additional decade in patient age. The caveat to those data is that older age also predicted in-hospital mortality in patients not treated with rt-PA, and the observational design of that study did not allow for direct comparison of the two groups [80].

Practitioners need to remember that once thrombolytics are administered, patients should be admitted to the intensive care unit or to an acute stroke unit. In addition, no invasive access, including arterial lines, central lines, or Foley catheters, should be placed for at least 2 hours following the completion of the thrombolytic dose.

Current thrombolytic guidelines stem from the original NINDS study and do not account for subsequent advances in imaging techniques, the variety of causative vascular lesions, and the judgment and experience of individual clinicians [85]. As knowledge and experience with particular vascular lesions increases, the accepted indications for thrombolysis will likely evolve. Clinical trials investigating longer time windows and the use of intra-arterial administration of thrombolytics are in progress at stroke centers around the country. Given the abysmal prognosis for basilar occlusion, some investigators use thrombolytics up to 48 hours after symptom onset [86]. Emergency physicians practicing in the community setting are well advised to develop protocols and working agreements with stroke centers to maximize the therapeutic options for these patients.

Dizziness

Dizziness is a common symptom in all age groups but is particularly prevalent in the elderly population. Approximately 50% of geriatric patients experience dizziness, and it is one of the most common presenting complaints in adults older than age 75 years [87,88]. The evaluation of the patient experiencing dizziness can be difficult, because patients use that word to describe a myriad of sensations, including fatigue, near-syncope, disequilibrium, and vertigo. Many elderly patients present with a mixed picture in which two or more forms of dizziness exist. The astute clinician must perform a careful history and physical examination to determine the source of symptoms and institute proper therapy. Although a complete review of the assessment of the patient experiencing dizziness goes beyond the scope of this article, it is well covered elsewhere [87,89,90]. This section focuses primarily on vertigo, because this includes most of the serious neurologic causes of dizziness.

Vertigo, or the illusory sense of motion, is usually peripheral, even in older patients. Peripheral vertigo is associated with acute onset of episodic, severe vertigo frequently associated with nausea, vomiting, tinnitus, and hearing loss. Common causes of peripheral vertigo include motion sickness, benign paroxysmal positional vertigo (BPPV), otitis media, vestibular neuronitis, Ménière disease, and toxic labyrinthitis from ototoxic medications. Vertigo that is positional and lasts for less than 30 seconds is almost always caused by BPPV. This diagnosis can be made by performing the Dix-Hallpike maneuver. Patients who have central vertigo experience less intense symptoms of longer duration. The differential diagnosis of central vertigo includes alcohol intoxication, temporal lobe seizures, migraine, head trauma, vertebrobasilar insufficiency, and posterior fossa masses or ischemia.

Although peripheral causes of vertigo tend to be "benign", the symptoms are, at a minimum, annoying and at times incapacitating to patients. The attendant nausea and vomiting may lead to dehydration that results in further morbidity. Simple treatments initiated in the ED can lead to significant clinical benefits. Recent data suggest that steroids improve outcomes in patients who have vestibular neuronitis [91]. Also, 80% to 85% of patients who have BPPV can be cured in the ED with a simple bedside maneuver, the modified Epley [92].

Distinguishing between peripheral and central causes of vertigo is critical [90], because many central etiologies require emergent treatment. Hearing loss strongly suggests a peripheral cause, because the colocation of hearing and balance occurs only in the peripheral nervous system. The presence of vascular risk factors (hypertension, diabetes, smoking) and abrupt onset of severe headache increase the likelihood of stroke. The presence of other neighborhood signs and symptoms of posterior circulation deficits (diplopia, dysarthria, ataxia, long tract problems) is another clue to serious central disease. Although patients who have peripheral vertigo may have difficulty walking, patients who have cerebellar stroke often cannot walk at all. Gait testing is therefore mandatory in all such patients. Nystagmus, when present, can help distinguish central from peripheral vertigo. Patients who have pure vertical or direction-changing nystagmus should be assumed to have a central cause until proven otherwise.

Vertigo is a concerning symptom in elderly patients, because they are at greater risk for serious CNS pathology. History and physical examination are not infallible in distinguishing central from peripheral disease. For example, infarction of vestibular nuclei from basilar artery branch occlusion can be indistinguishable from vestibular neuronitis by examination. Norrving conducted a small prospective study of 24 patients aged 50 to 75 years who presented with isolated acute vertigo and discovered that 6 of the 24 (25%) were having cerebellar ischemia [93]. Some of these events were cardioembolic; diagnosing such events provides physicians with the opportunity to initiate anticoagulation and prevent subsequent strokes. Unless the cause of vertigo is clearly benign, physicians must maintain a lower threshold for imaging and neurologic consultation in vertiginous elderly patients (Fig. 7).

Central nervous system infection

Meningitis and epidural abscess

Physicians must be alert to the higher likelihood and subtler presentation of infectious disease in the geriatric population [94]. Functional decline of immune cells associated with normal aging, termed immunosenescence, and other contributors such as malnutrition, result in increased susceptibility to infection. Presenting complaints in elderly patients are often nonspecific, such as confusion or frequent falls. In addition, older patients have a blunted fever response and may be normo- or even hypothermic.

Meningitis can occur at any age, but its largest spikes in incidence occur in infants and in people older than age 60 years. Geriatric incidence is estimated to be two to nine cases per 100,000 population [95]. Diagnosing meningitis in the geriatric population carries special clinical urgency, given the increased rate of serious complications and in-hospital mortality [96].

Unfortunately diagnostic and treatment delays are common in part because elderly patients are likely to present with an array of subtle, nonspecific signs and symptoms. The clinical triad of fever, nuchal rigidity, and altered mental status is rarely present in its entirety and has an abysmal 46% sensitivity among older patients. More than 99% have at least one of these findings, however, making the absence of all three useful in ruling out the diagnosis [97].

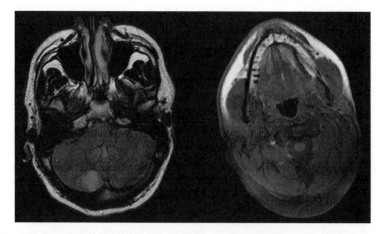

Fig. 7. The axial MRI on the left shows small areas of restricted diffusion in the right inferior cerebellum, indicating an acute right anterior inferior cerebellar artery (AICA) territory infarct. Signal changes in the right vertebral artery seen in the second image are consistent with thrombosis and dissection. This elderly patient presented with acute onset vertigo and ataxia.

Signs and symptoms of meningeal irritation are particularly unhelpful in aging patients. Nuchal rigidity, found in 92% of young patients who have meningitis, is less common and less specific in the elderly population. Neck stiffness is found in 57% of elderly patients who have meningitis [98], but in 35% of those without any evidence of CNS infection [99]. Rigidity may represent multiple other conditions in this age group, including Parkinson disease, osteoarthritis, or cervical spondylosis. Meningeal signs are also less reliable; 12% of healthy elderly people display a positive Kernig sign and 18% have a positive Brudzinski [99].

Further complicating clinical assessment is that 40% to 58% of elderly patients who have meningitis present with concomitant infections, such as pneumonias or urinary tract infections [100]. The discovery of a large infiltrate on a chest radiograph can distract clinicians from the presence of CNS infection and lead to premature closure of the diagnostic work-up.

Spinal epidural abscess is another dangerous infection more common in older patients. Any delay in diagnosis can be disastrous, because emergent surgical debridement in combination with antibiotics can prevent permanent paralysis and death. It is a difficult diagnosis to make in elderly patients, who frequently present to the ED with back pain from degenerative disease. In fact, diagnostic delays occur in up to 75% of patients, in part because more than 85% do not have the classic triad of spinal pain, fever, and neurologic deficits [101]. A lack of fever and leukocytosis does not rule out the diagnosis. Although MRI is the gold standard test (Fig. 8), some have advocated the use of inflammatory markers, such as erythrocyte sedimentation rate (ESR), as a screening tool for patients who have a lower pretest probability [101].

Patients who have suspected epidural abscess must be transferred to a center that offers MRI imaging and spinal surgery consultants. Antibiotic therapy should be administered before transfer. Patients who have suspected cervical abscesses should be monitored carefully in the ED and sent by ALS

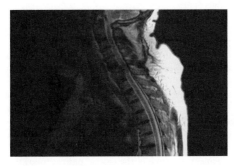

Fig. 8. Central nervous system infections can present without fever or neurologic signs in elderly patients. This is a sagittal MRI image of the spine in a 73-year-old woman who presented to the emergency department with a sole complaint of neck pain. This image reveals C6/7 osteomyelitis and discitis with epidural extension resulting in spinal cord compression.

if transferred, because they are at risk for respiratory decompensation. For safety, some patients may require intubation to undergo MRI or transfer.

Summary

Geriatrics is an important subspecialty within the field of emergency medicine and represents a burgeoning area of practice. The special vulnerability of the elderly population to neurologic disease and injury and the comparative subtlety of clinical presentation mean that physicians should have a lower threshold for laboratory studies, radiologic imaging, consultation, and admission. Transferring appropriate patients to tertiary centers that offer specialized trauma, neurologic, and neurosurgical care, greatly enhances survival and functional outcomes.

References

[1] Sanders AB. Care of the elderly in emergency departments: where do we stand? Ann Emerg Med 1992;21(7):792–5.

[2] McNamara RM, Rousseau E, Sanders AB. Geriatric emergency medicine: a survey of practicing emergency physicians. Ann Emerg Med 1992;21(7):796–801.

[3] Sacco RL, Wolf PA, Bharucha NE, et al. Subarachnoid and intracerebral hemorrhage: natural history, prognosis, and precursive factors in the Framingham Study. Neurology 1984; 34(7):847–54.

[4] Kassell NF, Torner JC, Haley EC Jr, et al. The International Cooperative Study on the Timing of Aneurysm Surgery. Part 1: overall management results. J Neurosurg 1990; 73(1):18–36.

[5] Jennett B, Bond M. Assessment of outcome after severe brain damage. Lancet 1975; 1(7905):480–4.

[6] Lanzino G, Kassell NF, Germanson TP, et al. Age and outcome after aneurysmal subarachnoid hemorrhage: why do older patients fare worse? J Neurosurg 1996;85(3):410–8.

[7] Sedat J, Dib M, Lonjon M, et al. Endovascular treatment of ruptured intracranial aneurysms in patients aged 65 years and older: follow-up of 52 patients after 1 year. Stroke 2002;33(11):2620–5.

[8] Andreoli A, di Pasquale G, Pinelli G, et al. Subarachnoid hemorrhage: frequency and severity of cardiac arrhythmias. A survey of 70 cases studied in the acute phase. Stroke 1987;18(3):558–64.

[9] Deibert E, Barzilai B, Braverman AC, et al. Clinical significance of elevated troponin I levels in patients with nontraumatic subarachnoid hemorrhage. J Neurosurg 2003;98(4): 741–6.

[10] Skultety FM, Nishioka H. Report on the Cooperative Study of Intracranial Aneurysms and Subarachnoid Hemorrhage. Section VIII, Part 2: the results of intracranial surgery in the treatment of aneurysms. J Neurosurg 1966;25:683–704.

[11] Kassell NF, Torner JC, Jane JA, et al. The International Cooperative Study on the Timing of Aneurysm Surgery. Part 2: surgical results. J Neurosurg 1990;73(1):37–47.

[12] Inagawa T. Management outcome in the elderly patient following subarachnoid hemorrhage. J Neurosurg 1993;78(4):554–61.

[13] Elliott JP, Le Roux PD. Subarachnoid hemorrhage and cerebral aneurysms in the elderly. Neurosurg Clin N Am 1998;9(3):587–94.

[14] Mayberg MR, Batjer HH, Dacey R, et al. Guidelines for the management of aneurysmal subarachnoid hemorrhage. A statement for healthcare professionals from a special writing group of the Stroke Council, American Heart Association. Stroke 1994;25(11):2315–28.

[15] Rose JC, Mayer SA. Optimizing blood pressure in neurological emergencies. Neurocrit Care 2004;1:287–300.

[16] Torbey MT, Hauser TK, Bhardwaj A, et al. Effect of age on cerebral blood flow velocity and incidence of vasospasm after aneurysmal subarachnoid hemorrhage. Stroke 2001; 32(9):2005–11.

[17] Taylor CL, Yuan Z, Selman WR, et al. Mortality rates, hospital length of stay, and the cost of treating subarachnoid hemorrhage in older patients: institutional and geographical differences. J Neurosurg 1997;86(4):583–8.

[18] Molyneux A, Kerr R, Stratton I, et al. International Subarachnoid Aneurysm Trial (ISAT) of neurosurgical clipping versus endovascular coiling in 2143 patients with ruptured intracranial aneurysms: a randomised trial. Lancet 2002;360(9342):1267–74.

[19] Wiebers DO. Neuroepidemiology of unruptured intracranial aneurysms: implications for decision making regarding patient management. Neurosurg Clin N Am 2005;16(2):309–12.

[20] Wiebers DO. Patients with small, asymptomatic, unruptured intracranial aneurysms and no history of subarachnoid hemorrhage should generally be treated conservatively. Stroke 2005;36(2):408–9.

[21] Chung RY, Carter BS, Norbash A, et al. Management outcomes for ruptured and unruptured aneurysms in the elderly. Neurosurgery 2000;47(4):827–32 [discussion: 832–3].

[22] Barker FG Jr, Amin-Hanjani S, Butler WE, et al. Age-dependent differences in short-term outcome after surgical or endovascular treatment of unruptured intracranial aneurysms in the United States, 1996–2000. Neurosurgery 2004;54(1):18–28 [discussion: 28–30].

[23] Jager TE, Weiss HB, Coben JH, et al. Traumatic brain injuries evaluated in US emergency departments, 1992–1994. Acad Emerg Med 2000;7(2):134–40.

[24] Mosenthal AC, Lavery RF, Addis M, et al. Isolated traumatic brain injury: age is an independent predictor of mortality and early outcome. J Trauma 2002;52(5):907–11.

[25] Vollmer DG, Torner JC, Jane JA, et al. Age and outcome following traumatic coma: why do older patients fare worse? J Neurosurg 1991;75:S37–49.

[26] Sterling DA, O'Connor JA, Bonadies J. Geriatric falls: injury severity is high and disproportionate to mechanism. J Trauma 2001;50(1):116–9.

[27] Helling TS, Watkins M, Evans LL, et al. Low falls: an underappreciated mechanism of injury. J Trauma 1999;46(3):453–6.

[28] Baker SP, O'Neill B, Haddon W Jr, et al. The injury severity score: a method for describing patients with multiple injuries and evaluating emergency care. J Trauma 1974;14(3):187–96.

[29] Hui T, Avital I, Soukiasian H, et al. Intensive care unit outcome of vehicle-related injury in elderly trauma patients. Am Surg 2002;68(12):1111–4.

[30] Meldon SW, Reilly M, Drew BL, et al. Trauma in the very elderly: a community-based study of outcomes at trauma and nontrauma centers. J Trauma 2002;52(1):79–84.

[31] Demetriades D, Sava J, Alo K, et al. Old age as a criterion for trauma team activation. J Trauma 2001;51(4):754–6 [discussion: 756–7].

[32] Zink BJ. Traumatic brain injury outcome: concepts for emergency care. Ann Emerg Med 2001;37(3):318–32.

[33] Scheetz LJ. Trauma center versus non-trauma center admissions in adult trauma victims by age and gender. Prehosp Emerg Care 2004;8(3):268–72.

[34] Ma MH, Mackenzie EJ, Alcorta R, et al. Compliance with prehospital triage protocols for major trauma patients. J Trauma 1999;46(1):168–75.

[35] Demetriades D, Karaiskakis M, Velmahos G, et al. Effect on outcome of early intensive management of geriatric trauma patients. Br J Surg 2002;89(10):1319–22.

[36] Mosenthal AC, Livingston DH, Lavery RF, et al. The effect of age on functional outcome in mild traumatic brain injury: 6-month report of a prospective multicenter trial. J Trauma 2004;56(5):1042–8.

[37] Fogelholm R, Waltimo O. Epidemiology of chronic subdural haematoma. Acta Neurochir (Wien) 1975;32:247–50.

[38] Iantosca MR, Simon RH. Chronic subdural hematoma in adult and elderly patients. Neurosurg Clin N Am 2000;11(3):447–54.

[39] Weiner HL, Constantini S, Cohen H, et al. Current treatment of normal-pressure hydrocephalus: comparison of flow-regulated and differential-pressure shunt valves. Neurosurgery 1995;37(5):877–84.

[40] Machulda MM, Haut MW. Clinical features of chronic subdural hematoma: neuropsychiatric and neuropsychologic changes in patients with chronic subdural hematoma. Neurosurg Clin N Am 2000;11(3):473–7.

[41] Yamamoto H, Hirashima Y, Hamada H, et al. Independent predictors of recurrence of chronic subdural hematoma: results of multivariate analysis performed using a logistic regression model. J Neurosurg 2003;98(6):1217–21.

[42] Lomoschitz FM, Blackmore CC, Mirza SK, et al. Cervical spine injuries in patients 65 years old and older: epidemiologic analysis regarding the effects of age and injury mechanism on distribution, type, and stability of injuries. Am J Roentgenol 2002;178(3):573–7.

[43] Touger M, Gennis P, Nathanson N, et al. Validity of a decision rule to reduce cervical spine radiography in elderly patients with blunt trauma. Ann Emerg Med 2002;40(3):287–93.

[44] Irwin ZN, Arthur M, Mullins RJ, et al. Variations in injury patterns, treatment, and outcome for spinal fracture and paralysis in adult versus geriatric patients. Spine 2004;29(7): 796–802.

[45] Spivak JM, Weiss MA, Cotler JM, et al. Cervical spine injuries in patients 65 and older. Spine 1994;19(20):2302–6.

[46] Johnston SC, Gress DR, Browner WS, et al. Short-term prognosis after emergency department diagnosis of TIA. JAMA 2000;284(22):2901–6.

[47] Lovett JK, Dennis MS, Sandercock PA, et al. Very early risk for stroke after a first transient ischemic attack. Stroke 2003;34(8):e138–40.

[48] Feinberg WM. Guidelines for the management of transient ischemic attacks. Ad Hoc Committee on Guidelines for the Management of Transient Ischemic Attacks of the Stroke Council, American Heart Association. Heart Dis Stroke 1994;3(5):275–83.

[49] Shah KH, Edlow JA. Transient ischemic attack: review for the emergency physician. Ann Emerg Med 2004;43(5):592–604.

[50] The National Institute of Neurological Disorders and Stroke rt-PA Stroke Study Group. Tissue plasminogen activator for acute ischemic stroke. N Engl J Med 1995;333(24):1581–7.

[51] Albers GW, Caplan LR, Easton JD, et al. Transient ischemic attack—proposal for a new definition. N Engl J Med 2002;347(21):1713–6.

[52] Ay H, Oliveira-Filho J, Buonanno FS, et al. 'Footprints' of transient ischemic attacks: a diffusion-weighted MRI study. Cerebrovasc Dis 2002;14(3–4):177–86.

[53] Kidwell CS, Alger JR, Di Salle F, et al. Diffusion MRI in patients with transient ischemic attacks. Stroke 1999;30(6):1174–80.

[54] Rovira A, Rovira-Gols A, Pedraza S, et al. Diffusion-weighted MR imaging in the acute phase of transient ischemic attacks. Am J Neuroradiol 2002;23(1):77–83.

[55] North American Symptomatic Carotid Endarterectomy Trial Collaborators. Beneficial effect of carotid endarterectomy in symptomatic patients with high-grade carotid stenosis. N Engl J Med 1991;325(7):445–53.

[56] Barnett HJ, Taylor DW, Eliasziw M, et al. Benefit of carotid endarterectomy in patients with symptomatic moderate or severe stenosis. North American Symptomatic Carotid Endarterectomy Trial Collaborators. N Engl J Med 1998;339(20):1415–25.

[57] Brott TG, Brown RD Jr, Meyer FB, et al. Carotid revascularization for prevention of stroke: carotid endarterectomy and carotid artery stenting. Mayo Clin Proc 2004;79(9): 1197–208.

[58] Yadav JS, Wholey MH, Kuntz RE, et al. Protected carotid-artery stenting versus endarterectomy in high-risk patients. N Engl J Med 2004;351(15):1493–501.

[59] EAFT (European Atrial Fibrillation Trial) Study Group. Secondary prevention in non-rheumatic atrial fibrillation after transient ischaemic attack or minor stroke. Lancet 1993;342(8882):1255–62.

[60] Al-Sadat A, Sunbulli M, Chaturvedi S. Use of intravenous heparin by North American neurologists: do the data matter? Stroke 2002;33(6):1574–7.

[61] Benavente O, Eliasziw M, Streifler JY, et al. Prognosis after transient monocular blindness associated with carotid-artery stenosis. N Engl J Med 2001;345(15):1084–90.

[62] Chang E, Holroyd BR, Kochanski P, et al. Adherence to practice guidelines for transient ischemic attacks in an emergency department. Can J Neurol Sci 2002;29(4):358–63.

[63] Baumlin KM, Richardson LD. Stroke syndromes. Emerg Med Clin North Am 1997;15(3): 551–61.

[64] Huff JS. Stroke mimics and chameleons. Emerg Med Clin North Am 2002;20(3):583–95.

[65] Moster ML, Johnston DE, Reinmuth OM. Chronic subdural hematoma with transient neurological deficits: a review of 15 cases. Ann Neurol 1983;14(5):539–42.

[66] Libman RB, Wirkowski E, Alvir J, et al. Conditions that mimic stroke in the emergency department. Implications for acute stroke trials. Arch Neurol 1995;52(11):1119–22.

[67] Scott PA, Silbergleit R. Misdiagnosis of stroke in tissue plasminogen activator-treated patients: characteristics and outcomes. Ann Emerg Med 2003;42(5):611–8.

[68] The National Institute of Neurological Disorders and Stroke (NINDS) rt-PA Stroke Study Group. A systems approach to immediate evaluation and management of hyperacute stroke. Experience at eight centers and implications for community practice and patient care. Stroke 1997;28(8):1530–40.

[69] Qureshi AI, Tuhrim S, Broderick JP, et al. Spontaneous intracerebral hemorrhage. N Engl J Med 2001;344(19):1450–60.

[70] Broderick JP, Adams HP Jr, Barsan W, et al. Guidelines for the management of spontaneous intracerebral hemorrhage: a statement for healthcare professionals from a special writing group of the Stroke Council, American Heart Association. Stroke 1999;30(4):905–15.

[71] Brott T, Broderick J, Kothari R, et al. Early hemorrhage growth in patients with intracerebral hemorrhage. Stroke 1997;28(1):1–5.

[72] Mayer SA. Ultra-early hemostatic therapy for intracerebral hemorrhage. Stroke 2003; 34(1):224–9.

[73] O'Neill PA, Bluth M, Gloster ES, et al. Successful use of recombinant activated factor VII for trauma-associated hemorrhage in a patient without preexisting coagulopathy. J Trauma 2002;52(2):400–5.

[74] Hankey GJ, Hon C. Surgery for primary intracerebral hemorrhage: is it safe and effective? A systematic review of case series and randomized trials. Stroke 1997;28(11):2126–32.

[75] Mendelow AD, Gregson BA, Fernandes HM, et al. Early surgery versus initial conservative treatment in patients with spontaneous supratentorial intracerebral haematomas in the International Surgical Trial in Intracerebral Haemorrhage (STICH): a randomised trial. Lancet 2005;365(9457):387–97.

[76] Sudlow CL, Warlow CP. Comparable studies of the incidence of stroke and its pathological types: results from an international collaboration. International Stroke Incidence Collaboration. Stroke 1997;28(3):491–9.

[77] American Academy of Emergency Medicine Work Group on Thrombolytic Therapy in Stroke. Statement on the Use of Intravenous Thrombolytic Therapy in the Treatment of Stroke. 2002. Available at: http://www.aaem.org/positionstatements/thrombolytictherapy. shtml. Accessed February 27, 2006.

[78] Ingall TJ, O'Fallon WM, Asplund K, et al. Findings from the reanalysis of the NINDS tissue plasminogen activator for acute ischemic stroke treatment trial. Stroke 2004;35(10): 2418–24.

[79] Wardlaw JM, Sandercock PA, Berge E. Thrombolytic therapy with recombinant tissue plasminogen activator for acute ischemic stroke: where do we go from here? A cumulative meta-analysis. Stroke 2003;34(6):1437–42.

[80] Heuschmann PU, Kolominsky-Rabas PL, Roether J, et al. Predictors of in-hospital mortality in patients with acute ischemic stroke treated with thrombolytic therapy. JAMA 2004;292(15):1831–8.

[81] Katzan IL, Furlan AJ, Llyod LE, et al. Use of tissue-type plasminogen activator for acute ischemic stroke: the Cleveland area experience. JAMA 2000;283(9):1151–8.

[82] Katzan IL, Hammer MD, Furlan AJ, et al. Quality improvement and tissue-type plasminogen activator for acute ischemic stroke: a Cleveland update. Stroke 2003;34(3):799–800.

[83] Asimos AW, Norton HJ, Price MF, et al. Therapeutic yield and outcomes of a community teaching hospital code stroke protocol. Acad Emerg Med 2004;11(4):361–70.

[84] Reed SD, Cramer SC, Blough DK, et al. Treatment with tissue plasminogen activator and inpatient mortality rates for patients with ischemic stroke treated in community hospitals. Stroke 2001;32(8):1832–40.

[85] Caplan LR. Treatment of acute stroke: still struggling. JAMA 2004;292(15):1883–5.

[86] Lindsberg PJ, Soinne L, Tatlisumak T, et al. Long-term outcome after intravenous thrombolysis of basilar artery occlusion. JAMA 2004;292(15):1862–6.

[87] Walker JS, Barnes SB. Dizziness. Emerg Med Clin North Am 1998;16(4):845–75 [vii.].

[88] Baloh RW. Dysequilibrium in older people. West J Med 1993;159(2):180.

[89] Davis EA. Emergency department approach to vertigo. Emerg Med Clin North Am 1987; 5(2):211–26.

[90] Baloh RW. Vertigo. Lancet 1998;352(9143):1841–6.

[91] Strupp M, Zingler VC, Arbusow V, et al. Methylprednisolone, valacyclovir, or the combination for vestibular neuritis. N Engl J Med 2004;351(4):354–61.

[92] Chang AK, Schoeman G, Hill M. A randomized clinical trial to assess the efficacy of the Epley maneuver in the treatment of acute benign positional vertigo. Acad Emerg Med 2004;11(9):918–24.

[93] Norrving B, Magnusson M, Holtas S. Isolated acute vertigo in the elderly; vestibular or vascular disease? Acta Neurol Scand 1995;91(1):43–8.

[94] Gavazzi G, Krause KH. Ageing and infection. Lancet Infect Dis 2002;2(11):659–66.

[95] Miller LG, Choi C. Meningitis in older patients: how to diagnose and treat a deadly infection. Geriatrics 1997;52(8):43–4, 47–50, 55.

[96] Gorse GJ, Thrupp LD, Nudleman KL, et al. Bacterial meningitis in the elderly. Arch Intern Med 1984;144(8):1603–7.

[97] Attia J, Hatala R, Cook DJ, et al. The rational clinical examination. Does this adult patient have acute meningitis? JAMA 1999;282(2):175–81.

[98] Choi C. Bacterial meningitis. Clin Geriatr Med 1992;8(4):889–902.

[99] Puxty JA, Fox RA, Horan MA. The frequency of physical signs usually attributed to meningeal irritation in elderly patients. J Am Geriatr Soc 1983;31(10):590–2.

[100] Rasmussen HH, Sorensen HT, Moller-Peterson J, et al. Bacterial meningitis in elderly patients: clinical picture and course. Age Ageing 1992;21(3):216–20.

[101] Davis DP, Wold RM, Patel RJ, et al. The clinical presentation and impact of diagnostic delays on emergency department patients with spinal epidural abscess. J Emerg Med 2004; 26(3):285–91.

[102] Kostanian V, Choi JC, Liker MA, et al. Computed tomographic characteristics of chronic subdural hematomas. Neurosurg Clin N Am 2000;11(3):479–89.

ELSEVIER
SAUNDERS

Emerg Med Clin N Am
24 (2006) 299–316

EMERGENCY
MEDICINE
CLINICS OF
NORTH AMERICA

Altered Mental Status in Older Emergency Department Patients

Scott T. Wilber, MD[a,b,*]

[a]*Emergency Medicine, Northeastern Ohio Universities College of Medicine,
4209 Street Route 44, Rootstown, OH 44272*
[b]*Emergency Medicine Research Center, Summa Health System,
41 Arch Street, Suite 519, Akron, OH 44309, USA*

Mental status abnormalities are a common reason for older patients to visit the emergency department (ED). The general term "mental status change" has numerous synonyms, including confusion, organic brain syndrome, change in mental status (Δ MS), decreased level of consciousness ($\downarrow$ LOC), or simply "not acting right." These terms are applied to a broad spectrum of conditions that are encompassed in the disease category of mental status abnormalities. Patients presenting to the ED with an altered mental status generally require an extensive work-up, including a detailed history that is difficult to obtain from the individual patient. For emergency physicians, this translates into a time consuming evaluation talking with patient families and caregivers, reviewing old medical records, obtaining laboratory and radiologic studies, and possibly specialty consultations. Often there is still diagnostic uncertainty after the ED evaluation and inpatient observation, and further testing is required to make a definitive diagnosis.

Emergency physicians can expect that older patients will make up an increasing number and proportion of their patients over the next 30 years [1]. Currently patients older than age 64 years account for 15% of ED visits nationally [2]. In 30 years, ED visits for elderly patients are predicted to increase to 25% to 30%. At least 25% of all ED patients over age 65 years have some form of altered mental status [3–6], and this percentage increases with age. The effects on patient care are substantial: from the need for rapid

Dr. Wilber is supported by a Dennis W. Jahnigen Career Development Scholars Award, funded by the American Geriatrics Society, the John A. Hartford Foundation, and the Atlantic Philanthropies.

* Emergency Medicine Research Center, Summa Health System, 41 Arch Street, Suite 519, Akron, OH 44309.

E-mail address: wilbers@summa-health.org

evaluation of comatose patients, to the recognition and management of delirium, to the recognition that older patients who have dementia may not follow discharge instructions. Adopting an organized approach to the evaluation of mental status is therefore important for the evaluation of all older ED patients.

This article reviews the significance of altered mental status in older ED patients. Specific diagnoses are discussed, including delirium, stupor and coma, and dementia, with a focus on delirium. Finally, an approach to all older patients is suggested that should result in increased clinician comfort with older patients, improved ability to communicate with other physicians, increased quality of care, and improved patient and family satisfaction.

Background

There are two main components to the category of altered mental status. The first consists of the level of consciousness, or arousal. The second consists of the content of consciousness, or cognition [7]. The distinction between these two components is important, because impairments of the content of consciousness are not necessarily accompanied by impairments in level of consciousness. This may help lead the physician to the appropriate diagnosis.

Determinations of the level of consciousness, or arousal, often can be made by simple observation of the patient during routine history and examination. A normal level of consciousness consists of a patient who is awake and attentive. This level of arousal depends on an intact reticular activating system, cerebral cortex, and communication between the two [7]. Coma is at the other end of the spectrum. Comatose patients have no response to external stimuli or awareness of the external environment [7]. In between these two extremes are the abnormalities of consciousness noted more commonly, including hyperalert or vigilant patients, lethargic patients, and stuporous patients.

Hyperalert or vigilant patients have a heightened level of awareness of their external environment [8]. They may have difficulty following normal conversation because of inattention and are excessively aware of external stimuli. For instance, the beeping of a monitor may occupy their attention, even when asked to ignore it. The sheets, gowns, and monitor leads may fascinate the patient. Often there is excessive psychomotor stimulation. These patients may be at increased risk for harming themselves by getting out of bed unattended.

Lethargic patients are those who are not awake and alert, but who can be prompted to awaken with minimal stimuli [8]. This group includes patients who seem to be asleep each time the physician enters the room, but with shaking their shoulder or speaking their name, they awaken. The patient then regresses to a sleeping level of consciousness when conversation ceases.

Stupor consists of a level of consciousness from which the patient can be aroused only with maximal stimuli [7,8]. This may consist of loud verbal stimuli, shaking, or noxious stimuli. The patient may not awaken to a normal level of consciousness, however, and conversation therefore may be impossible. Without continued application of the stimuli, the patient's level of consciousness regresses [7].

Attention is another component of the level of consciousness. Patients with a normal state of consciousness are attentive during the history and examination; they are able to focus, sustain, and shift attention appropriately [9]. Patients who are inattentive may be hyperalert or lethargic. As discussed later, inattention is a clue to the diagnosis of delirium [9].

The level of consciousness, especially in delirium, may be fluid. Patients at times may be awake and inattentive, then progress to a hyperalert state requiring constant supervision, and later may be lethargic. Although delirium may progress to stupor or coma, however, and the etiologies are similar, stupor and coma are exclusive diagnoses [9].

Content of consciousness, or cognition, can be measured using multiple tools, which are discussed later.

Epidemiology

Numerous studies have evaluated the epidemiology of cognitive impairment in older ED patients. Although the overall proportions of cognitively impaired patients in the studies vary somewhat, it is clear that cognitive impairment is common in this population. Approximately 10% to 20% of community dwelling persons have cognitive impairment [10,11], as do 48% of nursing home residents [12]. This increases with age, reaching a prevalence of nearly 50% in those over age 85 years [11]. Cognitively impaired persons may visit the ED more frequently, however, because up to 40% of ED patients are found to be cognitively impaired without delirium [3].

In a study of ED patients 65 years old and older with no prior history of dementia, Gerson and colleagues found that 34% of the patients had moderate cognitive impairment, and an additional 26% had minimal impairment, leaving only 40% of patients cognitively intact [3]. Naughton and colleagues performed two studies of ED patients aged 70 years or older [4,5]. Subjects were evaluated with the Glasgow coma scale, the Mini-Mental Status Examination (MMSE), and the Confusion Assessment Method (CAM, a validated delirium screening tool). In the first study, 8.5% of patients had impaired consciousness (stupor or coma), 9.6% of patients had delirium, 22% had cognitive impairment without delirium, and 60% were cognitively intact [4]. In the second study, 4.8% had impaired consciousness, 17% had delirium, 38% had cognitive impairment without delirium, and 40% were cognitively intact [5].

Delirium

Delirium is an acute, fluctuating change in cognition, accompanied by impaired attention and consciousness [9,13]. Delirium represents the most serious cause of altered mental status seen in older ED patients [14]. Approximately 10% of ED patients over age 65 years present with delirium [4–6,14–16]. Most often, however, these patients are not diagnosed by the emergency physician [6,14–16].

Epidemiology

Numerous studies have evaluated the epidemiology of delirium in older ED patients, with remarkably similar results. In addition to the two studies noted by Naughton [4,5], Lewis and colleagues found a prevalence of delirium of 10% [6], Elie 9.6% [15], Hustey 12% [16], and Kakuma 8.4% [14].

The mortality associated with delirium changes depending on whether or not the diagnosis is made in the ED (or in hospital). Lewis found a 3-month mortality rate in those patients discharged to home with delirium of 14% versus 8% for those without delirium, though this difference was not statistically significant ($P = .2$) [6]. Kakuma found a statistically significant association between delirium and mortality even after adjusting for confounders [14]. Subjects whose delirium was undetected in the ED had a 3-month mortality of 31%, which was significantly higher than that of those whose delirium was detected (12%), and non-delirious subjects (14%) [14]. These sobering statistics on mortality are consistent with other studies on the prognosis of delirium. The mortality rate for elders who develop delirium during hospitalization is 22% to 76%, and the 3-month mortality rate of delirium is 14 times higher than for other affective disorders [9]. Although many patients who have delirium recover fully, elderly patients are prone to a prolonged recovery period with increased likelihood of persistent cognitive deficits [9].

Diagnosis of delirium

Diagnostic criteria for delirium were first presented in the Diagnostic and Statistical Manual of Mental Disorders (DSM), 3rd Edition, in 1980 [17]. In 1987 the revision of the DSM-III expanded these to nine diagnostic criteria [17]. DSM-IV further refined and simplified the diagnostic criteria, making them easier to use, even by nonpsychiatric-trained professionals [13]. The DSM-IV criteria for delirium are:

A. Disturbance of consciousness (ie, reduced clarity of awareness of the environment) with reduced ability to focus, sustain, or shift attention.
B. A change in cognition (such as memory deficit, disorientation, language disturbance) or the development of a perceptual disturbance that is not better accounted for by a pre-existing, established, or evolving dementia.
C. The disturbance develops over a short period of time (usually hours to days) and tends to fluctuate during the course of the day [13].

The fourth criterion in the DSM-IV involves the etiology of delirium (caused by a general medical condition, substance induced, multiple etiologies, or not otherwise specified) [13].

The first criterion, disturbance in consciousness, may involve lethargy that does not reach the level of stupor or coma, inattention, or psychomotor stimulation (hyperalert). Overall approximately 25% of patients are lethargic, termed "hypoactive" delirium. Another 25% are hyperalert, termed "hyperactive" delirium. Approximately 35% of cases are mixed, with alterations between hyperactive and hypoactive. Finally, approximately 15% of patients who have delirium have normal psychomotor activity [18,19].

The second criterion involves cognition. The first deficit to appear is generally impairment of short-term memory, which is nearly universal in patients who have delirium [13]. Inouye and colleagues found impaired memory to be 100% sensitive and 33% specific for delirium [8]. Memory impairment can be tested easily with three-item recall. Disorientation to time or place may occur, though disorientation to self is uncommon [13]. The same study noted earlier found disorientation to be 89% sensitive and 63% specific [8]. Perceptual disturbances may include delusions, illusions, misperceptions, or frank hallucinations. Visual hallucinations are most common, though auditory, tactile, gustatory, or olfactory illusions or hallucinations may occur [9]. Overall, perceptual disturbances are less common than memory disturbances, occurring in only 23% of patients who have delirium. They are more specific for delirium, however (90% specific) [8].

The third criterion involves the rapidity of onset and fluctuation in impairment. Delirium occurs abruptly and is usually apparent within hours to days of onset [13]. Patients may have a prodrome of restlessness, impaired attention, and sleep disturbance that can last several days before the onset of frank delirium [9]. It is this criterion that differentiates delirium from dementia. It is important for the emergency physician to use all available data sources in confused elders to determine the onset of symptoms, because this has a major bearing on the workup, treatment, and disposition. When patients present from home, it is helpful to discuss the changes noted by family or caregiver. Live-in family may be able to provide a clearer history of the duration of symptoms than others who haven't seen the patient in many months. In nursing home patients, it is often helpful to contact the nurse who sent the patient to help determine the duration of symptoms. From clinical experience, it seems safe to assume that the duration of onset is acute if someone was concerned enough to have the patient seen in the ED.

Fluctuating course is sometimes difficult to evaluate during the ED stay. If family or other surrogates are available, one may be able to determine fluctuation from their history. These surrogates may describe, for example, that the patient seemed normal for the last 2 days but was anxious and confused at night. Occasionally one can determine fluctuation directly in the ED, especially in patients who have mixed symptoms. In these cases, one may have to wake the patient to do a history and examination, and later be told by the nurse that the patient is trying to climb out of bed or has pulled out the IV. Again, it would seem prudent to suspect delirium in the ED if the other criteria are present and fluctuation cannot be demonstrated by history or examination.

The Confusion Assessment Method (CAM)

The CAM was first described by Inouye in 1990 [8]. In developing this tool, the investigators operationalized the DSM-III criteria for delirium, to "enable nonpsychiatrically trained clinicians to identify delirium quickly and accurately in both clinical and research settings" [8]. This original study found a sensitivity of 96% and a specificity of 93%. The CAM has become one of the most widely used screening tools for delirium and has been studied extensively. Reports of the CAM's sensitivity and specificities have varied widely, with sensitivities ranging from 13% to 100% and specificities ranging from 89% to 100% [20]. Although frequently used in research studies on older ED patients [4–6,15,16], only one study has evaluated the use of the CAM by lay-interviewers in the ED compared with a gold-standard CAM assessment. In this study, the agreement between raters was substantial (kappa 0.91), as were the sensitivity (86%) and specificity (100%) [21].

The CAM requires the presence of acute onset *and* fluctuating course *and* inattention, and *either* disorganized thinking *or* altered level of consciousness [8]. Memory impairment and disorientation are not incorporated into the CAM, though they performed well in the CAM validation study. Disorganized thinking is defined as "rambling or irrelevant conversation, unclear or illogical flow of ideas, or unpredictable switching from subject to subject" [8]. This criterion is more subjective than memory impairment and disorientation (when measured using validated scales), though the authors of the original study found perfect agreement between different raters (albeit academic geriatricians) on this item [8].

Despite the CAM's relative simplicity, recommendations for its use in textbooks of emergency medicine [22,23], and use in clinical research in emergency medicine [4–6,15,16], the overall sensitivity of ED physician diagnosis for delirium has not changed substantially since it has become widely recommended. In a study conducted in 1992, Lewis found that ED physicians correctly identified delirium in 17% of older patients in whom it was present [6]. In a study done in 2001, Hustey found that ED physicians correctly identified delirium in 16% of older patients in whom it was present [16]. Two studies from academic EDs in Canada do show higher rates of detection (25% and 56%) [14,15].

Differential diagnosis

The primary differential diagnosis for patients who have delirium is dementia, because both may cause impaired cognition. One of the key elements of the history is the onset of the symptoms; in delirium the symptoms are acute, whereas in dementia the onset is longer and more subtle. Additionally, patients who have dementia generally do not have impairment in their level of consciousness [18]. Delirium may be superimposed on dementia in 22% to 89% of patients who have dementia [24]. To detect these cases, the physician must quantify changes in cognition and their onset. Again, physicians must be aware that those who know the patient well, such as family or nursing home staff, can better detect a change in the patient's cognition than the physician can. One therefore should take these complaints seriously in patients who have dementia.

Other differential diagnoses for patients presenting with delirium include primary psychiatric disorders, such as acute psychosis. The term "pseudodelirium" has been suggested to identify this condition [18]. This diagnosis, however, should be made only in patients without a prior history of psychiatric disease after extensive evaluation, rather than in the ED [18].

Other symptoms of delirium

In addition to the diagnostic criteria listed previously, patients may manifest other symptoms of delirium. Altered sleep–wake patterns occur in 60% to 70% of patients [25]. This usually is manifested as daytime drowsiness and nighttime agitation and disorientation, often referred to as sundowning. This symptom in particular may be trying for caregivers, who become exhausted from caring for patients at night or are concerned about the patient's safety. Emotional disturbances may occur and may fluctuate from anxiety, fear, irritability, and anger to depression and apathy. Nonfocal neurologic deficits may occur, such as speech and language deficits (dysarthria, dysnomia, dysgraphia, or aphasia) [9].

Many of the physical signs and symptoms that can occur are associated with specific etiologies of delirium. For example, asterixis is associated with hepatic and renal disease. Nystagmus and cerebellar abnormalities may suggest alcohol or drug intoxication. Pupillary abnormalities also can suggest drug intoxication (eg, miosis with narcotics). Alcohol or sedative–hypnotic withdrawal is associated with coarse tremors, tachycardia, and low-grade fever. Because of the frequency of anticholinergic medications causing delirium, one should be alert for symptoms consistent with an anticholinergic toxidrome (dry mouth, urinary retention, tachycardia, fever).

Etiology

Delirium is a manifestation of various medical disorders of cerebral metabolism or neurotransmission, and as such the etiologies are broad [17,18]. The etiologies can be divided into four categories: (1) primary intracranial diseases, (2) systemic diseases that affect the brain secondarily, (3) exogenous toxins, and (4) withdrawal from substances [18]. Within these broad categories there are numerous causes, as noted in Table 1. In the elderly

Table 1
Common and serious etiologies of delirium in older patients

Primary CNS disease	Cerebrovascular accident
	Acute or chronic subdural hematoma
	Encephalitis
	Meningitis
	Seizures
	Nonconvulsive status epilepticus
	Postictal state
	Hypertensive encephalopathy
Systematic diseases	Infections
	Pneumonia
	Urinary tract infections
	Skin and soft tissue infections
	Cardiopulmonary disorders
	Acute myocardial infarction
	Congestive heart failure
	Arrhythmia
	Cardiogenic shock
	Acute or chronic respiratory failure
	Hypoxia
	Hypercarbia
	Uremia
	Hepatic encephalopathy
	Fluid or electrolyte abnormalities
	Dehydration
	Hypernatremia
	Hypoglycemia
	Hyper- or hypocalcemia
Medications	Anticholinergic medications
	Antihistamines
	Antiemetics
	Antiparkinsonian medications
	Antispasmodics (gastrointestinal)
Withdrawal	Alcohol
	Sedative–hypnotics

patient, determination of a single etiology may be difficult, and often more than one etiology contributes to the delirium [18].

Common etiologies in elderly patients include infections, medications, and primary CNS disorders. One study of delirium in community-dwelling elders implicated infections in 43% of cases, primary intracranial diseases in 25%, cardiovascular disorders in 18%, and medications in 12% [26].

Many medications can cause delirium, including medications available over the counter and those commonly prescribed to elders. The most common category of medications to cause delirium is drugs with anticholinergic properties: antihistamines, antiemetics, antipsychotics, antiparkinsonian drugs, antidepressants, and gastrointestinal antispasmodics [27]. Antihistamines particularly should be searched for, because often they are combined in over-the-counter medications, such as cold tablets and sleep aids. Patients and families should be questioned about these medications in the case of acute delirium without a clear etiology. Medications with more obvious CNS activities include narcotics, sedative–hypnotics, and alcohol. Meperidine has toxic metabolites that may accumulate, leading to delirium in older patients, especially those who have renal disease [27]. Older patients are also susceptible to delirium from fentanyl patches because of accumulation of active drug over time [27]. Other medications in common use and implicated in causing delirium in the elderly patient include corticosteroids, antibiotics (fluoroquinolones, beta-lactams, trimethoprim-sulfamethoxazole), muscle relaxants, antihypertensives, and H2 blockers [27]. Although this medication list is extensive, additional medications may cause delirium. Consequently a thorough history of new medications, including over-the-counter medications, is essential. It is imperative to review the side-effect profile of any new medication and to assume that new medications may have precipitated the patient's symptoms if alternative explanations are not available.

Diagnostic testing

Diagnostic testing in patients who have delirium is directed at discovering the etiology of the patient's symptoms. Given the large number of causes of delirium, the workup of an older patient who has delirium can be extensive. Sometimes a presumed etiology can be determined from the history and physical examination. This may be difficult, however, if a history from a surrogate is not available and the patient is unable to cooperate with the examination. Also, the possibility of multiple etiologies of delirium exists [9]. Consequently algorithms for diagnostic testing are not available, and the evaluation in each patient may be different. The work-up of the individual patient should be based on a careful clinical assessment and tailored diagnostic tests rather than a shotgun approach [28].

Most older patients who present to the ED with delirium require at least a complete blood count, electrolytes, BUN, creatinine, glucose, and EKG. Because infections are a common cause of delirium in older patients and because these infections may present without fever or elevated WBC count [29], additional work-up for infection may be helpful. Common infections in older patients include pneumonia and urinary tract infections; chest radiograph and urinalysis therefore may be helpful. Lumbar puncture should be performed if signs of meningitis are present. If the EKG shows new abnormalities, cardiac enzymes should be measured. Hepatic function tests and serum ammonia levels can be reserved for those patients who have a history of hepatic problems or those who have physical findings of hepatic disease (scleral icterus, jaundice, asterixis). Patients who have a history of chronic lung disease and who present with delirium should have an arterial blood gas study performed, because hypercarbia caused by respiratory failure may present with delirium.

The routine use of computed tomography (CT) of the brain in patients who have delirium is not recommended [9,28]. Naughton and colleagues studied the use of CT in delirious ED patients aged 70 years and older. They found substantial inconsistency in the use of CT by emergency physicians in the evaluation of delirium. Furthermore, only 15% of the scans had acute findings, and all but one of these was in patients who had substantially impaired consciousness or new focal neurologic findings [5]. It is therefore appropriate to limit initial CT scanning to those who have stupor, coma, or new focal neurologic findings. If no plausible etiology of the delirium has been determined after a thorough history, examination, and the laboratory studies mentioned, however, CT should be considered in other patients who have delirium.

Treatment

Treatment of delirium usually is directed at the underlying cause of the delirium. Some patients who have delirium, however, require interventions aimed at treating the symptoms of delirium. These may involve environmental interventions, such as turning off the lights, bringing families to the bedside, or providing the patient with glasses or hearing aids to reduce sensory impairments [9]. Physical restraints should be avoided if possible, because they may increase the patient's agitation and the severity of the delirium. When physical restraints are used, the patient should be observed closely to reduce the risk for injury from the restraints, and the restraints should be removed as soon as possible.

Pharmacologic treatment of the symptoms of delirium is preferred over physical restraint. Of the available drugs to treat the symptoms of delirium in older ED patients, the antipsychotic haloperidol is recommended most frequently [9,18,30]. Although antipsychotic drugs are implicated in causing delirium, haloperidol has limited anticholinergic effects [18]. Doses of haloperidol for this indication are lower than for other patients in need of chemical restraint; the usual recommended doses are 0.5 to 1.0 mg orally, intramuscularly, or intravenously [18,31]. This can be repeated every 30 minutes until the desired effect is achieved [32]. Droperidol also has been used successfully for delirium; however, it is more likely to cause hypotension, sedation, and extrapyramidal effects [32]. Furthermore, given the recent controversy over the black box warning because of prolongation of the QT interval and arrhythmia [33], haloperidol seems to be a safer choice. Newer generation antipsychotics, such as risperidone and olanzapine, also have been studied to treat the symptoms of delirium in older patients [30].

Benzodiazepines, especially lorazepam, are used commonly to treat the symptoms of delirium [31]. They are especially beneficial for specific conditions, such as the treatment of delirium caused by alcohol or sedative hypnotic withdrawal or seizures [9,30]. The risk for paradoxic central nervous system reactions that may worsen the patient's condition, however, is higher in older patients [32]. One randomized trial found that lorazepam was ineffective at reducing delirium symptoms, whereas haloperidol produces rapid improvement in symptoms [9]. The American Psychiatric Association Practice Guideline for the Treatment of Delirium recommends avoiding benzodiazepines except in the conditions noted previously [30].

Disposition

Delirium has many causes; all are potentially serious. The mortality associated with delirium is high, especially if unrecognized [14]. Furthermore, delirious patients are at risk for injuring themselves and require continuous supervision to prevent injury. Consequently older ED patients should be admitted to the hospital for evaluation unless there is a single, clear, and reversible etiology of the delirium, such as intoxication from a short-acting medication. In the latter case, the patient should be observed until the symptoms of delirium have resolved and be discharged with family or friends who can observe the patient.

Tests for cognitive impairment

Cognitive impairment from dementia or delirium is common, yet frequently it is not diagnosed by emergency physicians. Given the complexity of evaluating older patients who have even simple complaints, emergency physicians must maintain a high index of suspicion for cognitive impairment in older ED patients. When cognitive impairment is relevant to the reason a patient is in the ED, an evaluation of their mental status is warranted. The standard mental status screen since 1975 has been the Mini Mental Status Exam (MMSE) [34]. This 20-question test is familiar to most emergency physicians. It is comprehensive, testing orientation, registration, recall, calculation, and ability to follow commands. Certain features, however, make it undesirable for routine ED use. First, it is not memorized or scored easily, making the use of instructions and scoring sheets a must. Furthermore, it requires intact vision, hearing, and the ability to write. Any of these may be limited in older ED patients, who may have left their glasses at home or who may be unable to write because of the presence of IVs or injuries in the writing arm. Finally, it takes a median of 6 minutes and a maximum of 14 minutes to complete [35]. These issues limit the suitability of the MMSE for routine ED use.

Many other mental status screens have been developed and validated. Screens studied for ED use include the Orientation Memory Concentration Test (OMCT), the Clock-Drawing Test (CDT), the Mini-Cog, and the Six-Item Screener (SIS).

Orientation Memory Concentration Test

The OMCT has been used in ED-based research studies to evaluate mental status in older ED patients [3,16]. Consisting of six questions, including temporal orientation, counting backward from 20, saying the months in reverse order, and short-term memory, the test takes 2 to 5 minutes to perform. The scoring is weighted, and the memory phrase is somewhat awkward, making a scoring sheet or pocket card a must for administration. Recently, Huff and colleagues evaluated this tool in the ED using a different weighting system and have published norms for this scoring system [36,37].

Clock-Drawing Test

The CDT uses a different approach than the other tests. The CDT evaluates many different cognitive functions, including long-term memory, concentration, and abstract thinking [38]. There is no uniformity in the instructions for or scoring of the CDT. One simple approach, however, is to instruct patients to draw the face of a clock, placing the hands at 10 minutes after 11. The clinician then evaluates the clocks for four features: (1) a complete circle, (2) numbers correctly placed, (3) one hand larger than the other, and (4) hands read the correct time. If any of these features are absent, the CDT is scored as abnormal [39]. Using this simple approach, the CDT takes a median of 2 minutes to perform [35]. Although the scoring is somewhat subjective, studies have shown that emergency physicians with only brief training in scoring agree on whether the CDT is normal or abnormal [35]. Similar to the MMSE, however, the CDT requires intact vision and the ability to write, which, as noted, may be limited in ED patients. Fig. 1 shows the results of clock tests in older ED patients.

Mini-Cog

The Mini-Cog was developed as a brief screen for use in primary care settings [40]. It incorporates a clock-drawing test with three-item recall. Patients are first given a three-item recall list (such as "pencil, car, boat") and then are asked to draw the face of a clock and place the hands at ten after eleven. The clock is normal if all numbers are present in the correct order and position, and the hands show the correct time. After drawing the clock, the patients are asked to repeat the three items. One point is given

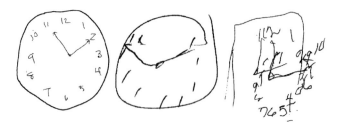

Fig. 1. Clock-drawing tests in older ED patients.

for each correct answer. Normal cognition consists of a score of 3 or a score of 1 or 2 with a normal clock. Abnormal cognition is defined as a score of 0 or a score of 1 or 2 with an abnormal clock [40]. In a recent ED study, the authors found the Mini-Cog to be 77% sensitive and 85% specific for cognitive impairment when compared with the MMSE as gold standard [41].

Six-Item Screener

The SIS is a rapid, easily remembered, and easily scored mental status test [42]. The SIS consists of three-item recall and temporal orientation (Fig. 2); scoring is the sum of correct answers. The SIS was developed and validated on two patient samples, a community sample and an Alzheimer patient clinic sample. Overall sensitivity and specificity were very good when compared with the MMSE. The authors recently studied the SIS in ED patients 65 years and older and found the SIS (using a cutoff of 4 abnormal/5 normal) had a sensitivity of 94% and a specificity of 85% when compared with the MMSE as gold standard (with a 23/24 cutoff) [41]. The SIS takes a median of 1 minute to administer [35] and can be incorporated into the physical examination, so it is unlikely to substantially increase the time to evaluate an older patient. Furthermore, its simplicity makes it easy to remember and score without scoring sheets or pocket cards. Finally, the SIS tests two core components of cognition: short-term memory and orientation. Both of these are important to evaluate for delirium and represent early cognitive deficits (memory) and later deficits (orientation) [13].

Instructions for the patient: I would like to ask you some questions that ask you to use your memory. I am going to name three objects. Please wait until I say all three words, then repeat them. Remember what they are because I am going to ask you to name them again in a few minutes. Please repeat these words for me: APPLE – TABLE – PENNY. (*May repeat names 3 times if necessary, repetition not scored.*)

Did the patient correctly repeat all three words?   Yes   No

    1. What year is this?   _____ (1)
    2. What month is this?   _____ (1)
    3. What is the day of the week?   _____ (1)

What are the three objects I asked you to remember?
    4. Apple   _____ (1)
    5. Table   _____ (1)
    6. Penny   _____ (1)

Total Score: _____ **(6)**

Fig. 2. Six-item screener. *From* Callahan CM, Unverzagt FW, Hui SL, et al. Six-item screener to identify cognitive impairment among potential subjects for clinical research. Med Care 2002;40(9):771–81; with permission.

Stupor and coma

As noted, the impairment in consciousness in patients who have delirium does not reach the level of stupor or coma [9]. Delirium, however, if untreated, may progress to stupor, coma, and eventually death. Most cases of coma (85%) are caused by systemic disease rather than by primary CNS abnormalities, and the etiologies are similar to those of delirium [43]. Consequently there is substantial overlap between the discussion of delirium and that of stupor or coma. Although comatose patients require a more rapid evaluation, the evaluation is similar to that of delirious patients.

It is helpful to use validated scales to evaluate the level of consciousness in patients who have stupor and coma. Two scales commonly are used. The first can be remembered by the mnemonic AVPU, which stands for *a*lert, responsive to *v*erbal stimuli, responsive to *p*ainful stimuli, or *u*nresponsive [44]. This classification is overly simplistic, however, because it doesn't include the level of response to the stimuli. For instance, patients who respond to painful stimuli by answering a question differ substantially from those whose response is posturing. To improve the description of the level of consciousness, the Glasgow Coma Scale (GCS) may be used. The GCS rates eye opening and motor response to verbal and painful stimuli, and verbal response. Patients who have coma do not open their eyes, obey commands, or have understandable conversation [4]. Rather than focus on the overall score, it is important to document the patient's response to stimuli.

Dementia

Dementia is characterized by the gradual and progressive development of multiple cognitive deficits, especially memory [13]. It is rare for an emergency physician to be confronted with the need to diagnose dementia. Most patients who have a gradual cognitive decline without acute change can be referred for evaluation as an outpatient. Chronic cognitive impairment, however, may affect the patient's ED care in many ways, from limiting the reliability of the medical history to reducing his or her understanding of and compliance with discharge instructions [45]. Consequently it is important to recognize this chronic impairment so that appropriate measures can be undertaken to improve the history and the patient's treatment.

General approach

Based on all of this information, a general approach to evaluating mental status in older ED patients can be developed. This approach should be used to evaluate mental status in *all* older ED patients, because the recognition of delirium is difficult [6,14–16] and the consequences of missed delirium are serious [14]. To be used this widely, however, the approach must be rapid, simple, and easy to incorporate into the routine history and examination, without substantially increasing the time needed to evaluate the patient.

The first item to assess is the level of consciousness, which corresponds to item A of the DSM-IV-R criteria for the diagnosis of delirium [13]. Normal consciousness is alert and attentive. Abnormal levels of consciousness include alert and inattentive, hyperalert, lethargic, stuporous, or comatose. In patients who have stupor or coma, it is important to document the patient's response to verbal and painful stimuli by the AVPU scale or the GCS. This information can be obtained during the routine history and examination, though the physician must observe the patient's level of attention during the interview.

The second item assessed is cognition. Rather than rely on orientation alone, short-term memory should be tested to improve the recognition of cognitive impairment. The use of validated scales is recommended. The most rapid and simplest scale is the SIS (Fig. 2). The advantages include its simplicity; it is easy to memorize and score. A cut-off of three or more errors had similar sensitivity and specificity for a diagnosis of dementias as did a cut-off score of 23 on the MMSE [42]. Furthermore, it tests temporal orientation and short-term memory, which correspond to item B of the DSM-IV-TR criteria [13]. Finally, it takes a median of 1 minute to perform in the ED [35] and can be incorporated into the history and examination, so the time needed to evaluate the patient is not prolonged. An alternative is the OMCT, which also assesses memory and orientation [3]. Cognition should be assessed in all patients who are not in stupor or coma. If uncertainty exists about the patient's cognitive status, the clock drawing test can be added (see Fig. 1).

After assessing these two items, patients can be termed "normal mental status" if their level of consciousness is normal and their cognition is normal. Patients who are stuporous or comatose are diagnosed as such, and evaluation of the etiology and treatment proceeds. If the patient has impaired consciousness or impaired cognition or both, evaluation of the acuity of onset of the symptoms must be investigated. All possible sources of information, including family, friends, and nursing home staff, should be used. For those whose onset of symptoms is acute (hours to days), delirium should be the working diagnosis and further testing is warranted. If the symptoms are chronic and progressive, however, dementia is more likely.

Using this approach allows emergency physicians to improve their ability to recognize delirium and to communicate their findings to other physicians without substantially altering the time to evaluate the patient. Recognition of cognitive impairment should improve the quality of patient care [46].

Summary

Mental status abnormalities are common in older emergency department patients and may be present in up to 40% of ED patients. These abnormalities may be chronic, from dementia, or acute, from delirium. Making the diagnosis of delirium in the ED is challenging and requires a systematic approach to patients who have an altered mental status. Gerson and colleagues found that 60% of geriatric ED patients had some degree of cognitive impairment. The challenge is to identify those geriatric patients who have acute changes. The mortality for patients who have delirium that is not diagnosed in the ED or in the hospital is significantly higher than the mortality for patients in whom the delirium is diagnosed. Consequently the recognition of delirium is essential for the provision of quality emergency department care. An approach to older ED patients that focuses on appropriately categorizing mental status impairment without substantially increasing the time to evaluate the patient has been presented in this article, and it is hoped that adoption of this approach should result in improvement in the care of older ED patients.

References

[1] US Census Bureau. Population Division, Population Projections Branch. US interim projections by age, sex, race, and Hispanic origin. Available at: http://www.census.gov/ipc/www/usinterimproj/. Accessed January 31, 2005.

[2] McCaig LF, Burt CW. National Hospital Ambulatory Medical Care Survey: 2002 Emergency Department Summary. Advance data from vital and health statistics; no 340. Hyattsville, MD: National Center for Health Statistics; 2004.

[3] Gerson LW, Counsell SR, Fontanarosa PB, et al. Case finding for cognitive impairment in elderly emergency department patients. Ann Emerg Med 1994;23:813–7.

[4] Naughton BJ, Moran MB, Kadah H, et al. Delirium and other cognitive impairment in older adults in an emergency department. Ann Emerg Med 1995;25:751–5.

[5] Naughton BJ, Moran M, Ghaly Y, et al. Computed tomography scanning and delirium in elder patients. Acad Emerg Med 1997;4:1107–10.

[6] Lewis LM, Miller DK, Morley JE, et al. Unrecognized delirium in ED geriatric patients. Am J Emerg Med 1995;13:142–5.

[7] Plum F, Posner JB. The pathologic physiology of signs and symptoms of coma. In: Plum F, Posner JB, editors. The diagnosis of stupor and coma. Philadelphia: FA Davis; 1980. p. 1–59.

[8] Inouye SK, van Dyck CH, Alessi CA, et al. Clarifying confusion: the confusion assessment method. A new method for detection of delirium. Ann Intern Med 1990;113(12):941–8.

[9] American Psychiatric Association. Practice guideline for the treatment of patients with delirium. Am J Psychiatry 1999;156:1–20.

[10] Unverzagt FW, Gao S, Baiyewu O, et al. Prevalence of cognitive impairment: data from the Indianapolis Study of Health and Aging. Neurology 2001;57(9):1655–62.

[11] Boustani M, Peterson B, Hanson L, et al. Screening for dementia in primary care: a summary of the evidence for the US Preventive Services Task Force. Ann Intern Med 2003;138:927–37.

[12] Magaziner J, German P, Zimmerman SI, et al. The prevalence of dementia in a statewide sample of new nursing home admissions aged 65 and older: diagnosis by expert panel. Epidemiology of Dementia in Nursing Homes Research Group. Gerontologist 2000;40(6):663–72.

[13] American Psychiatric Association. Diagnostic and statistical manual of mental disorders. 4th edition. Text revision. Washington, DC: American Psychiatric Association; 2000.

[14] Kakuma R, du Fort GG, Arsenault L, et al. Delirium in older emergency department patients discharged home: effect on survival. J Am Geriatr Soc 2003;5:443–50.

[15] Elie M, Rousseau F, Cole M, et al. Prevalence and detection of delirium in elderly emergency department patients. CMAJ 2000;163:977–81.

[16] Hustey FM, Meldon SW. The prevalence and documentation of impaired mental status in elderly emergency department patients. Ann Emerg Med 2002;39(3):248–53.

[17] Murphy BA. Delirium. Emerg Med Clin North Am 2000;18(2):243–52.

[18] Lipowski ZJ. Delirium in the elderly patient. N Engl J Med 1989;320(9):578–82.

[19] Delirium. In: Beers MH, Berkow R, editors. The Merck Manual of Geriatrics. 3rd edition. Whitehouse Station, NJ: Wiley; 2004.

[20] Laurila JV, Pitkala KH, Strandberg TE, et al. Confusion assessment method in the diagnostics of delirium among aged hospital patients: would it serve better in screening than as a diagnostic instrument? Int J Geriatr Psychiatry 2002;17(12):1112–9.

[21] Monette J, Galbaud du Fort G, Fung SH, et al. Evaluation of the Confusion Assessment Method (CAM) as a screening tool for delirium in the emergency room. Gen Hosp Psychiatry 2001;23(1):20–5.

[22] Sanders AB. The elder patient. In: Tintinalli JE, Kelen GD, Stapcynski JS, editors. Emergency medicine, a comprehensive study guide. New York: McGraw-Hill; 2004. p. 1896–900.

[23] Bernstein E. Functional assessment, mental status, and case finding. In: Sanders AB, editor. Emergency care of the elder person. St. Louis, MO: Beverly Cracom Publications; 1996. p. 97–116.

[24] Fick DM, Agostini JV, Inouye SK. Delirium superimposed on dementia: a systematic review. J Am Geriatr Soc 2002;50(10):1723–32.

[25] Cole MG, McCusker J, Dendukuri N, et al. Symptoms of delirium among elderly medical inpatients with or without dementia. J Neuropsychiatry Clin Neurosci 2002;14(2):167–75.

[26] Rahkonen T, Makela H, Paanila S, et al. Delirium in elderly people without severe predisposing disorders: etiology and 1-year prognosis after discharge. Int Psychogeriatr 2000;12(4):473–81.

[27] Anonymous. Drugs that may cause cognitive disorders in the elderly. Med Lett Drugs Ther 2000;42(1093):111–2.

[28] Inouye SK. The dilemma of delirium: clinical and research controversies regarding diagnosis and evaluation of delirium in hospitalized elderly medical patients. Am J Med 1994;97(3):278–88.

[29] Wilber ST. Geriatric pneumonia. In: Ma O, Meldon S, Woolard R, editors. Geriatric emergency medicine. 1st edition. New York: McGraw-Hill; 2004.

[30] Cook IA. Guideline watch: practice guideline for the treatment of patients with delirium. Arlington, VA: American Psychiatric Association; 2004.

[31] Carnes M, Howell T, Rosenberg M, et al. Physicians vary in approaches to the clinical management of delirium. J Am Geriatr Soc 2003;51(2):234–9.

[32] Fish DN. Treatment of delirium in the critically ill patient. Clin Pharm 1991;10(6):456–66.

[33] Kao LW, Kirk MA, Evers SJ, et al. Droperidol, QT prolongation, and sudden death: what is the evidence? Ann Emerg Med 2003;41(4):546–58.

[34] Folstein MF, Folstein SE, McHugh PR. Mini-Mental State: a practical method for grading the cognitive state of patients for the clinician. J Psychiatr Res 1975;12(3):189–98.

[35] Wilber ST, Blanda M, Gerson LW. Three screening tests for cognitive impairment in older emergency department patients [abstract]. Acad Emerg Med 2004;11:475.

[36] Huff JS, Farace E, Brady WJ, et al. The quick confusion scale in the ED: comparison with the mini-mental state examination. Am J Emerg Med 2001;19(6):461–4.

[37] Irons MJ, Farace E, Brady WJ, et al. Mental status screening of emergency department patients: normative study of the quick confusion scale. Acad Emerg Med 2002;9(10):989–94.

[38] Lorentz WJ, Scanlan JM, Borson S. Brief screening tests for dementia. Can J Psychiatry 2002;47:723–33.

[39] Powlishta KK, Von Dras DD, Stanford A, et al. The clock drawing test is a poor screen for very mild dementia. Neurology 2002;59(6):898–903.

[40] Borson S, Scanlan J, Brush M, et al. The Mini-Cog: a cognitive 'vital signs' measure for dementia screening in multi-lingual elderly. Int J Geriatr Psychiatry 2000;15:1021–7.

[41] Wilber ST, Lofgren SD, Mager TG, et al. An evaluation of two screening tools for cognitive impairment in older ED patients. Acad Emerg Med 2005;12(7):612–6.

[42] Callahan CM, Unverzagt FW, Hui SL, et al. Six-item screener to identify cognitive impairment among potential subjects for clinical research. Med Care 2002;40(9):771–81.

[43] Wolfe RE, Brown DFM. Coma and depressed level of consciousness. In: Marx JA, editor. Rosen's emergency medicine concepts and clinical practice. St. Louis, MO: Mosby; 2002. p. 137–44.

[44] Kalbfleisch N. Altered mental status. In: Sanders AB, editor. Emergency care of the elder person. St. Louis, MO: Beverly Cracom Publications; 1996. p. 97–116.

[45] Wilber ST. Geriatric emergency medicine. In: Solomon DH, LoCicero J, Rosenthal RA, editors. New frontiers in geriatrics research: an agenda for surgical and related medical specialties. 1st edition. New York: American Geriatrics Society; 2004.

[46] Sanders AB. Missed delirium in older emergency department patients: a quality-of-care problem. Ann Emerg Med 2002;39:338–41.

ELSEVIER
SAUNDERS

Emerg Med Clin N Am
24 (2006) 317–338

EMERGENCY
MEDICINE
CLINICS OF
NORTH AMERICA

Pulmonary Emergencies in the Elderly

Jason Imperato, MD, MBA[a],*,
Leon D. Sanchez, MD, MPH[b]

[a]Department of Emergency Medicine, Mount Auburn Hospital,
330 Mount Auburn Street, Cambridge, MA 02138, USA
[b]Department of Emergency Medicine, Beth Israel Deaconess Medical Center,
One Deaconess Road, Boston, MA 02115, USA

In the United States, the proportion and absolute number of elderly persons is ever increasing. These individuals become more susceptible to medical ailments because of the physiologic changes that are a part of the aging process. Not only are pulmonary disorders more prevalent in elderly persons, differences in the disease process can make the identification and management of pulmonary disorders challenging for the clinician. Specifically, differences in the presenting symptoms, interpretation of diagnostic studies, and treatment modalities make pulmonary disorders in the elderly more demanding than in younger individuals.

In this article, we will first review the physiologic changes in the respiratory system that occur during aging and attempt to relate these changes to the development of pulmonary disease in this population. Later, we will discuss specific pulmonary ailments that are common in the elderly population. Specifically, pulmonary embolism, pneumonia, chronic obstructive pulmonary disease (COPD), asthma, and tuberculosis (TB) will be discussed. Particular emphasis will be placed on the differences between these disease processes in older patients as compared with younger patients.

Pulmonary function in the elderly

The changes in general respiratory function that occur during the aging process play an important role in the differences in disease manifestations in geriatric patients. The entire respiratory system from the chest wall to the alveoli undergoes anatomic changes with aging. As a result, it has been established that even in the absence of disease pulmonary function deteriorates with age.

* Corresponding author.
E-mail address: Jimperat@mah.harvard.edu (J. Imperato).

With age there is a reduction in bronchiole airway size secondary to alterations in the supporting connective tissue leading to decreased elastic recoil, decreased diameter, early closure, and increased airflow resistance [1]. The alveolar ducts and sacs dilate and may coalesce due to changes in the relative proportions of decreased elastic tissues and increased collagen that occur during aging [2]. This leads to a smaller number of alveoli and a resultant diminished alveolar surface area necessary for gas exchange.

The supporting muscles of respiration are also altered during the aging process. Age related kyphoscoliosis, calcifications of the intercostal cartilages, and arthritis of the costovertebral joints lead to an increased rigidity of the thoracic cage and resultant decreased chest wall compliance. As a result, elderly patients rely more on the diaphragm and abdominal muscles and less so on the thoracic muscles to breathe [2]. Because of reduction in muscle strength with age, including that of the diaphragm and accessory respiratory muscles, elderly patients are more susceptible to fatigue when the work of breathing is increased by cardiopulmonary insult [3].

The structural changes of both the lungs and the chest wall produce the predictable decline in pulmonary function seen in elderly patients. Measurements of airflow that are decreased in age include the forced vital capacity (FVC), forced expiratory volume in one second (FEV1), and the ratio of FEV1 to FVC. These changes are due to increased rigidity of the chest wall, loss of elastic recoil of the lung, and decreased force generated by the muscles of respiration [1,2]. Increased alveolar diameter and subsequent air trapping in the distal airways increases the residual volume. The combination of the above findings results in a relatively constant total lung capacity.

The changes described may result in the altered gas-exchange functions seen in the elderly. Ventilation-perfusion mismatching occurs secondary to the collapse of peripheral bronchioles leading to a decrease in alveolar ventilation in the dependent areas of the lung. This, combined with decreases in alveolar surface area, contributes to alterations in the total pulmonary diffusing capacity.

The response to hypoxic and hypercapnic stimuli is diminished in older patients compared with younger patients [4]. There is also a reduced effectiveness of cough and compromised mucociliary clearance with age altering defense mechanisms [3]. This makes geriatric patients more susceptible to pulmonary infections, and their response to cardiopulmonary insult is reduced compared with the general population.

Pulmonary embolism in the elderly

Pathophysiology and risk factors

Pulmonary emboli most often begin as clots that originate in the deep veins of the lower extremities. These thromboemboli can then travel to the pulmonary vasculature of the lungs, resulting in a wide range of responses, from asymptomatic to cardiogenic shock.

The risks for development of thrombus formation can be described by Virchow's triad, including venous stasis, endothelial injury, and hypercoagulability. Although it is unclear if advanced age is an independent risk factor for thromboemboli, elderly patients typically have a higher incidence of risk factors for clot formation [5]. In one study of patients over 65 years old diagnosed with pulmonary embolism, greater than 70% had more than one risk factor for thrombus formation [6].

Venous stasis, most typically from immobility, has been found to be the most common risk factor for the development of pulmonary embolism in all age groups [7]. Older patients have an increased incidence of immobility secondary to comorbid medical conditions such as stroke, hip and pelvic fractures, and other chronic diseases. One study showed 65% of patients older than 65 years old diagnosed with pulmonary embolism were at bed rest for over 4 days [8].

Endothelial injury leads to clot formation through the activation of the coagulation cascade and promotion of platelet adhesion and aggregation. Endothelial injury may result from certain vasoconstrictive or chemotherapeutic agents, burns, trauma, or surgical procedures [9]. Hypercoagulability in the elderly can be attributed in part to increases in fibrinogen and other procoagulant levels and decreases in antithrombin levels seen in aging [2]. It remains unclear whether or not age alone is an independent risk factor for venous thrombosis or if it is confounded by associated diseases and the prolonged bed rest that often accompanies it [10]. Regardless, it is clear the geriatric patients are more susceptible to developing venous thrombosis and pulmonary embolism.

Signs and symptoms

The clinical presentation of pulmonary embolism is often nonspecific, making the diagnosis notoriously difficult in patients of all ages. One study showed pulmonary embolism was an incidental finding in 63% of autopsy cases, and that in 70% of cases when the patient died from a pulmonary embolism there was no antemortem suspicion for the diagnosis [11]. Making the diagnosis of pulmonary embolism is even more challenging in elderly patients; therefore, an even higher index of suspicion is essential to avoid missing the diagnosis [6].

Common symptoms of pulmonary embolism include dyspnea, pleuritic chest pain, cough, palpitations, leg swelling, hemoptysis, anxiety, and syncope, while common signs include tachycardia and tachypnea. There are varying opinions about the frequency at which these symptoms and signs are seen in elderly patients as opposed to younger patients. Although some report that common symptoms are less frequently reported by the elderly [12,13], others report a similar rate of signs and symptoms with the exception of hemoptysis, which is see less frequently in the elderly [7].

There are several reasons for the difficulty in diagnosing older patients with pulmonary embolism. The diagnosis may not be considered in patients presenting with dyspnea or chest pain, as these symptoms can often be attributed to alternative diagnoses such as myocardial ischemia, congestive heart failure, COPD, or asthma. Elderly patients may also delay seeking medical care secondary to the blunted perception of dyspnea seen during the aging process [14,15].

Diagnostic testing

The testing used to diagnose pulmonary embolism in the elderly is similar to that used in younger patients. Modalities used when investigating the presence of a pulmonary embolism may include chest radiograph, electrocardiogram, arterial blood gas, D-dimer concentration, lung scanning, and spiral computerized tomography. Although the testing modalities may be similar, the interpretation of test results differs with the aging process.

Chest radiographs are useful to rule out other diagnoses that can mimic pulmonary embolism such as congestive heart failure, pneumothorax, or pneumonia. A normal chest radiograph in the setting of dyspnea or chest pain should raise the clinician's suspicion for pulmonary embolism. In elderly patients a normal chest radiograph is seen less frequently. One study revealed that 82% of patients with pulmonary embolism over age 70 had abnormal films [16].

Electrocardiographic findings in pulmonary embolism are nonspecific. Classic findings of right heart strain such as a new right bundle branch block and an S1Q3T3 pattern occur infrequently, and as a result, an electrocardiogram is rarely diagnostic in pulmonary embolisms. Electrocardographic abnormalities specific to a pulmonary embolism occur with nearly equal frequency in both younger and older patients [7].

Arterial blood gas findings are also nonspecific in making the diagnosis. Classic findings including hypoxia, a widened alveolar–arterial gradient, and respiratory alkalosis can be suggestive but not diagnostic. Because the aging process leads to a decrease in the partial pressure of arterial oxygen and an increase in the alveolar–arterial gradient, arterial blood gas abnormalities can be particularly difficult to interpret in the geriatric population [17].

D-dimer testing in the evaluation of patients with suspected pulmonary embolism has gained recent popularity. The D-dimer concentration is not specific for the diagnosis of pulmonary embolism [18], as it can be elevated in other clinical situations such as cancer, postsurgical, or congestive heart failure. The usefulness of the test in the general population is that the D-dimer is highly sensitive, and has a strong negative predictive value when below a certain threshold [19]. The utility of the test in advanced age is reduced because D-dimer values in the elderly are rarely below the negative predictive value threshold [20].

Imaging studies play an important role in the diagnosis of pulmonary embolism. Echocardiography is a noninvasive study that may reveal right ventricular strain in response to a pulmonary embolism suggesting the diagnosis. In the elderly, however, right ventricular dysfunction is more common and nonspecific secondary to preexisting disease such as COPD or valvular heart disease. A study of patients greater than 65 years of age with echocardiograms at the time of pulmonary embolism diagnosis found right ventricular dilatation and pulmonary artery systolic hypertension was present in more than half of the patients [8].

Ventilation-perfusion lung scanning can be a useful diagnostic imaging test when considering pulmonary embolism. Interpretation criteria have been derived from the PIOPED study, which assigned probabilities to lung scan patterns based on how likely they were at be associated with angiographically diagnosed pulmonary embolism [21]. The interpretation of such scans can be particularly difficult in the elderly as ventilation-perfusion lung scanning is frequently nondiagnostic when there is underlying cardiopulmonary disease [22]. Abnormal scans can be seen in COPD, congestive heart failure, pneumonia, interstitial lung disease, and lung cancer, all of which are seen more frequently with advanced age.

Spiral computerized tomography (CT) scans have recently become the study of choice in some institutions for clinically suspected pulmonary embolism. Several studies have shown that CT scans are both sensitive and specific in making the diagnosis in patients of all ages, and is useful in identifying alternative diagnoses [23–25]. The only limitation of CT scans in the elderly is the contrast load that may adversely affect patients with renal insufficiency, which is seen more frequently with advanced age.

Treatment

Emergency treatment of pulmonary embolism consists of stabilization of cardiopulmonary function and prevention of further embolization via anticoagulation. Parenteral administration of unfractionated heparin is the treatment of choice for pulmonary embolisms in patients of all ages, and should be initiated when the diagnosis is suspected. Bleeding secondary to heparin administration is a concern, particularly in the elderly, who are at increased bleeding risk compared with younger patients [26]. Because the response to unfractionated heparin varies from patient to patient, close monitoring of the activated partial thromboplastin time is necessary. More recently, low molecular weight heparin has been used to achieve anticoagulation in the treatment of pulmonary embolism because it does not require monitoring of laboratory tests and is clinically effective [27].

Oral anticoagulation with warfarin represents the long-term treatment of pulmonary embolism and venous thromboembolism. Like unfractionated heparin, the dose response to warfarin varies from patient to patient, and as a result, close monitoring of the international normalized ratio is necessary.

of pneumonia is only found in less than 50% of patients [37]. Moreover, the causative organisms are often different in elderly.

The location in which the elderly patient resides also affects the type of organism that causes pneumonia, and antimicrobial therapy should be based on the residence of the individual at time of infection. Typically, the disease is classified into one of three types that include CAP, long-term care facility (LTCF) pneumonia, and nosocomial or hospital-acquired pneumonia.

Common causes of CAP in the elderly include the following [30,38]:

Streptococcus pneumoniae
Haemophilus influenzae
Enteric Gram-negative bacilli
Staphylococcus aureus
Aspiration (anaerobes and aerobes)
Influenza and other viruses
Mycoplasma pneumoniae
Chlamydia pneumoniae
Legionella pneumonphila

S pneumoniae is by far the most common bacterial cause of CAP in elderly patients accounting for 30% to 50% of cases. The likelihood of other common causative agents was shown in one study where *S pneumoniae* accounted for 43%, enteric Gram-negative bacilli for 37%, *H influenzae* for 20%, and *S aureus* for 14% of cases [39]. *S aureus* pneumonia can sometimes be seen as a postinfluenza pneumonia or in those with diabetes or chronic renal failure [29]. This is covered in more detail in the chapter on Infectious Emergencies in the Elderly.

Patients that reside in long-term care facilities, like nursing homes or skilled nursing facilities, are infected by slightly different organisms compared with those seen in the community. The causes of pneumonia in elderly patients in LTCF include the following [30,38]:

Streptococcus pneumoniae
Enteric Gram-negative bacilli
Staphylococcus aureus
Aspiration (anaerobes and aerobes)
Haemophilus influenzae
Moraxella catarrhalis
Enterococci
Influenza and other viruses

Although *S pneumoniae* is still the leading cause of infection in these patients, there is an increased rate of infection from Gram-negative organisms, *S aureus*, and anaerobes [39].

The pathogens responsible for hospital-acquired pneumonia include the following [30,38]:

Enteric Gram-negative bacilli
Aspiration (anaerobes and aerobes)
Streptococcus pneumoniae
Staphylococcus aureus
Legionella pneumophila
Moraxella catarrhalis
Influenza and other viruses

Unlike CAP and LTCF pneumonia where *S pneumoniae* is the most common causative organism, nosocomial pneumonia is most often due to enteric Gram-negative bacilli with *Pseudomonas aeuruginosa* and *Klebsiella pneumoniae* being most common [39].

Treatment

Emergency treatment of pneumonia consists of stabilizing pulmonary function, maintaining adequate oxygenation, reversing dehydration, and antimicrobial therapy.

Empiric antimicrobial therapy in the emergency department should be based on the patient's age, presence of comorbid illnesses, severity of pneumonia, and the residence of the patient at time of infection [35]. Multiple algorithms have been proposed for empiric treatment of CAP. Appropriate therapeutic agents may include (1) a second-generation cephalosporin (cefuroxime) plus a macrolide (azithromycin or clarithromycin), (2) a third-generation cephalosporin (ceftriaxone or cefotaxime) plus a macrolide (azithromycin or clarithromycin), or (3) an antipneumococcal fluoroquinolone (levofloxacin or gatifloxacin) alone. Such regimens have been shown to lower 30-day mortality in elderly patients with CAP [40]. Empiric therapy for hospital-acquired pneumonia should be based on those pathogens that are historically seen in a particular health care facility.

Timely administration of antimicrobial therapy is essential in improving patient outcomes. In one large study, approximately 75% of patients received their first dose of antibiotics within 8 hours upon arrival to the hospital, and those patients had significantly lower 30-day mortality than patients who received their first dose of antibiotics at a later time [41].

Obstructive pulmonary disease in the elderly

Definitions and pathophysiology

COPD is a clinical spectrum that encompasses a number of disease states characterized by a reduction in expiratory flow. These include asthma, chronic bronchitis, and emphysema. Following a brief discussion of chronic bronchitis, this section will focus on emphysema, as it is a disease of primarily the elderly population. Asthma will be discussed in more detail in the next section.

Chronic bronchitis is historically defined as a chronic productive cough for at least 3 months of the year for at least 2 successive years. Pathologic changes seen in chronic bronchitis include hypertrophy of the mucous glands of the larger airways and inflammation. Eventually airflow obstruction develops, and can lead to hypoventilation and hypercapnia. Patients with chronic bronchitis are often referred to as "blue bloaters" because both cyanosis and right heart failure are common [42].

Emphysema is an anatomic disorder characterized by enlargement of the distal air spaces and destruction of the alveolar walls. The changes seen as emphysema develops are in large part due to the degradation of elastin, which leads to decreased lung elasticity, lung hyperinflation, and air trapping from premature closure of the smaller airways. Emphysema patients are often labeled as "pink puffers" because oxygenation is generally preserved as it is offset by hyperventilation [42].

Chronic bronchitis and emphysema typically coexist in the majority of COPD patients, as only a small percentage of patients may have a relatively "pure form" of either condition [42]. Cigarette smoking is the leading cause of COPD. Other risk factors include male gender, occupational exposures, air pollution, and alpha-1-antitrypsin deficiency.

Signs and symptoms

The patient with an acute exacerbation of COPD will often complain of shortness of breath, cough, or wheezing. Although these symptoms are common in many pulmonary disorders seen in the elderly, a past history of COPD should lead the clinician to the proper diagnosis.

On examination, the clinician may notice tachypnea, tachycardia, increased anteroposterior diameter of the chest, and use of the accessory muscles of respiration. Percussion of the patient's chest may reveal limited excursion of the diaphragm, consistent with hyperinflation of the lungs. During auscultation of the chest a prolonged expiratory phase is often noted. Expiratory wheezes are often heard, but decreased or absent breath sounds are common secondary to limited air movement, which may not produce wheezing. As symptoms progress, the patient may develop cyanosis, confusion, stupor, or coma secondary to severe hypoxemia and hypercapnia.

In severe cases of COPD pulmonary artery hypertension may develop, leading to right ventricular enlargement, which is referred to as cor pulmonale. Signs of cor pulmonale include jugular venous distention, tender hepatomegaly, and peripheral edema.

Diagnostic testing

The diagnosis of an acute exacerbation of COPD is primarily clinical. Diagnostic studies may aid in making the diagnosis, excluding other diagnoses, and determining the severity of the disease presentation. Chest radiographs are commonly performed. Other studies that may be indicated include electrocardiogram, pulmonary function testing, arterial blood gas, routine blood tests, brain natriuretic peptide (BNP), and sputum and blood cultures.

A chest radiograph is useful to rule out alternative diagnoses such as pneumonia, congestive heart failure, and pneumothorax. It may also reveal some characteristic changes seen in emphysema, including flattening of the diaphragms, hyperinflation of the lungs with decreased peripheral vascular markings, increased retrosternal airspace, or the presence of bullae [1].

An EKG may be useful in the setting of COPD exacerbation. The EKG can show signs of right ventricular hypertrophy from cor pulmonale, but may be more useful in identifying other diagnoses such as myocardial ischemia or pulmonary embolism. A sudden deterioration of a COPD patient should further raise concerns for alternative diagnoses such as pneumothorax or pulmonary embolism.

Bedside pulmonary function tests such as the peak expiratory flow rate can provide an early objective assessment of the patient's general condition. Flow data is particularly useful if performed sequentially before and after treatments to allow the clinician to determine if the patient is improving or deteriorating. Elderly patients may have difficulty using the airflow measuring device leading to unreliable flow data.

The use of pulse oximetry may help identify hypoxia, but it does not reveal hypercapnia or acid-base disturbances, which are common during acute COPD exacerbations. Arterial blood gas (ABG) determinations can be useful in evaluating hypercapnia and hypoxemia, and can help differentiate acute versus chronic disease as uncompensated respiratory acidosis is characteristic of acute ventilatory failure [1].

Routine blood work is often not diagnostic in COPD, but is typically included in patient evaluation. BNP may help differentiate COPD from congestive heart failure. Additionally, sputum cultures, when available, may help guide antibiotic selection in both chronic bronchitis and emphysema.

Treatment

The emergency treatment of COPD should be directed at reversing hypoxemia and airflow obstruction. The mainstays of therapy include supplemental oxygen, bronchodilators, and corticosteroids. Treatment of such patients requires frequent reevaluation for response to therapy, as patients with severe disease may need mechanical ventilation secondary to respiratory failure.

The benefits of supplemental oxygen therapy include increasing tissue oxygen delivery, decreasing bronchoconstriction, and reversing hypoxia-induced pulmonary hypertension [1]. The goal is to maintain an arterial oxygen pressure (PaO_2) of greater than 60 mmHg or an arterial oxygen saturation (SaO_2) of greater than 90%. Several devices can be used to accomplish this goal, including a nasal cannula, simple face mask, Venturi mask, or nonrebreather mask. The clinician must be careful because some patients rely on their hypoxic drive for ventilatory stimulation, and depression of the respiratory center can lead to hypercapnia and CO_2 narcosis. Repeated clinical evaluations after supplemental oxygen is the most important measure of response to therapy, but, repeat ABGs may also be helpful in more severe cases.

Inhaled β2-adrenergic agonists such as albuterol are the initial pharmacologic treatment of choice during an acute exacerbation of COPD as they promote bronchodilation and improve mucociliary clearance. Although these medications can be delivered by oral and parenteral routes, inhaled therapy is preferred by administration via a metered dose inhaler with a spacing device or a compressor-driven nebulizer. Treatments may be administered every 15 to 20 minutes or on a continuous basis depending on the clinical situation [43].

There is evidence that the therapeutic response to inhaled β2-adrenergic agonists decreases with advanced age [44], which is consistent with the findings that the number of β2-receptors declines with age [45]. However, a more recent study showed that younger patients and elderly patients responded equally well to inhaled albuterol [46].

The aerosolized route achieves topical administration of a relatively small dose of drug, producing local effects with minimal systemic absorption and thus few side effects. Although generally safe in the elderly, β2-adrenergic agonists are not without side effects. Skeletal muscle tremor is most common, but other adverse effects may include tachycardia, hypertension, palpitations, anxiety, or headache. These medications can also cause a dose-dependent drop in serum potassium and increase in the QT interval on the electrocardiogram, so caution must be taken, especially in elderly patients with cardiac disease.

Inhaled anticholinergic agents such as ipratropium bromide should be used in conjunction with β2-adrenergic agonists as first-line therapy for acute COPD exacerbations. In COPD, vagally mediated cholinergic tone is increased, leading to constriction of the proximal airways [47]. Anticholinergic agents block muscarinic receptors in the airways, and as a result decrease both bronchial smooth muscle tone and release of mucous secretions.

Patients with COPD may respond to inhaled anticholingerics despite a lack of response to inhaled β2-agonists [48]. Because these agents affect the larger airways and β2-agonists affect the smaller airways, the medications may show synergism when used together. The combined effects of these agents has been shown to be superior to either agent used alone [49–51]. Another advantage of ipratropium bromide is that it has an excellent safety profile with few side effects, dry mouth being most common, and rarely a metallic taste being described. These medications are longer acting than β2-agonists, and can be given every 4 hours.

Patients with acute COPD exacerbations often have a history of congestive heart failure. Although diagnostic tests such as the chest radiograph and BNP concentration can help differentiate between the two conditions, it is often necessary to initially treat these patients for both conditions simultaneously until diagnostic information is available.

Although corticosteroids act too slowly to alter the immediate emergency department course, they do play a role in the treatment of COPD. Studies have shown that steroids help decrease the relapse rate of acute exacerbations and reduce treatment failures [43,52–54]. Further discussion of corticosteroids in pulmonary disease takes place in the following section on asthma.

Antibiotic therapy in the setting of COPD exacerbations may also be of some benefit, particularly in those patients who complain of cough with sputum production. A small clinical benefit for empiric antibiotics in the setting of COPD exacerbations was shown in a meta-analysis of nine randomized, placebo-controlled trials [55].

Asthma in the elderly

Historically, asthma has been described as a disease of younger patients and its prevalence is often underestimated in the elderly. Because of this, asthma is often overlooked and underdiagnosed in the elderly population. Factors that may account for this underestimation include the overlap of asthma symptoms with those of chronic bronchitis and emphysema and the coexistence of other cardiopulmonary conditions that may mimic asthma [2,56].

Definition and pathophysiology

Asthma is an inflammatory disease of the airways, characterized by increased responsiveness of the tracheobronchial tree to various stimuli leadings to diffuse airway narrowing. In susceptible individuals this can cause recurrent episodes of wheezing, shortness of breath, chest tightness, and cough. These symptoms are usually associated with widespread but variable airflow narrowing that is at least partially reversible either spontaneously or with treatment [57].

The cardinal features of asthma include bronchial hyperresponsiveness and airway obstruction. Bronchial hyperresponsiveness is an exaggerated bronchoconstrictive response by the airways to a variety of stimuli such as aeroallergens, histamine, methacholine, cold air, and environmental irritants. It is thought that airway inflammation is the stimulus for bronchial hyperresponsiveness, as it can be induced by a number of inciting events including viral respiratory infections, allergic reactions, and noxious agents [57].

Airway obstruction is another cardinal feature of asthma, and may be caused by acute bronchoconstriction, mucus plugging of the airways, bronchial wall edema, inflammatory cell infiltration, smooth muscle hypertrophy, and uncoupling of elastic recoil forces. This airway obstruction results in the predictable decline in pulmonary function testing seen in both elderly and younger patients with asthma [57].

Signs and symptoms

The signs and symptoms of asthma are similar in patients of all age groups. The most common symptoms reported are cough, wheezing, and shortness of breath. These symptoms can be mimicked in other diseases that commonly afflict elderly patients such as emphysema, bronchitis, congestive heart failure, pneumonia, or gastroesophageal reflux disease. As a result, while the clinician must consider an expanded differential diagnosis in this clinical setting, he must be certain to contemplate asthma to make the diagnosis.

One significant difference in presentation is that elderly patients are symptomatic longer than younger patients before seeking medical attention. In one study of hospital admissions for asthma, 65% of patients over age 65 years had symptoms for more than 14 days compared with 29% of patients under 40 years [58]. Proposed explanations for the delay in seeking treatment are a blunted perception of breathlessness in elderly patients or that the elderly patient may assume that their symptoms are due to deconditioning or to normal aging [15,59].

On examination, typical findings may include tachycardia, tachypnea, hypoxia, and expiratory wheezes on auscultation of the lungs. The clinical response to an exacerbation of asthma may be blunted in elderly patients, making it difficult for the clinician to make the diagnosis. In one study older patients had a larger than predicted decrease in pulmonary function compared with younger patients even though physician assessed severity of pulmonary function was similar in both groups [60].

Diagnostic testing

The diagnosis of asthma is primarily clinical. However, because the presentation of asthma may mimic other cardiopulmonary diseases in the elderly, diagnostic tests are often needed to rule out alternative causes of the patients symptoms.

Chest radiographs in the setting of asthma are often nonspecific, and not typically recommended in the setting of asthma. However, a chest film may be of use in elderly patients with shortness of breath or cough to rule out congestive heart failure, pneumonia, pneumothorax, or lung cancer. Chest radiographs should always be obtained in those patients who do not respond to therapy, and who require hospital admission because they are at risk for pulmonary complications [61]. An electrocardiogram may be performed, because myocardial ischemia and pulmonary embolism should be considered as possible causes of the shortness of breath.

Laboratory studies are not routine in cases of asthma exacerbations if the clinician is certain of the diagnosis, as complete blood counts and serum electrolytes are rarely helpful in confirming the diagnosis. In addition, ABGs are only needed in the most severe cases of asthma that do not respond to standard therapy.

Pulmonary function testing such as peak flow measurements may aid in making the diagnosis, as there is a predictable decrease in such measurements during an acute asthma exacerbation. Lung function testing is especially important in this age group because there is an age-related reduction in the perception of bronchoconstriction in the elderly [15].

Treatment

Asthma therapy in the elderly is similar to that for younger patients. The goals of treatment for acute asthma exacerbations are to reverse airflow obstruction, ensure adequate oxygenation, and relieve inflammation. Treatment should generally follow the recommendations of the National Asthma Education and Prevention Program [62], and should include inhaled bronchodilators in mild cases and the addition of corticosteroids in more severe cases.

Like in COPD, inhaled β2-adrenergic agonists such as albuterol are the initial treatment of choice during an acute exacerbation of asthma. Although these medications can be delivered by oral and parenteral routes, inhaled therapy is the preferred method of treatment during asthma exacerbations. As seen earlier, the clinician must be aware of the common side effects of these medications such as skeletal muscle tremor, tachycardia, hypertension, palpitations, anxiety, and headache.

Epinephrine and terbutaline are β2-adrenergic agonists that can be given subcutaneously. Both can produce tachycardia, hypertension, dysrhythmias, and vasoconstriction, especially in patients with preexisting heart disease. As a result, these medications should not be used in elderly patients, who more commonly suffer from cardiac abnormalities [63].

Inhaled anticholinergic agents such as ipratropium bromide produce bronchodilation by reducing vagal tone, and may be a good adjunct therapy in cases of more severe asthma [64,65]. This is because anticholinergic agents affect larger, central airways while β2-adrenergics dilate small airways. The medication is poorly absorbed from the mucosal surfaces of the lung, and as a result, it has an excellent safety profile with few side effects.

Anti-inflammatory agents such as corticosteroids are another mainstay in the treatment of acute asthma exacerbations. Corticosteroids act by preventing migration and activation of inflammatory cells, interfering with the production of prostaglandins and leukotrienes, and enhancing the action of β-adrenergic receptors on airway smooth muscle [57]. Corticosteroids should be administered in patients in whom airway obstruction is not immediately relieved after the first nebulized bronchodilator treatment, or who have had prolonged duration of symptoms. Acceptable routes of administration in the acute setting include 40 to 60 mg prednisone orally or 60 to 125 mg methylprednisolone intravenously [66].

The side effects of chronic steroid use are particularly concerning in the elderly. Chronic steroid use can lead to osteoporosis, hyperglycemia, hypertension, impaired immune response, and cataracts. These disorders are all problems that are typically seen in the elderly population without the use of chronic steroids, and chronic steroid use will worsen these conditions.

Pulmonary tuberculosis in the elderly

Epidemiology and pathophysiology

TB in humans is caused by any one of three pathogenic mycobacteria with *Mycobacerium tuberculosis* (MTB) being the most common agent. TB infection can manifest as disease in any one of multiple organ systems. This section will focus on pulmonary TB and its manifestations.

In the United States, over half of all TB cases occur in people over the age of 65 years [67]. TB cases are fourfold higher in residents of nursing homes compared with elderly patients living at home [68]. The exact mechanism for the age distribution of TB cases is not clear. It is commonly believed that the high rates of active infection in the elderly are due to the large proportion of the elderly population having been previously infected and subsequently reactivating latent infection [69]. Moreover, this reactivation is thought to result from a reduction in host defenses that occur during the aging process.

Signs and symptoms

As with many other diseases, the symptoms of tuberculosis are often atypical in elderly patients. As a result, pulmonary TB in the elderly frequently goes unrecognized [70]. The classic symptoms of pulmonary TB include fever, night sweats, weight loss, fatigue, cough, and hemoptysis. Additional symptoms may include pleuritic chest pain, shortness of breath, anorexia, weakness, or failure to thrive.

It has been suggested that because of differing symptomatology pulmonary TB in the elderly might differ from the disease presenting in younger patients. One study showed that the cardinal symptoms were significantly less likely in patients greater than 65 years old [71]. A meta-analysis showed several clinical differences between older and younger patients with pulmonary TB. Older patients were less likely to have fever, sweating, and hemopytsis, and were more likely to have shortness of breath [72].

The physical examination for TB is largely nonspecific and nondiagnostic. Examination of the chest is unlikely to help with the diagnosis, as it may range from normal to a few scattered bronchial breath sounds. Other nonspecific findings include fever, pallor, and evidence of weight loss.

Diagnostic testing

Because the history and physical for tuberculosis in the elderly is usually nonspecific, diagnostic testing is almost always needed to establish the presence of a TB infection. Useful studies available to the clinician include routine laboratory tests, chest radiographs, tuberculin skin tests, and microbiology testing.

The chest radiograph is the most useful study in making a presumptive diagnosis of TB, as primary TB infections usually have distinct radiographic findings. Classic findings of TB on the chest radiograph are a pneumonic infiltrate with enlarged hilar or mediastinal nodes. Typically, the infiltrate involves a single lobe, and is classically in one of the upper lobes. In contrast, mid-zone and lower zone infiltrates may predominate in the elderly patient making the diagnosis even more elusive in this population [2].

A normal chest radiograph has a high negative predictive value and is therefore a useful screening test in the emergency department. However, there is a false-negative rate in approximately 1% of immunocompetent patients, so depending on the clinical circumstances, the chest radiograph does not always rule out the diagnosis [73].

If the clinical picture or chest radiograph findings suggest the diagnosis of pulmonary tuberculosis, the emergency physician should initiate mycobacteriologic studies of the patient's sputum. Spontaneously produced sputum collected under direct supervision is the ideal method of collection, but nebulizer induction of sputum and gastric aspiration of swallowed respiratory secretions are alternative methods in patients not able to produce sputum [74]. Direct microscopic examination of a stained sputum specimen is the most rapid test to support a diagnosis of TB because it can detect acid fast bacillus (AFB). Because of limited sensitivity, a negative AFB smear does not rule out the diagnosis of pulmonary TB. It is recommended that three specimens be obtained on three different days and retested [74]. The presumptive diagnosis of TB based on smear testing is usually confirmed by isolating the organism in culture. Because of the amount of time it takes for positives cultures to manifest, they have a limited role in the emergency department.

Tuberculin skin testing

The tuberculin skin test remains the standard method for detecting latent MTB infection. The tuberculin test is based on the principle that MTB infection induces sensitivity to certain antigens of the bacillus. These antigens are contained in the preparation called purified protein derivative (PPD), which is administered intradermally and then read 48 to 72 hours after administration. The largest diameter of palpable induration is measured in millimeters and recorded. Current Centers for Disease Control and Prevention guidelines use 15 mm of induration as a positive test for people without TB risk factors but 10 mm of induration should be used in residents of long-term facilities such as nursing homes [75].

False negative skin tests may occur in immunosuppressed persons, whose delayed-type hypersensitivity responses may decrease or disappear. This condition is known as anergy, and is thought to be more common in the elderly population. In men, PPD reactivity drops from 50% in patients who are between 65 and 74 years of age to 10% in patients who are older than 95 years of age, and in women, the rate drops from 40% to about 5%, respectively, in the same age groups [76]. This increased prevalence of anergy in the elderly has been attributed to a decline in cellular immunity with age, eradication of the dormant infecting organism from within the host, or a combination of both [77,78]. Absence of a reaction to a tuberculin skin test does not rule out the diagnosis, especially in the elderly [79].

Treatment

The treatment for tuberculosis does not vary much among differing age groups. Medical therapy regimens are divided into treatment of latent TB infections and treatment of active disease.

Latent TB treatment is used to prevent the development of active TB disease in persons known or likely to be infected with *M tuberculosis*, as demonstrated by a positive PPD test. Current recommendations are treatment with isoniazid for 9 months [79,80]. Treatment for active TB infections are targeted against multidrug-resistant TB, and the initial drug regimen should consist of the four-drug regimen of isoniazid, rifampin, ethambutol, and pyrazinamide for 4 months, followed by isoniazid and rifampin for an additional 4 months [79,81]. Treatment must be tailored to the particular resistance profile of the infecting organism.

Summary

The aging process results in changes in pulmonary physiology that make the elderly population more susceptible to pulmonary disease. These physiologic changes also alter the clinical presentation of such diseases, making the diagnosis and treatment of pulmonary disorders particularly challenging for the clinician. It is important for the clinician to have a high index of suspicion for pulmonary disorders to make the proper diagnosis. It is essential to keep in mind the subtle differences between pulmonary diseases in the elderly compared with younger patients.

References

[1] Williams JM, Evans TC. Acute pulmonary disease in the aged. Clin Geriatr Med 1993;9: 527–45.
[2] Chan E, Welsh C. Geriatric respiratory medicine. Chest 1998;114:1704–33.
[3] Sevransky JE, Haponik EF. Respiratory failure in elderly patients. Clin Geriatr Med 2003; 19:205–24.

[4] Kronenberg R, Drage C. Attenuation of the ventilatory and heart rate responses to hypoxia and hypercapnia with aging in normal men. J Clin Invest 1973;52:1812–9.

[5] Hansson P, Welin L, Tibblin G, et al. Deep vein thrombosis and pulmonary embolism in the general population: The study of men born in 1913. Arch Intern Med 1997;157: 1665–70.

[6] Busby W, Bayer A, Pathy J. Pulmonary embolism in the elderly. Age Ageing 1988;17:205–9.

[7] Stein P, Gottschalk A, Saltzman H, et al. Diagnosis of acute pulmonary embolism in the elderly. J Am Coll Cardiol 1991;18:1452–7.

[8] Masotti L, Ceccarelli E, Cappelli R, et al. Pulmonary embolism in the elderly: clinical, instrumental and laboratory aspects. Gerontaology 2000;46:205–11.

[9] Berman AR. Pulmonary embolism in the elderly. Clin Geriatr Med 2001;17:107–30.

[10] Berman AR, Arnsten JH. Diagnosis and treatment of pulmonary embolism in the elderly. Clin Geriatr Med 2003;19:157–75.

[11] Stein P, Henry J. Prevalence of acute pulmonary embolism among patients in a general hospital and at autopsy. Chest 1995;108:978–81.

[12] Taubman L, Silverstone F. Autopsy proven pulmonary embolism among the institutionalized elderly. J Am Geriatr Soc 1986;34:752–6.

[13] Goldhaber S, Hennekens C, Evans D, et al. Factors associated with correct antemortem diagnosis of major pulmonary embolism. Am J Med 1982;73:822–6.

[14] Altose M, Leitner J, Cherniack N. Effects of age and respiratory efforts on the perception of resistive ventilatory loads. J Gerontol 1985;40:147–53.

[15] Connolly M, Crowley J, Charan N, et al. Reduced subjective awareness of bronchoconstriction provoked by methacholine in elderly asthmatic and normal subjects as measured on a simple awareness scale. Thorax 1992;47:410–3.

[16] Elliot C, Goldhaber S, Visani L, et al. Chest radiographs in acute pulmonary embolism: results from the International Cooperative Pulmonary Embolism Registry. Chest 2000;118: 33–8.

[17] Campbell E, Lefrak S. How aging affects the structure and function of the respirator system. Geratrics 1978;33:68–74.

[18] Bounameaux H, de Moerloose P, Perrier A, et al. Plasma measurement of D-dimer as diagnostic aid in suspected venous thromboembolism: an overview. Thromb Haemost 1994;71: 1–6.

[19] Goldhaber S, Simons G, Eliott C, et al. Quantitative plasma D-dimer levels among patients undergoing pulmonary angiography for suspected pulmonary embolism. JAMA 1993;270: 2819–22.

[20] Tardy B, Tardy-Poncet B, Viallon A, et al. Evaluation of D-dimer ELISA test in elderly patients with suspected pulmonary embolism. Thromb Haemost 1998;79:38–41.

[21] Investigators PIOPED. Value of the ventilation/perfusion scan in acute pulmonary embolism: results of the prospective investigation of pulmonary embolism diagnosis (PIOPED). JAMA 1990;263:2753–9.

[22] Lesser B, Leeper K, Stein P, et al. The diagnosis of acute pulmonary embolism in patients with chronic obstructive pulmonary disease. Chest 1992;102:17–22.

[23] Van Rossum A, Treurniet F, Kieft G, et al. Role of spiral volumetric computed tomographic scanning n the assessment of patients with clinical suspicion of pulmonary embolism and an abnormal ventilation/perfusion lung scan. Thorax 1996;51:23–8.

[24] Mayo J, Remy-Jardin M, Muller N, et al. Pulmonary embolism: prospective comparison of spiral CT with ventilation-perfusion scintigraphy. Radiology 1997;205:447–52.

[25] Remy-Jardin M, Remy J, Deschildre F, et al. Diagnosis of pulmonary embolism with spiral CT: comparison with pulmonary angiography and scintigraphy. Radiology 1996;200: 699–706.

[26] Jick H, Slone D, Borda I, et al. Efficacy and toxicity of heparin in relation to age and sex. N Engl J Med 1968;279:284–6.

[27] Simmonneau G, Sors H, Charbonnier B, et al. A comparison of low-molecular-weight heparin with unfractionated heparin for acute pulmonary embolism. N Engl J Med 1997;337:663–9.

[28] Gurwitz J, Avorn J, Ross-Degnan D, et al. Aging and anticoagulation response to warfarin therapy. Ann Intern Med 1992;116:901–4.

[29] Niederman MS, Ahmed QAA. Community-acquired pneumonia in elderly patients. Clin Geriatr Med 2003;19:101–20.

[30] Feldman C. Pneumonia in the elderly. Med Clin North Am 2001;85:1441–59.

[31] Puchelle E, Zahm J, Bertrand A. Influence of age on mucociliary transport. Scand J Respir Dis 1979;60:307–13.

[32] Metlay J, Schulz R, Li Y, et al. Influence of age on symptoms at presentation in patients with community acquired pneumonia. Arch Intern Med 1997;157:1453–9.

[33] Harper C, Newton P. Clinical aspects of pneumonia in the elderly veteran. J Am Geriatr Soc 1989;37:867–72.

[34] Venkatesan P, Gladman J, MacFarlane J, et al. A hospital study of community acquired pneumonia in the elderly. Thorax 1990;17:254–8.

[35] Niederman M, Bass J, Campbell G, et al. Guidelines for the initial management of adults with community-acquired pneumonia: diagnosis, assessment of severity, and initial antimicrobial therapy. Am Rev Respir Dis 1993;148:1418–26.

[36] Hash R, Stephens J, Laurens M, et al. The relationship between volume status, hydration, and radiographic findings in the diagnosis of community-acquired pneumonia. J Fam Pract 2000;49:833–7.

[37] Granton JT, Grossman RF. Community-acquired pneumonia in the elderly patient: clinical features, epidemiology, and treatment. Clin Chest Med 1993;14:537–53.

[38] Marrie TJ. Pneumonia. Clin Geriatr Med 1992;8:721–34.

[39] Garb J, Brown R, Garb J, et al. Differences in etiology of pneumonias in nursing home and community patients. JAMA 1978;240:2169–72.

[40] Gleason P, Meehan T, Fine J, et al. Associations between initial antimicrobial therapy and medical outcomes for hospitalized elderly patients with pneumonia. Arch Intern Med 1999;159:2562–72.

[41] Meehan T, Fine M, Krumholz H, et al. Quality of care, process, and outcomes in elderly patients with pneumonia. JAMA 1997;278:2080–4.

[42] Mahler DA, Barlow PB, Matthay RA. Chronic obstructive pulmonary disease. Clin Geriatr Med 1986;2:285–311.

[43] Cydulka RK, Khandelwal S. Chronic obstructive pulmonary disease. In: Tintinalli JE, Kelen GD, Stapczynski JS, editors. Emergency medicine: a comprehensive study guide. 5th ed. New York: McGraw-Hill; 2000. p. 485–90.

[44] Ullah M, Newman G, Saunders K. Influence of age on response to ipratopium and salbutamol in asthma. Thorax 1981;36:523–9.

[45] Schocken D, Roth G. Reduced β-adrenergic receptor concentration in ageing man. Nature 1977;267:856–8.

[46] Kradjan W, Driesner N, Abuan T, et al. Effect of age on bronchodilator response. Chest 1992;101:1545–51.

[47] Petty TL. Definitions in chronic obstructive pulmonary disease. Clin Chest Med 1990;11:363–74.

[48] Bruan S, McKenzie W, Copeland C, et al. A comparison of the effect of ipratropium and albuterol in the treatment of chronic obstructive airway disease. Ann Intern Med 1989;149:544–7.

[49] Combivent Inhalation Aerosol Study Group. In chronic obstructive pulmonary disease, a combination of ipratropium bromide and albuterol is more effective than either agent alone. An 85-day multicenter trial. Chest 1994;105:1411–9.

[50] Combivent Inhalation Solution Study Group. Routine nebulized ipratropium and albuterol together are better than either alone in COPD. Chest 1997;112:1514–21.

[51] Gross N, Tashkin D, Miller R, et al. Inhalation by nebulization of albuterol–ipratopium combination (Dey combination) is superior to either agent alone in the treatement of chronic obstructive pulmonary disease. Dey Combination Solution Study Group. Respiration (Herrlisheim) 1998;65:354–62.

[52] Murata G, Gorby M, Chick T, et al. Intravenous and oral corticosteroids for the prevention of relapse after treatment of decompensated COPD. Effect on patients with a history of multiple relapses. Chest 1990;98:845–9.

[53] Emerman C, Connors A, Lukens T, et al. A randomized controlled trial of methylprednisolone in the emergency treatment of acute exacerbations of COPD. Chest 1989;95: 563–7.

[54] Thompson W, Nielson C, Carvahlo P, et al. Controlled trial of oral prednisone in outpatients with acute COPD exacerbations. Am J Respir Crit Care Med 1996;154:407–12.

[55] Saint S, Bent S, Vittinghoff E, et al. Antibiotics in chronic obstructive lung disease exacerbations: a meta-analysis. JAMA 1995;273:957–60.

[56] Banarjee D, Lee G, Malik S, et al. Underdiagnosis of asthma in the elderly. Br J Dis Chest 1987;81:23–9.

[57] Braman SS. Asthma in the elderly. Clin Geriatr Med 2003;19:57–75.

[58] Petheram I, Jones D, Collins J. Assessment and management of acute asthma in the elderly: a comparison with younger asthmatics. Postgrad Med J 1982;58:149–51.

[59] Braman S. Asthma in the elderly. Contemp Intern Med 1995;7:13–24.

[60] Bailey W, Richards J, Brooks C, et al. Features of asthma in older adults. J Asthma 1992;29: 21–8.

[61] Pickup C, Nee P, Randall P. Radiographic features in 1016 adults admitted to hospital with acute asthma. J Accid Emerg Med 1994;11:234–7.

[62] National Asthma Education and Prevention Program Expert Panel Report 2: guidelines for the diagnosis and management of asthma. Bethesda (MD): National Institutes of Health (NIH), NIH Publication; 1997. No. 97-4051:1–146.

[63] Nowak R, Tokarski G. Asthma. In: Marx JA, Hockberger RS, Walls RM, editors. Rosen's emergency medicine: concepts and clinical practice. 5th ed. St. Louis (MO): Mosby; 2002. p. 938–56.

[64] Rodrigo G, Rodrigo C, Burschtin O. A meta-analysis of the effects of ipratropium bromide in adults with acute asthma. Am J Med 1999;107:363–70.

[65] Stoodley R, Aaron S, Dales R. The role of ipratropium bromide in the emergency management of acute asthma exacerbation: a meta-analysis of randomized clinical trials. Ann Emerg Med 1999;34:8–18.

[66] Cydulka RK, Khandelwal S. Acute asthma in adults. In: Tintinalli JE, Kelen GD, Stapczynski JS, editors. Emergency medicine: a comprehensive study guide. 5th ed. New York: McGraw-Hill; 2000. p. 476–85.

[67] Dutt AK, Stead WW. Tuberculosis in the elderly. Med Clin North Am 1993;77:1353–68.

[68] Stead W, Lofgren J, Warren E, et al. Tuberculosis as an endemic and nosocomial infection among the elderly in nursing homes. N Engl J Med 1985;312:1483–7.

[69] Stead W. Pathogenesis of a first episode of chronic pulmonary tuberculosis in man: recrudescence of the residuals of primary infection or exogenous reinfection. Am Rev Respir Dis 1967;95:729–45.

[70] Fulton J, McCallioin J. Tuberculosis: diagnostic difficulty in the elderly. J Clin Exp Gerontol 1987;82:602–6.

[71] Korzeniewska M, Krysl J, Muller N, et al. Tuberculosis in young adults and the elderly. Chest 1994;106:28–32.

[72] Perez-Guzman C, Vargas M, Torres-Cruz A, et al. Does aging modify pulmonary tuberculosis?: a meta-analytical review. Chest 1999;116:961–7.

[73] Leung A. Pulmonary tuberculosis: the essentials. Radiology 1999;210:307–22.

[74] Chan D. Tuberculosis. In: Marx JA, Hockberger RS, Walls RM, editors. Rosen's emergency medicine: concepts and clinical practice. 5th ed. St. Louis (MO): Mosby; 2002. p. 1903–24.

[75] CDC: guidelines for preventing the transmission of *Mycobacterium tuberculosis* in health-care facilities. MMWR 1994;43(RR-13):1–141.

[76] Dorken E, Grzybowski S, Allen E. Significance of the tuberculin test in the elderly. Chest 1987;92:237–40.

[77] Nissar M, Williams C, Ashby D, et al. Tuberculin testing in residential homes for the elderly. Thorax 1993;48:1257–60.

[78] Crossley KB, Peterson PK. Infections in the elderly. Clin Infect Dis 1996;22:209–15.

[79] Zevallos M, Justman JE. Tuberculosis in the elderly. Clin Geriatr Med 2003;19:121–38.

[80] American Thoracic Society/Centers for Disease Control. Targeted tuberculin testing and treatment of latent tuberculosis infection. Am J Respir Crit Care Med 2000;161:S221–47.

[81] Bass J, Farer L, Hopewell P, et al. Treatment of tuberculosis and tuberculosis infection in adults and children. American Thoracic Society and The Centers for Disease Control and Prevention. Am J Respir Crit Care Med 1994;149:1359–74.

ELSEVIER
SAUNDERS

Emerg Med Clin N Am
24 (2006) 339–370

EMERGENCY
MEDICINE
CLINICS OF
NORTH AMERICA

Cardiovascular Emergencies in the Elderly

Rohit Gupta, MD[a],*, Seth Kaufman, MD[b]

[a]*Department of Emergency Medicine, Advocate Christ Medical Center, 4440 West 95th Street, Oak Lawn, IL 60453, USA*
[b]*Section of Emergency Medicine, University of Chicago, 5841 South Maryland Avenue, Chicago, IL 60637, USA*

According to the US Census bureau, the number of people in the United States over the age of 65 will double from the 35 million in 2000 to more than 70 million by 2030. As the population ages, the volume and proportion of geriatric patients presenting to acute care facilities will also increase. To prepare for the coming flood, emergency physicians must become comfortable dealing with this population. Geriatric patients are at high risk for cardiovascular emergencies with significant pathology and severe morbidity and mortality. This article discusses five common cardiovascular emergencies: acute coronary syndrome, congestive heart failure, dysrythmias, aortic dissection, and ruptured abdominal aortic aneurysm. The discussion focuses on the differences in presentation, management, and outcomes that characterize each disease among the elderly. As a rule, the elderly have significantly worse outcomes than younger patients. Although the graver prognosis is certainly due in part to the elderly being sicker with less physiologic reserve, it is also due to delays in diagnosis and under use of therapy on the part of providers.

Acute coronary syndrome

Coronary heart disease is the leading killer in America claiming 1,000,000 lives annually. The incidence of coronary heart disease increases with age. It is the largest killer among geriatric patients. With a few exceptions, the diagnosis and management of acute coronary syndrome (ACS) in the elderly is similar to that in younger patients. The goals of care focus on accurate, early diagnosis and aggressive therapy.

---

* Corresponding author.
E-mail address: rogu@alum.mit.edu (R. Gupta).

Definition

The term ACS applies to a spectrum of ischemic heart disease ranging from unstable angina (UA), through non-ST segment elevation myocardial infarction (MI) (NSTEMI), to ST segment elevation MI (STEMI). The term has evolved to encompass a range of high-risk diagnoses that mandate aggressive therapy, but that cannot always be distinguished at initial presentation.

The definition of acute myocardial infarction (AMI) is evolving. The consensus definition proposed in 2000 by the European Society of Cardiology, American College of Cardiology (ACC), and American Heart Association (AHA) requires either pathologic findings of MI at autopsy; or a typical rise and fall in troponin or creatine kinase-MB (CK-MB) with ischemic symptoms, development of pathologic Q waves, EKG changes indicative of ischemia, or coronary artery intervention [1].

In contrast, UA is marked by active ischemia without infarction. The diagnosis is made in patients with clinical symptoms of ischemia, EKG evidence of ischemia, or proven coronary artery disease, but without cardiac enzyme elevation.

Epidemiology

ACS is the leading cause of death in America. Accounting for 6 million visits annually, chest pain is the second most common chief complaint evaluated in emergency departments (EDs). ACS is the cause in 20% to 25% of cases [2]. It is particularly common in the elderly. Patients over the age of 65 account for 60% to 65% of MIs [3] and 80% of deaths. One study of 600 ED patients with chest pain has shown that ACS increased from <7% in patients <40 years to >71% in patients >80 years [4]. Among all patients with ACS, approximately 30% have STEMI, 25% have NSTEMI, and 38% have UA [5]. The elderly tend to have a higher rate of NSTEMI and less UA.

History and physical examination

A careful history is the cornerstone of evaluation. A careful history is the most informative and discriminatory evaluation tool. The classic history consists of crushing, substernal chest pain that radiates to the arm, neck, or jaw. Chest pain, considered a hallmark feature, is classically diffuse, hard to localize, and described as a crushing, throbbing, or pressure.

Unfortunately, atypical presentations are common. Data from the GRACE registry analyzing 20,881 patients with ACS show that 1763 (8.4%) presented without chest pain [6]. Of the patients with atypical presentations, 23.8% were not initially recognized as having an ACS. After reviewing medicare records of 434,877 patients with confirmed AMI, Canto et al [7] found that 33% of patients did not have chest pain. The sensitivity of chest pain was only 67%. A second study by Canto et al analyzing 4167 patients with UA reported that >50% presented with atypical symptoms, defined as the absence of any chest pain, and the absence of pain that was a squeezing, tightness, aching, crushing, dullness, or exacerbated by exercise and relieved by rest [8]. In each of these studies, risk factors for atypical presentations included being elderly, being female, or having congestive heart failure (CHF) or diabetes mellitus (DM).

When dealing with the elderly, the emergency physician (EP) should maintain a very high index of suspicion and actively seek out an ACS even in seemingly noncardiac patients. In the GRACE Registry, the dominant atypical symptoms were dyspnea (49.3%), diaphoresis (26.2%), nausea or vomiting (24.3%), and syncope (19.1%) [6]. A similar distribution was reported in Canto's study of UA [8]. In 1977, Bean reported 10 "masqueraders of MI": (1) CHF; (2) classic angina pectoris without a particularly severe or prolonged attack; (3) cardiac arrhythmia; (4) atypical location of the pain; (5) central nervous system manifestations resembling stroke; (6) apprehension and nervousness; (7) sudden mania, psychosis, confusion, or change in mental status; (8) syncope; (9) overwhelming weakness; and (10) acute indigestion [9].

Although extremely important, no element or combination of elements in the history can effectively confirm or eliminate the diagnosis. Several excellent articles report the positive and negative likelihood ratios of various features of the history and physical examination [2,10,11]. Often derived on younger patients with typical presentations, the results of these studies may not be applicable to the elderly, and should be interpreted with caution.

Traditional risk factors for coronary artery disease (CAD) include smoking, hypertension, hyperlipidemia, and DM. Age is an important independent risk factor. Although traditional risk factors adequately assess for lifetime risk, they are less useful in predicting an ACS.

The physical examination is also less useful in diagnosing ACS. Patients with hypotension, crackles, peripheral edema, and other stigmata of CHF are at high risk. Rarely, an ACS may be ruled out on physical examination by identifying other definitive causes of chest pain, such as trauma or tension pneumothorax.

Diagnostic tests

EKG

The single most important test to diagnose an ACS remains the EKG. It should be performed within 10 minutes of presentation. A low threshold should be maintained to obtain an EKG in the elderly. The sensitivity and specificity of the EKG depend on the interpretation criteria employed. With strict criteria (new ST elevation of 0.1 mV in two contiguous leads or a new left bundle branch block), the EKG lacks sensitivity (61%) but is highly specific (95%) for AMI [2]. Specific criteria are appropriate when deciding to treat invasively because they do not unnecessarily expose large numbers of patients to the risks of treatment. In contrast, with liberal criteria (any ST or T-wave abnormalities), the EKG is highly sensitive (94–99%) but not specific (23%) for AMI [2]. Other ischemic changes include Q waves,

ST segment depression, T-wave inversion, dynamic changes, and changes confined to territorial distributions.

Although a normal EKG reduces the risk of an ACS, it does not rule it out definitively. In one series, 37% of patients with an initially normal EKG had a final diagnosis of UA [2]. The EKG modifies pretest probability of ACS in conjunction with the history; it cannot be used to risk stratify the patient by itself.

Interpretation of the EKG in the elderly can be challenging. The elderly tend to have abnormal baseline EKGs. Prior MI, left ventricular hypertrophy (LVH), preexistent bundle branch blocks, nonspecific ST-T changes, and atrial fibrillation (AF) often make reading the EKG difficult. An old EKG for comparison should be obtained. Up to 25% of missed MIs may be attributable to errors in reading diagnostic EKGs [12].

Cardiac enzymes

Biochemical markers provide useful diagnostic and prognostic information in the elderly. Released after myocardial cell necrosis, enzyme elevation distinguishes AMI from UA. As more sensitive enzymes that identify microinfarction become available, patients previously diagnosed with UA will be diagnosed with MI. Of the myriad of biomarkers studied, the most sensitive and specific are CK-MB and troponin.

CK-MB is a cardiac-specific subform of creatine kinase, a protein found in both cardiac and skeletal muscle. The sensitivity of CK-MB varies with time, first appearing in the circulation within 3 hours of infarction, peaking at 12 to 24 hours, and normalizing by 3 to 4 days. The sensitivity of a single measurement is only 47%, but rises to >90% with serial testing until at least 8 hours after symptom onset. The specificity is high (>95%) [2].

Troponin I and T are contractile proteins found only in cardiac myocytes. Being exquisitely sensitive and reasonably specific for AMI, troponins are the new "gold standard" for the diagnosis of MI. Troponins, also time dependent, appear within 6 hours of infarction and remain elevated for 4 to 8 days. Sensitivity is only 50% when measured within 4 hours of symptom onset, but rises to >95% after 8 hours [13]. The specificity is high, but may be lowered by renal failure. At least one study suggests that the specificity is lower in the elderly versus younger patients (94% versus 83%) [14]. Troponins are also useful in identifying elderly patients with atypical presentations of ACS with nondiagnostic EKGs. In addition to diagnostic utility, troponins also have prognostic value. An elevated troponin increases the odds of short-term mortality three- to eightfold [15].

Risk stratification

The immediate goal of any evaluation is to rapidly decide whether a patient is having an ACS. The decision is not an easy one. Missed or mistreated ACS is the leading cause of malpractice payout against EPs.

Consequently, most EPs make the decision conservatively. Only 30% of patients admitted to hospitals for evaluation of chest pain wind up having acute cardiac ischemia. The cost of negative workups is estimated to be $5 billion. After the initial evaluation, patients should be placed into one of four categories: definite ACS, probable ACS, probably not ACS (but still requiring workup to rule out ACS), or definitely not ACS.

With a working diagnosis of probable or definite ACS, the EP must further risk stratify to optimally treat. Patients with STEMI are in the highest risk group. The UA/NSTEMI patients can be further risk stratified using clinical criteria. High-risk features include: recurrent or persistent ischemic pain, elevated troponin, dynamic EKG changes, concomitant CHF, high-risk findings on stress testing, hemodynamic instability, and a history of primary coronary intervention (PCI) or coronary artery bypass graft (CABG). Numerical scores that objectively guide risk stratification have been developed and validated [16,17]. Accurate risk stratification is important, as it guides the speed, type, and invasiveness of therapy.

Therapy

Detailed guidelines have been published by the ACC and AHA for UA/NSTEMI in 2002 [18] and STEMI in 2004 [19]. The guidelines are up to date, evidence based, and widely available. Consequently, specific treatment recommendations will only be discussed briefly. Rather, the discussion will focus on differences in therapy between elderly and younger patients. Table 1 summarizes the classification of recommendations in the guidelines.

Overview of therapy

All patients with suspected ACS should be managed aggressively. Geriatric patients should be treated as aggressively as younger patients employing anti-ischemic, antiplatelet, anticoagulation, and reperfusion therapy. As in younger patients, reperfusion is the priority. PCI is the preferred therapy when available rapidly. Door-to-balloon times should be less than 90 minutes. When PCI is not available, reperfusion should be instituted with fibrinolysis. Door-to-drug times should be less than 30 minutes. Antiplatelet,

Table 1
Classification of recommendations by AHA/ACC

Class I	There is evidence or general agreement that the treatment is useful and effective
Class II	There is a conflicting evidence of divergence of opinion
IIa	The weight of evidence favors utility-efficacy
IIb	Utility-efficacy is less well established
Class III	There is evidence or general agreement that the treatment is neither useful nor effective and may be harmful

Abbreviations: AHA, American Heart Associations; ACC, American College of Cardiology.

anti-ischemic, and anticoagulation therapy should be initiated along with re-perfusion. Patients should be admitted to the coronary care unit (CCU) when clinically appropriate.

High-risk elderly patients with UA/NSTEMI should also be treated aggressively. The main caveat is that reperfusion with fibrinolytics is not indicated for patients in this category. Maximal anti-ischemic and anticoagulation should be started. Antiplatelet therapy with ASA or Plavix is indicated. Further antiplatelet therapy with Glycoprotein (GP) IIb/IIIa inhibitors may be started in conjunction with cardiology. Patients should be admitted to the CCU when clinically appropriate. Early invasive management is recommended.

Treatment algorithms for low- to moderate-risk UA/NSTEMI patients have not been formalized. A wide variety of approaches are employed including basic anti-ischemic and antiplatelet therapy, and various risk stratification schemes including inpatient telemetry admission, chest pain observation units, and expedited ED evaluations with ED initiated stress testing. Institution specific protocols for treatment should be formalized.

Specific therapeutic agents

Anti-ischemic therapy

Anti-ischemic therapy aims to increase oxygen supply and decrease cardiac workload. Oxygen therapy is recommended in patients with O_2 saturation <90% (Class I). Nitrates reduce ischemia by dilating coronary arteries, increasing blood flow, and decreasing preload and afterload. Although no studies have demonstrated direct survival benefit in the elderly, nitrates reduce anginal symptoms; their use is considered standard of care. Morphine sulfate may reduce cardiac workload by decreasing heart rate and systolic blood pressure. Its use, also not supported by evidence, is recommended because it reduces pain, a primary goal in the management of ACS.

Based on compelling evidence, beta-blockers are the best anti-ischemic therapy. Beta-blockers prevent recurrent ischemia and life-threatening ventricular arrythmias. Their use is strongly recommended (Class I for UA/NSTEMI/STEMI) in all patients without a contraindication [18,19]. Beta-blockers decrease mortality to a similar or greater extent than aspirin. Data from the first international study of infarct survival (ISIS-1) showed a 15% absolute reduction in short-term mortality attributable to atenolol use. The reduction was even greater (23%) among the elderly [20]. Beta-blockers also reduce the incidence of heart failure in the elderly after MI.

Antiplatelet therapy

The data supporting the use of ASA is irrefutable. Composite data from 287 studies demonstrate a 22% relative risk reduction from 13.2% to 10.7% with the use of ASA [21]. The benefits of aspirin extend across all age groups. Its use is strongly recommended (Class I for UA/NSTEMI/STEMI) [18,19].

The superiority of primary PCI over fibrinolysis for reperfusion is clear in younger patients. One small randomized trial demonstrated that the benefit of PCI extends to patients over 75 years, reducing death, reinfarction, or stroke versus fibrinolysis (9% versus 29%, respectively) [28]. Because its efficacy is less dependent on time, PCI is preferred when there is a delay in presentation. PCI is also preferred in high-risk presentations (ie, cardiogenic shock), with a high risk of bleeding, and when thrombolysis fails [19].

Evidence of under treatment in the elderly

Despite clear guidelines that advocate for treatment in the elderly, evidence suggests that elderly patients are frequently undertreated. After reviewing records of 2409 patients with AMI, McLaughlin et al [29] reported that the elderly were less frequently treated with ASA and beta-blockers (6% and 15–35%, respectively) compared with younger patients <65 years. The evidence for underuse of reperfusion is even stronger. In one study, only 25% of ideal, eligible, elderly candidates received primary PCI or fibrinolysis [30]. Another study reported that among ideal eligible patients, 80% of patients <65 years of age received reperfusion, compared with 76% of those 65 years to 75 years, and only 49% of those above age 75 years. A Canadian study by Boucher et al [27] demonstrated similar results. The odds of being treated compared with the youngest group (<65 years) was 0.7 for patients 65 years to 75 years, 0.4 for those aged 75 years to 84 years, and 0.1 for those >85 years.

Prognosis

The prognosis for elderly patients with ACS is significantly worse than for younger patients. Mortality is higher for the elderly (19% versus 5%) [31]. In a recent review of Canadian patients with AMI, mortality rates increased dramatically from 2.1% in patients <55 years to 26.3% in patients >85 years [27]. Age was the most important predictor of in-hospital mortality.

Congestive heart failure

Causing 900,000 admissions annually, decompensated CHF is the most common reason for admission in the elderly population [32]. Improved survival after MI and a growing elderly population has resulted in an increase in the prevalence of CHF. Despite major advances in diagnosis and treatment, the survival rate has not improved in recent decades [33]. The pathophysiology, variable clinical presentation, rapid ED diagnosis, and aggressive ED management of decompensated CHF in the elderly are discussed.

Pathophysiology

The cardiocirculatory changes that lead to CHF are a product of mechanical and neurohormonal dysfunction [34,35]. Decreased elasticity of the aorta and great vessels in the elderly causes increased afterload, left ventricular hypertrophy, and increased coronary oxygen consumption. When oxygen requirements exceed supply, subendocardial ischemia, myocardial interstitial fibrosis, and eventually, systolic and diastolic failure develop. Decreased cardiac output causes renal hypoperfusion, activates the renin–angiotensin pathway, and increases circulating catecholamines. Subsequent potent vasoconstriction and increased renal sodium absorption maintain perfusion in the short term, but exacerbate heart failure over time. Worsening intravascular fluid retention, vasoconstriction, sympathetic resistance, and ventricular hypertrophy lead to the syndrome of CHF.

Triggers of decompensation

Major causes of decompensation in the elderly are listed in Table 3. Often due to lack of education, medication and dietary noncompliance are the most common causes [36–38]. In an interview-based study by Cline et al [38], only 55% of elderly patients could correctly name their medications. In a similar study, only 26% of older patients were aware of the need for fluid restriction [36]. Arrhythmias such as AF, sick sinus syndrome, and ventricular dysrhythmias increase with age and can trigger decompensation [37]. Anemia causes a physiologic increase in cardiac output with a decrease in coronary oxygen supply, resulting in decreased cardiac contractility [39]. Infectious diseases, such as influenza and pneumonia, are physiologic stressors, and can cause a patient to decompensate and develop CHF. Last, medications such as nonaspirin nonsteroidal anti-inflammatory drugs and Beta-blockers can exacerbate CHF, especially when taken incorrectly.

Clinical presentation

The most common signs and symptoms of decompensated CHF are worsening dyspnea on exertion, orthopnea, and lower extremity edema. Unfortunately, the clinical presentation in the elderly is often atypical [40]. Older patients may present with nonspecific symptoms such as confusion and decreased exercise tolerance. If dyspnea is present in the older patient, it is

Table 3
Causes of acutely decompensated congestive heart failure (CHF)

Nonadherence
Medication
Diet
Cardiac ischemia
Arrhythmia
Renal failure
Pulmonary embolism
Uncontrolled hypertension
Adverse effects of medications
Infection

a marker of more advanced disease. The initial assessment of airway, breathing, and circulation may underestimate the severity of illness. Being less sensitive to hypoxia and hypercapnea, geriatric patients may not be tachypneic. Resting tachycardia is uncommon because of sympathetic resistance [41].

Searching for the trigger is as important as evaluating the severity of the exacerbation. The patient and family should be asked about recent weight gain, medication adherence, recent medication adjustments, and any change in urinary output. Chest pain or angina equivalents such as nausea and epigastric discomfort may represent underlying myocardial ischemia. The presence of syncope and palpitations may provide the clue to an underlying tachyarrhythmia.

A complete physical examination in the ED is warranted. Auscultating crackles, cardiac wheezes, and decreased breath sounds may represent pulmonary edema or pleural effusion. Jugular venous distension is one of the most sensitive clinical markers [42]. An S3 gallop or a displaced apical impulse indicate left ventricular hypertrophy and are common in CHF. A new murmur may represent valvular pathology or papillary muscle ischemia. With extremely low interrater reliability, these findings are difficult to detect; in the elderly, they can be extremely subtle.

Laboratory and radiographic evaluation

In the elderly population, the EP must often rely on laboratory and imaging studies to diagnose and assess the severity of a CHF exacerbation. A thorough evaluation includes a complete blood count, electrolyte panel, cardiac markers, EKG, echocardiography, chest radiography, and increasingly, specialized testing such as serum B-type natriuretic peptide (BNP).

Basic laboratory tests

Anemia is an independent prognostic factor in older patients with CHF. Anemic patients are at significantly higher risk of mortality despite adjusting for comorbidities [43]. Hypokalemia and other electrolyte abnormalities, often from diuretic therapy, are common and potentially fatal [44].

EKG and cardiac markers

CHF complicating UA or MI greatly increases morbidity and mortality. An EKG and cardiac enzymes must be obtained in almost every patient to assess for and exclude ischemia. Additionally, troponin has prognostic value independent of its utility in diagnosing MI. In elderly patients with decompensated CHF, an elevated troponin correlates with the severity, mortality, and length of hospitalization [45].

Echocardiography

By enabling rapid measurement of the ejection fraction (EF), echocardiography is a valuable tool in the initial assessment of CHF. The AHA/ACC guidelines strongly advocate using echocardiography in critically ill patients because it can help diagnose other reversible etiologies such as pericardial tamponade and pulmonary embolism [46].

Chest Radiography

Chest x-ray (CXR) may confirm the diagnosis of CHF, and may demonstrate or suggest other important clinical entities such as pneumonia, pneumothorax, and aortic dissection. The CXR may be normal early in the course of congestive heart failure, and CHF should not be ruled out based on CXR alone.

B-type natriuretic peptide

BNP is an endogenous hormone released during ventricular stretching. Two studies, Breathing Not Properly and REDHOT, established its utility in the acute setting [47,48]. Breathing Not Properly demonstrated that the BNP was more sensitive then clinical judgment alone (90% versus 49%) for diagnosing CHF. REDHOT illustrated the value of the BNP as an important predictor of mortality at 90 days. The role of the BNP in elderly patients is less clear. The BNP is significantly lower (413 pg/mL versus 821 pg/mL) in patients with diastolic versus systolic dysfunction resulting in decreased sensitivity and accuracy [49]. In addition, the BNP is lower in elderly patients independent of their EF [50]. Despite these differences, earlier diagnosis and treatment, facilitated by BNP use, may reduce the length of hospitalization and the need for intensive care unit (ICU) admission [48].

Management

The keys to managing decompensated CHF are to establish a definitive airway, aggressively support respiration, and rapidly administer pharmacologic agents to improve cardiac output. With greater comorbidities and less reserve, the elderly often require aggressive management. Pharmacologic therapy focuses on correcting volume overload with diuretics, improving hemodynamics by reducing preload and afterload, and augmenting cardiac contractility with inotropic agents.

Airway management

Airway and breathing must be aggressively managed. Decompensated CHF often results in acute respiratory distress and hypoxia that is refractory to supplemental oxygen, noninvasive ventilatory support, and diuresis. Indications for establishing a definitive airway with endotracheal intubation include apnea, impending apnea, severe fatigue, or inability to handle secretions. Carrying a significant risk of nosocomial infection and ventilator associated injury, endotracheal intubation, especially in the elderly, is not benign [51].

Many patients with cardiogenic pulmonary edema can be managed with noninvasive ventilatory support. Continuous positive airway pressure

(CPAP) decreases the rate of endotracheal intubation [52] and may also improve survival. The data supporting bilevel positive airway pressure (BiPAP) use is not as clear. Sharon et al [53] compared nitrate therapy versus BiPAP in 40 patients with acute respiratory failure from pulmonary edema and found a statistically significant increase in the rate of MI in patients who received BiPAP. Until larger studies establish the safety of BiPAP, CPAP should be used preferentially.

Nitrates

Nitrates are considered first-line therapy for decompensated CHF. Nitrates improve hemodynamics by causing arterial and venous dilation that reduce afterload and preload, and to a lesser extent, by directly dilating coronary arteries. Risks of therapy include life-threatening hypotension, especially in the setting of cardiac tamponade, right heart failure, right heart MI, or in patients who have taken erectile dysfunction agents such as sildenafil (Viagra). Given as a sublingual tablet or spray, transdermal paste, or intravenously, nitrates should be used aggressively and titrated rapidly to achieve therapeutic goals. Intravenous sodium nitroprusside should be reserved for patients with persistent hypertension refractory to other treatments.

Diuretics

Although diuretics are considered a mainstay of treatment, they are not always the most optimal therapy. Diuresis reduces intravascular volume, causes vasodilation, and may result in worsening hemoperfusion. Loop diuretics should be used with caution. In general, they are effective in the elderly and decrease the length of hospitalization [54]. Nesiritide, BNP, is one of the newest diuretics. The VMAC trial demonstrated that nesiritide improves hemodynamics and dyspnea when added to conventional therapy [55]. Studies evaluating its use in the ED (PROACTION) are in progress.

Angiotensin converting enzyme inhibitors

Angiotensin converting enzyme inhibitors (ACEI) reduce afterload and preload and are useful in chronic CHF patients. They may have a role in the treatment of acute pulmonary edema as well. Intravenous (IV) enalaprilat has been shown to cause rapid improvement in cardiac output and stroke volume in patients with severe CHF. Sublingual captopril has been shown to lead to a decrease in the need for intubation and ICU admission in pulmonary edema patients. ACEI may be an acceptable alternative to IV nitroglycerin in pulmonary edema patients with contraindications to nitrates, such as sildenafil (Viagra) use or severe aortic stenosis [56,57].

Inotropes

B-agonists such as dobutamine and phosphodiesterase inhibitors such as amrinone and milrinone are used in patients with severe decompensation. In combination with afterload reducing agents, inotropes improve cardiac output and symptoms [58,59]. Dobutamine carries a greater risk of ventricular ectopy and tachycardia compared with the phosphodiesterase inhibitors [58].

Prognosis and disposition

According to Framingham data, mortality in patients with CHF increases 27% per decade of advancing age in men and 61% in women [33]. A study of 112 patients discharged from the ED with CHF showed that within 3 months of the initial visit, more than 60% of patients experienced a recurrent visit, hospitalization, or death [60]. The Agency for Health Care Policy and Research defined criteria for admission based on the presence of myocardial ischemia, severe respiratory distress, hypoxia (O_2 saturation <90%), anasarca, hypotension (systolioc blood pressure <80), syncope, inadequate social support, severe comorbid illnesses, or failed outpatient therapy. Older patients present in more advanced stages; acute care physicians underestimate the severity of their illness [61]. With such high morbidity and mortality, the prudent EP should maintain a low threshold for admission in older patients with any degree of decompensated CHF.

Dysrhythmias

Conduction abnormalities cause significant mortality. Many of the 300,000 deaths each year from AMI are a result of ventricular tachyarrythmias (VT) [62]. The incidence of dysrythmias is increasing as the population is aging. AF is the most common sustained tachyarrhythmia in elderly patients. It causes approximately 20% of all stroke-related deaths [62]. Prehospital cardiac arrest and three common dysrhythmias: ventricular arrhythmias, atrioventricular (AV) blockade, and AF in the elderly are reviewed.

Out-of-hospital cardiac arrest

Aggressive efforts to perform early defibrillation as part of the AHA's "Chain of Survival" have improved morbidity and mortality in patients with ventricular fibrillation (VF) [63]. Several studies have evaluated these guidelines exclusively in the elderly. Older patients have similar survival rates to hospital discharge (14–24%) and similar neurologic outcomes as younger patients [64,65]. Bunch et al [66] showed that although older patients who survive to hospital discharge from VF have a favorable 5-year survival rate (66%), their survival rate is lower than the age-matched controls. Overall, out-of-hospital cardiac arrest has a poor but not dismal outcome [67,68]. Elderly patients should receive the same level of aggressive resuscitation with rapid response and early defibrillation as younger victims.

Ventricular tachycardia and ventricular fibrillation

Advancing age is an independent risk factor for life-threatening ventricular arrhythmias [69]. Sustained VT is defined as a wide QRS complex (>0.12 seconds) of five or more ventricular beats in succession and a heart rate over 100 beats per minute. Premature ventricular contractions and asymptomatic nonsustained VT are common in older patients, and may be a sign of subclinical coronary heart disease [70,71]. VT is most commonly caused by cardiac ischemia resulting in fibrotic changes and a reentrant circuit [72,73]. Other etiologies include medication-induced VT (digoxin, tricyclic antidepressants, antiarrhythmics), electrolyte disorders, and cardiomyopathies [74].

During the initial assessment, the presence of hemodynamic instability requires immediate cardioversion, or in the case of pulseless ventricular arrhythmias, emergent defibrillation as set out by the Advanced Cardiac Life Support guidelines [75]. With such a high prevalence of bundle branch blocks in elderly patients, identifying the pathologic rhythm may be difficult. Brugada and others [76,77] have created formulas based on the presence of AV dissociation, capture beats, fusion beats, and other EKG changes to decipher supraventricular tachycardia (SVT) with aberrancy from monomorphic VT. Many studies have shown that emergency physicians cannot reliably interpret the EKG using these formulas [78,79]. In the absence of old EKGs, all wide-complex ventricular arrhythmias should be presumed to be VT. In these situations, AV nodal blocking agents such as verapamil and adenosine are absolutely contraindicated.

In a stable patient with sustained, monomorphic VT, pharmacologic therapy may augment cardioversion [80,81]. Amiodarone is the initial choice for patients with an impaired ejection fraction. In all others consider procainamide [75]. Reversible causes such as medication toxicity and electrolyte abnormalities should be sought and corrected.

In elderly patients with VT or VF, definitive therapy often mandates placement of an automated implantable cardioverter-defibrillator (AICD). With a 2-year mortality rate of 30% after MI, AICDs are common in elderly patients. The MADIT and AVID trials demonstrated that AICDs are superior to pharmacologic therapy alone [82,83].

Atrioventricular blockade

AV blockade refers to impaired conduction between the atrium and ventricles. First-degree AV block is defined as prolonged AV conduction (PR interval >0.2 seconds) without loss of ventricular depolarization. Second-degree AV block refers to impaired conduction with a patterned loss of ventricular impulse. Third-degree block refers to the absence of all atrial conduction. Second-degree AV block is subdivided into Mobitz Type I (Wenckebach), marked by progressive lengthening of the PR interval until an impulse is blocked from causing ventricular depolarization, and

Mobitz Type II, in which a pattern of dropped impulses is present with a fixed PR interval.

As with VT, fibrosis of the conduction system from age-related changes and chronic ischemia are the most common etiologies. Other causes include calcification of the aortic and mitral valves and medication effects. Although the use of AV-nodal blocking agents is commonly seen as the etiology of AV blocks in elderly patients, the recurrence rate after the drug is discontinued is high and other etiologies are often found [84]. Elderly patients with first-degree or second-degree Mobitz type I are often asymptomatic. Those with higher degree blocks may present with presyncope or syncope, decreased exercise tolerance, increased falls, new-onset congestive heart failure, or signs of an ACS [85].

Emergent management in these patients depends solely on the presence of adequate perfusion. Bradycardia with hypotension requires emergent treatment first with pharmacologic agents followed by transcutaneous or transvenous pacing. Atropine, being safe and effective, is considered first-line therapy [86]. In the presence of AV-nodal blocking agents, glucagon may be effective. Patients with Mobitz Type II second-degree or third-degree heart block require cardiology consultation to consider a permanent pacemaker. In the elderly, pacemaker placement carries a significant risk of complications [87].

Atrial fibrillation

AF is the most common serious sustained cardiac arrhythmia in the elderly with a prevalence of 5% in patients over 65 years old [88]. The incidence doubles with each decade of life. and is independently associated with mortality [89]. AF is caused by ectopic atrial foci, resulting in disorganized depolarization and loss of atrial contraction. The resulting rapid ventricular rate causes a decrease in diastolic filling and hypotension. Elderly patients may present with symptoms of hemodynamic collapse such as lightheadedness, syncope, or falls, or may present with symptoms of the underlying trigger such as cardiac ischemia, pulmonary embolism, infection, or electrolyte abnormalities.

In the ED, the management is based on the degree of hemodynamic compromise and the etiology. In hypotensive patients, immediate cardioversion is required. Cardioversion is safe in elderly patients, and carries a similar success, complication, and failure rate as younger patients [90]. In all other patients, anticoagulation and rate control are the mainstays of treatment. Rate control agents are selected based on the patient's ejection fraction. In normal patients without heart failure, B-blockers such as metoprolol and calcium channel blockers such as diltiazem are preferred to accomplish rate control. In patients with impaired cardiac function, amiodarone is the preferred rate control agent. Causing less hypotension, it is safe in elderly patients [91]. Alternative agents in patients with impaired EF include digoxin and diltiazem, but beta-blockers and verapamil should be avoided.

The value of anticoagulation to prevent embolic stroke in the elderly population is controversial. Many physicians fear anticoagulation with coumadin because of concerns about frequent falls, medication compliance and gastrointestinal bleeding [92,93]. Several studies have validated significant bleeding complications in elderly patients especially from supratherapeutic anticoagulation (INR > 3.5) [94,95]. However, the benefit in appropriate patients far outweighs the risk. According to Framingham data, the attributable risk of stroke in patients 80 to 90 years of age with AF is 23% [96]. Anticoagulation decreases this risk by approximately 60% [97]. Many studies show that bleeding risk is independent of age; therefore, age should not be a factor in the clinical decision making [93,98].

In stable patients with new-onset AF of less than 48 hours, electrical cardioversion is safe. Although the AFFIRM trial showed that conversion to sinus rhythm is not associated with improved survival [99], the recently published RACE study suggested that conversion to sinus rhythm may be associated with an improved quality of life [100]. In patients with longstanding AF, the decision to rate control and anticoagulate or to cardiovert is an individual decision based on the risk of major bleeding complications. It should be made in conjunction with the patient, primary care physician, and cardiologist.

Aortic dissection

Aortic dissections are an infrequent but extremely high-risk cardiovascular emergency. Rapid diagnosis and aggressive therapy greatly improve prognosis. Unfortunately, antemortem diagnosis is difficult, and dissections are frequently missed. The emergency physician must maintain a high index of suspicion and skillfully use the history, physical examination, and CXR to reliably diagnose this elusive entity without initiating too many unnecessary and expensive workups.

Definition and pathophysiology

The normal aortic wall consists of three layers: the intima, the media, and the adventitia. An aortic dissection refers to the separation of the layers of the aortic wall, with entry of blood into the aortic media, and the creation of a false lumen. The dissection usually originates from a tear in the aortic intima. It can then propagate proximally or distally, leading to many of the clinical features of dissection. Factors that increase medial degeneration such as increasing age predispose one to develop the disease. Intramural hematoma without intimal tear is a distinct pathologic lesion that is being observed more frequently and may progress to dissection.

Classification

Aortic dissections are classified by the portion of the aorta involved. In the Stanford system, a type A dissection involves the ascending aorta, either alone or with the descending aorta, and a type B dissection is confined to the descending aorta [101]. Classification by site is important, carrying both therapeutic and prognostic significance. Dissections are also classified temporally as acute, if present less than 2 weeks, and as chronic, if present longer than 2 weeks. The majority are acute.

Epidemiology

Due to misdiagnosis, lack of detection, and immediate death without autopsy diagnosis, the exact incidence of aortic dissection is unknown. The estimated incidence is 5 to 30 cases per million; undoubtedly, it is rare. In one study, only 0.003% of patients presenting to an ED with acute back, chest, or abdominal pain were found to have aortic dissection [102]. Ascending dissections are twice as common as isolated descending dissections and have higher morbidity and mortality [103].

Important risk factors for aortic dissection include increasing age, aortic abnormalities, male gender, family history, and hypertension. The peak age of occurrence is between 60 and 80 years [104]. Aortic abnormalities such as connective tissue diseases, congenital heart disease, and bicuspid aortic valve significantly increase the risk. Up to 44% of patients with Marfan's syndrome develop an aortic dissection, accounting for the majority of cases under the age of 40 years. Marfan's, however, is distinctly uncommon among the elderly [105]. The ratio of men to women ranges from 2:1 to 5:1 in various series, but appears to equalize in the elderly [105]. Chronic systemic hypertension is present in most patients. Other recognized risk factors include cocaine use, cardiac surgery, and aortic catheterization.

History and physical examination

Aortic dissection classically presents with pain that is severe, of sudden onset, sharp, ripping, or tearing in quality, and that radiates to the back. Data from 464 patients in the International Registry of Acute Aortic Dissection (IRAD) confirm that severe pain, present in 95% of cases, is the most common presenting symptom [103]. Chest pain (73%) exceeds back pain (53%) and abdominal pain (30%). The onset is abrupt in 85% of patients [103]. Unfortunately, the classic presentation is less common in the elderly (76.5% versus 88.5%) [105]. Migratory pain, often considered a hallmark, and painless presentations are rare. The location of pain can localize the site of dissection: anterior pain suggests proximal dissection, pain in the jaw or throat suggests aortic arch dissection, back pain suggests descending dissection, and abdominal pain suggests dissection below the diaphragm. Symptoms associated with the onset of the acute, excruciating pain include anxiety, syncope, diaphoresis, and vomiting.

Many patients with aortic dissection have secondary organ involvement, most commonly cardiac (30%) or neurologic (18–30%) [106]. Syncope, the primary presentation in 12% to 13%, is more commonly associated with

Type A dissections. Depending on the extent of dissection, the vessels involved, and the degree of flow obstruction, patients with an aortic dissection can present with an acute stroke (5–10%), acute paraplegia (10%), acute cardiac ischemia, a cold, pulseless extremity, or cardiac tamponade [106]. Aortic dissection should be considered in any patient with chest pain and neurologic symptoms.

On the physical examination, the vital signs, peripheral pulse exam, and neurologic examination are useful. Most patients with aortic dissection are initially hypertensive, but up to 25% may be hypotensive [103]. Hypotension is more common in the elderly [105], but extremely uncommon in Type B dissections [107]. Measurement of the blood pressure in both arms and the thigh demonstrates a systolic pressure differential >20 mmHg in 20% to 40% of patients. Although a discrepant pulse or pressure is insensitive, it is specific with a likelihood ratio + of 5.7 (CI 1.4–23.0) [108]. Similarly, focal neurologic deficits are insensitive, but highly specific with a LR + of 6.6 (CI 1.6–28.0) in one study and 33 (CI 2.0–549.0) in another [108]. Bilateral weakness or paraplegia suggestive of a spinal cord lesion is present in 10% to 15% of patients with distal dissections. Auscultation of the heart for a diastolic murmur is not helpful [108].

Initial diagnostic tests

EKG

Although normal in only 30% of aortic dissections, no EKG findings are pathognomonic. The EKG is important to assess for cardiac ischemia. New Q waves or ST segment elevations, present in 7% of patients [108], are more common in the elderly [105].

CXR

The CXR is abnormal in 85% to 90% of patients. Mediastinal widening (>8 cm) is the most common finding, occurring in 63% of Type A dissections and 56% of Type B dissections [103]. Other common CXR findings include: (1) separation of calcium (>5 mm) from the edge of the aortic wall, (2) a blurred aortic knob, (3) a left pleuroapical cap, (4) a left pleural effusion, (5) deviation of the paraspinous line, (6) shift and elevation of the right mainstem bronchus, (7) deviation of the trachea or esophagus to the right.

Risk assessment

Aortic dissection is a diagnostic challenge. Physicians frequently do not suspect the diagnosis and diagnostic delay is common. Autopsies reveal that dissections are missed in more than 10% of patients [109]. Deciding when to pursue the diagnosis is challenging. Like other entities in which intervention can greatly improve outcome, the threshold to obtain definitive diagnostic testing must be kept low. Frequent negative workups may be tolerable. On the other hand, time consuming and expensive workups cannot be initiated in every patient. In particular, definitive treatment of much more common diagnoses (ie, cardiac ischemia) cannot be delayed chasing this relatively rare diagnosis.

According to a study by Von Kodolitsch, three indicators from the history, physical examination, and CXR can be combined to calculate the risk of aortic dissection [102]. Von Kodolitsch developed his risk stratification tool after examining 26 clinical and radiographic features in over 250 patients. The indicators are: (1) chest pain that is immediate in onset, of a ripping or tearing character; or both; (2) pulse differentials, blood pressure (BP) differentials, or both; and (3) a widened mediastinum, aortic silhouette, or both on CXR. The probability of aortic dissection is high ($>80\%$) when there is a pulse or BP differential or all three features are present. The probability is intermediate (30–40%) when there is aortic pain or widening on the CXR. The probability is low ($<7\%$) when none of the three features are present. The tool confirms the highly specific nature of pulse and BP differentials for the diagnosis.

Initial management

As soon as the diagnosis of aortic dissection is suspected, the patient should be monitored, receive two large-bore IVs, and start receiving fluid resuscitation with normal saline. Blood should be sent to the blood bank and for type and crossmatch. The airway should be managed aggressively with early intubation in hemodynamically unstable patients.

The initial management of all patients with suspected aortic dissection is medical with aggressive heart rate and BP control. In hypertensive patients, therapy begins with a beta-blocker, such as esmolol or metoprolol, with the goal of lowering the heart rate to a target of 60 bpm. Subsequently, a potent, IV vasodilator, such as nitroprusside, is added and titrated to a goal SBP of 100 to 120 mmHg. Monotherapy with IV labetolol is being increasingly used. Pain should be controlled with IV narcotics. Hypotensive patients must be aggressively resuscitated with normal saline. Inotropic agents should be avoided, as they increase shear stress. Other, more common causes of hypotension should be excluded. Even in the presence of cardiac ischemia, when aortic dissection is a serious consideration, anticoagulation and fibrinolytic therapy must be withheld, as the iatrogenic consequences of such therapy can be devastating. Cardiac ischemia should be treated with nitrates and beta-blockers until a definitive diagnosis is made.

The strategy employed to confirm diagnosis and classify the type of dissection depends on the resources that are available, the patient's clinical condition, the pretest suspicion, and the EKG findings. Definitive diagnosis of aortic dissection is complicated. Most patients require multiple imaging tests [103]. Unstable patients with a high pretest probability must not leave the ED except to go to the operating room. In such patients, cardiology and vascular surgery must be consulted immediately so that a transesophageal echocardiogram (TEE) can be performed at the bedside. Patients with new ST elevation consistent with AMI must be differentiated immediately. AMI is far more common than aortic dissection; delays in revascularization must be minimized. In such cases, the patient should receive an immediate TEE in the ED or be transferred to a catheterization lab, where the diagnosis can be made by aortography. Lower risk patients with intermediate to low risk of aortic dissection and stable vital signs can be definitively diagnosed using TEE, CT, or MRI scans of the chest and abdomen. These patients must be closely supervised by appropriate personnel throughout the diagnostic workup.

Specific diagnostic tests

CT

In IRAD, the CT scan was the initial diagnostic test in 61% of patients [103]. It is fast, universally available, noninvasive, not operator dependent, and highly accurate. The CT scan has a sensitivity of 94% and a specificity of 87% to 100% [110]. Additionally, it provides information about other potential diagnoses. Unfortunately, the CT scan usually cannot provide all of the information needed to make an operative decision, and a second study is frequently required. Other disadvantages include the contrast dye load, and the need to leave the ED.

TEE

In IRAD, echocardiography was the initial diagnostic procedure in 33% of patients [103]. The TEE is the ideal diagnostic test for an aortic dissection. It is quick, portable, does not require exposure to contrast, and can be performed in the ED. In experienced hands it is highly accurate. with a sensitivity that is as high as 98%, and a specificity that is between 63% to 96% [110]. It can provide all of the information needed to make an operative decision including: the entry site of the dissection, the presence of thrombus in a false lumen, the involvement of coronary and arch vessels, the presence and hemodynamic significance of a pericardial effusion, and the presence and severity of aortic regurgitation. The main disadvantage is its lack of universal availability.

Aortography

Historically, aortography was the gold standard but has been supplanted by CT scanning and TEE [103]. Aortography has a sensitivity of 87% and a specificity of 75% to 94% [111]. Disadvantages are that it is invasive, time consuming, and exposes patients to contrast dye. When performed in the angiography suite, it may be useful in moderate-or low-risk patients with STEMI in whom aortic dissection must be ruled out before definitive therapy.

MRI is an extremely accurate diagnostic modality for the diagnosis—its use will likely increase in the future. Transthoracic echocardiography is generally considered inadequate to assess the aorta.

Definitive management and disposition

Further management is determined by the type of dissection and complications. Proximal dissections are a surgical emergency. Data from the IRAD show that 72% of patients with Type A dissections are treated operatively [103]. Poor prognostic factors for surgical success include hypotension, renal failure, age >70 years, abrupt onset of pain, pulse deficit, and abnormal EKG, particularly ST elevation [112]. These factors have been combined into a predictive instrument [112]. Operative mortality at experienced centers varies from 7% to 36% [103]. Age alone should not exclude patients from surgery. Nonetheless, operative management is less common in the elderly. One study revealed that the elderly are managed operatively much less frequently (64% versus 86%) than younger patients [105]. Although their operative mortality rate is higher than younger patients (38% versus 23%), it is lower than in patients managed medically (38% versus 54%) [105].

Type B dissections are usually managed nonoperatively. In the IRAD, of 384 patients with Type B dissections, 73% of patients were treated medically [107]. Poor prognostic factors include hypotension, absence of chest/back pain, and branch vessel involvement [107]. Indications for surgery include: propagation (increasing aortic diameter), increasing size of hematoma, compromise of major branches of the aorta, impending rupture, or bleeding into the pleural cavity. Given the high morbidity and mortality and need for close monitoring, all patients must be managed in the ICU.

Prognosis

The diagnosis of aortic dissection carries a grave prognosis, particularly in the elderly. Many patients die before reaching the hospital. With the high rate of missed diagnosis, treatment is frequently delayed. Untreated dissections, especially proximal dissections, are highly lethal causing death in 40% to 50% patients within 48 hours and 90% within 1 year [108]. With aggressive diagnosis and modern treatment, survival improves dramatically. In the IRAD, the overall in-hospital mortality rate was 27.4% [103]. The in-hospital mortality was 33% for Type A, and 10% for Type B dissections [105,107]. The in-hospital prognosis for patients with Type A dissections is considerably worse for the elderly (mortality: 43% versus 28%) [105]. Ten-year survival for Type A dissections treated with surgery is 55%, and for Type B dissections is 56% [108]. Just as in younger patients, the elderly derive long-term benefit from aggressive management of aortic dissection [113].

Ruptured abdominal aortic aneurysm

Abdominal aortic aneurysms (AAA) are relatively frequent, especially in the elderly. The greatest risk of an AAA is rupture. A ruptured AAA is a true cardiovascular emergency with extremely high morbidity and mortality.

Emergency physicians should suspect the diagnosis of AAA in any patient with hypotension or syncope in combination with abdominal or back pain. Patients with high-risk presentations require emergent vascular surgery consultation.

Definition

An aortic aneurysm is a true aneurysm of the aorta in which all three layers of the aortic wall become dilated. An AAA is defined as an aortic diameter 1.5 times the diameter at the level of the renal arteries. A diameter greater than 3 cm is considered aneurismal in most patients.

Epidemiology and risk factors

The incidence of AAA is 36 cases per one hundred thousand person years and is increasing [114]. The incidence increases exponentially with age. Present in only 1% of men between the ages of 55 and 64, clinically significant aneurysms (>4 cm), increase in frequency by 3% to 4% per decade thereafter [115]. Besides age, other risk factors include smoking, male gender, White race, family history, and, to a lesser degree, hypertension [116]. Smoking, the most significant risk factor in some studies, promotes formation and growth of aortic aneurysms [116]. Males, with a rate that is four to five times higher than women, and whites, with a rate twice as high as blacks, are affected disproportionately.

The risk of rupture increases dramatically with the size of the aneurysm. In small aneurysms, <4 cm, the rate of rupture is low; for 4- to 5-cm aneurysms the rate is 1%; for 5- to 6-cm aneurysms the rate is 11%; and for aneurysms >6 cm the rate is 25% [117]. Multiple studies confirm that the risk of rupture increases dramatically as the size of the aneurysm exceeds 5 cm [118]. The risk of rupture is also greater in aneurysms that are growing rapidly.

The annual incidence of ruptured AAA, estimated from autopsy data in Sweden between 1971 and 1986, is 60 cases per million [119]. US estimates of patients that reach the hospital alive are 31 to 37 cases per million [120]. The incidence of ruptured AAA increases dramatically with age occurring in 0.01, 0.37, and 1.36 per 1000 people <60 years, 70 to 80 years, and >90 years, respectively [121].

History and physical examination

Unruptured abdominal aortic aneurysm

Most unruptured AAAs are asymptomatic, and are diagnosed incidentally on tests performed for other indications. Some unruptured aortic aneurysms may cause back, flank, or abdominal pain, especially if they are increasing rapidly in size. Symptomatic aneurysms are at increased risk of rupture.

An excellent review, summarizing the utility of the physical examination, suggests that the only maneuver of demonstrated value is abdominal palpation to detect a widened aortic pulsation [122]. Pooled data reveal that the sensitivity of abdominal palpation increases from 29% for small AAAs that are <4 cm, to 50% for AAAs between 4 and 5 cm, to 76% for AAAs that are >5 cm [122]. Obviously, obesity decreases sensitivity. Other findings including bruits, thrills, quality of pulsation, and quality and discrepancy of the femoral pulses proved to be inaccurate in diagnosis.

Ruptured abdominal aortic aneurysm

When an AAA ruptures or leaks, it becomes symptomatic. The classic triad of back pain, hypotension, and a pulsatile abdominal mass is rarely present, but most patients manifest at least one or two features. Pain, the most common finding, is located in the abdomen, back, or flank, is acute and severe, and may radiate to chest, thigh, or groin. Nausea, vomiting, diaphoresis, and syncope often accompany initial hemorrhage. Ruptured AAA should be the working diagnosis in any patient with a known AAA who presents with any of the classic features, and should be considered in any elderly patient with back pain. Cardiac arrest may be the presentation in 25% of cases.

On physical examination, the vital signs and abdominal exam are most revealing. Hypotension is present in one half to two thirds of patients. Tachycardia from pain and hemorrhage is usually present. Because most ruptured AAAs are large, a palpable abdominal mass is frequently present.

Being a relatively rare cause of abdominal and back pain, ruptured AAAs are frequently misdiagnosed. Common misdiagnoses include: renal colic, pyelonephritis, pancreatitis, cardiac ischemia, intestinal ischemia, and musculoskeletal back pain. The EP should consider ruptured AAA when diagnosing these other conditions in the elderly.

Diagnostic tests

Abdominal ultrasound

Ultrasound is an excellent tool to diagnose and monitor AAAs. In trained hands, ultrasound is nearly 100% sensitive [123]. It is also inexpensive, rapid, and requires no contrast or radiation. Ultrasound can be performed at the bedside by a trained ED physician, obviating the need to leave a monitored setting. Unfortunately, ultrasound cannot reliably detect rupture [124].

CT

A CT scan is also nearly 100% accurate for the detection of an AAA. Emergent evaluations with or without contrast have high utility [123]. The sensitivity of CT for detecting retroperitoneal hemorrhage is 77% to 100% [125]. Another major advantage of CT is that it thoroughly evaluates the abdomen for other diagnoses. Its disadvantages are that it is time consuming, requires contrast dye to properly assess alternative diagnoses, and requires potentially unstable patients to leave the ED.

Management

Ruptured abdominal aortic aneurysms

A ruptured, leaking, or symptomatic AAA must be managed aggressively. When the diagnosis is suspected, continuous monitoring, two large-bore IVs, and saline resuscitation should be initiated immediately. The patient should be typed and crossmatched for at least 10 units of blood. Resuscitation with saline and blood products should continue to a level that maintains cerebral and end organ perfusion—an systolic blood pressure of 90 to 100 mmHg is the goal in most patients. Overly aggressive elevation of blood pressure can lead to rupture of a contained hematoma. Surgery should be notified early and be involved throughout the evaluation. Definitive management is immediate surgical repair. Surgery should not be delayed for resuscitation or unnecessary testing.

The diagnostic strategy employed to confirm the diagnosis depends on the patient's condition. Hypotensive patients should get a bedside ultrasound. Although the ultrasound cannot reliably detect a ruptured AAA, the finding of a normal aortic diameter effectively excludes the diagnosis. The finding of an AAA in a hemodynamically unstable patient virtually confirms the diagnosis and mandates immediate surgery with no further imaging. Patients without hypotension should get an expedited CT scan to confirm rupture. Emergent surgery that reveals an intact, symptomatic aneurysm carries a much higher mortality than elective repair (26% versus 5%) [126].

Surgical repair of ruptured AAAs is risky. Although declining at a rate of 3.5% per decade, operative mortality is still >40% [127]. The biggest predictor is hypotension. Operative success is greater at experienced centers. Consideration should be given to transferring the patient to a regional center with expertise. No clear criteria exist that preclude surgery. Because ruptured AAA is uniformly fatal without repair, surgery is the only potentially life-saving option. Age is not a contraindication. Nonetheless, the elderly are managed operatively less frequently than younger patients [128].

Unruptured abdominal aortic aneurysms

Patients with an unruptured, nonleaking, asymptomatic AAA should be referred for outpatient management. Strategies for management are evolving, but most experts advise surgical repair for aneurysms that are >5 cm or growing rapidly. Several excellent articles offer a full discussion [115,129].

Prognosis

The survival rate after a ruptured AAA is dismal. Many patients (50–80%) die before reaching the hospital. Of those that are aggressively treated, immediate operative mortality is 40% to 50% [120,130]. Of those that survive the initial day of hospitalization, subsequent mortality is close to 30% [130]. The overall mortality exceeds 90% [121]. Outcomes are significantly worse in the elderly. In one study, the operative mortality was >50% for patients >65 years and <50% for patients <65 years of age [120].

Summary

Geriatric patients are at increased risk for cardiovascular emergencies. As the geriatric population grows, providing care to this high risk population will occupy an increasingly important part of every shift. This article discussed five common cardiovascular emergencies: ACS, CHF, dysrythmias, aortic dissection, and ruptured AAA. The geriatric population is challenging, especially in the rapid pace of the ED. Atypical presentations, complicated medical histories, and unclear information from a poor historian can make the already challenging art of diagnosis virtually impossible. The EP must be vigilant, maintaining a low threshold to test and actively seek a cardiovascular emergency. After a diagnosis is made, aggressive therapy must be implemented. With only a few caveats, management of the elderly patient is similar to that of younger patients. As a rule, across the entire spectrum of cardiovascular emergencies, the elderly have significantly worse prognosis than younger patients. Although the graver prognosis is certainly due in part to the elderly being sicker with less physiologic reserve, it is also due to delays in diagnosis and under use of therapy on the part of providers.

References

[1] Alpert JS, Thygesen K, Antman E, et al. Myocardial infarction redefined—a consensus comment of the joint ESC/ACC committee for the redefinition of myocardial infarction. J Am Coll Cardiol 2000;36:959–69.

[2] Pope JH, Selker HP. Diagnosis of acute cardiac ischemia. Emerg Med Clin North Am 2003; 21(1):27–59.

[3] Goldberg RJ, McCormick D, Gurwitz JH, et al. Age-related trends in short and long term survival after acute myocardial infarction. Am J Cardiol 1998;82:1311–7.

[4] Lee TH, Cook F, Weisberg M, et al. Acute chest pain in the emergency room: identification and examination of low-risk patients. Arch Intern Med 1985;145:65–9.

[5] Steg PG, Oldberg RJ, Gore JM, et al. Baseline characteristics, management practices, and in-hospital outcomes of patients hospitalized with acute coronary syndromes in the Global Registry of Acute Coronary Events (GRACE). Am J Cardiol 2002;90(4):358–63.

[6] Brieger D, Eagle K, Goodman S, et al. Acute coronary syndromes without chest pain, an underdiagnosed and undertreated high-risk group. Chest 2004;126:461–9.

[7] Canto JG, Shlipak MG, Rogers WJ, et al. Prevalence, clinical characteristics, and mortality among patients with myocardial infarction presenting without chest pain. JAMA 2000; 283(24):3223–9.

[8] Canto JG, Fincher C, Kiefe CI, Allison JJ, et al. Atypical presentations among Medicare beneficiaries with unstable angina pectoris. Am J Cardiol 2002;90(3):248–53.

[9] Bean WB. Masquerades of myocardial infarction. Lancet 1977;14:1044–6.

[10] Panju AA, Hemmelgarn BR, Guyatt GH, et al. The rational clinical examination: is this patient having a myocardial infarction? JAMA 1998;280(14):1256–63.
[11] Goodacre S, Locker T, Morris F, et al. How useful are clinical features in the diagnosis of acute, undifferentiated chest pain? Acad Emerg Med 2002;9(3):203–8.
[12] McCarthy B, Beshansky J, D'Agostino R, et al. Missed diagnoses of acute myocardial infarction in the emergency department: results from a multicenter study. Ann Emerg Med 1993;22:579–82.
[13] Antman EM, Grudzien C, Sacks DB. Evaluation of a rapid bedside assay for detection of serum cardiac troponin T. JAMA 1995;273(16):1279–82.
[14] Noeller TP, Medon SW, Peacock WF, et al. Troponin T in elders with suspected acute coronary syndromes. Am J Emerg Med 2003;21:293–7.
[15] Heidenreich PA, Alloggiamento T, Melsop K, et al. The prognostic value of troponin T in patients with non-ST elevation acute coronary syndromes: a meta-analysis. J Am Coll Cardiol 2001;38(2):478–85.
[16] Granger CB, Goldberg RJ, Dabbous O, et al. Predictors of hospital mortality in the global registry of acute coronary events. Arch Intern Med 2003;163:2345–53.
[17] Antman EM, Cohen M, Bernink PJ, et al. The TIMI risk score for unstable angina/non-ST elevation MI: a method for prognostication and therapeutic decision making. JAMA 2000; 284:835–42.
[18] Braunwald E, Antman EM, Beasley JW, et al. ACC/AHA guideline update for the management of patients with unstable angina and non-ST segment elevation myocardial infarction—2002: summary article: a report of the American College of Cardiology/American Heart Associaiton Task Force on s (Committee on the Management of Patients with Unstable Angina). Circulation 2002;106(14):1893–900.
[19] Antman EM, Anbe DT, Armstrong PW, et al. ACC/AHA guidelines for the management of patients with ST-elevation myocardial infarction—executive summary: a report of the ACC/AHA task force on practice guidelines. Circulation 2004;110:588–636.
[20] Randomised trial of intravenous atenolol among 16027 cases of suspected acute myocardial infarction: ISIS-1. First international study of Infarct Survival Collaborative Group. Lancet 1986;2:57–66.
[21] Fox K. Management of acute coronary syndromes: an update. Heart 2004;90:698–706.
[22] Yusuf S, Zhao F, Mehta SR, et al. Clopidogrel in unstable angina to prevent recurrent events trial investigators. Effects of clopidogrel in addition to aspirin in patients with acute coronary syndromes without ST-segment elevation. N Engl J Med 2001;345:494–502.
[23] Topol EJ, Neumann FJ, Montalescot G. A preferred reperfusion strategy for acute myocardial infarction. J Am Coll Cardiol 2003;42:1886–9.
[24] Krumholz HM, Hennen J, Ridker RM, et al. Use and effectiveness of intravenous heparin therapy for treatment of acute myocardial infarction in the elderly. J Am Coll Cardiol 1998; 31:973–9.
[25] Cohen M, Demers C, Gurfinkel EP, et al. A comparison of low-molecular weight heparin with unfractionated heparin for unstable angina and silent ischemia. N Engl J Med 1997; 337(7):447–52.
[26] Collins R. Optimizing thrombolytic therapy of acute myocardial infarction: age is not a contraindication. Circulation 1991;84:II230.
[27] Boucher JM, Racine N, Thanh T, et al. Age related differences in in-hospital morality and the use of thrombolytic therapy for acute myocardial infarction. CMAJ 2001;164(9): 1285–90.
[28] De Boer MJ, Ottervanger JP, van't Hof AW, et al. Reperfusion therapy in elderly patients with acute myocardial infarction: a randomized comparison of primary angioplasty and thrombolytic therapy. J Am Coll Cardiol 2002;39:1723–8.
[29] Mclaughlin TJ, Soumerai S, Willison D, et al. Adherence to national guidelines for drug treatment of suspected acute myocardial infarction: evidence for undertreatment in women and the elderly. Arch Intern Med 1996;156(7):799–805.

[30] Krumholz HM, Murillo JE, Chen J, et al. Thrombolytic therapy for eligible elderly patients with acute myocardial infarction. JAMA 1997;277(21):1683–8.

[31] Paul SD, O'Gara PT, Mahjoub ZA, et al. Geriatric patients with acute myocardial infarction: cardiac risk factor profiles, presentation, thrombolysis, coronary interventions, and prognosis. Am Heart J 1996;131:710–5.

[32] American Heart Association. 2002 Heart and stroke statistical update. Dallas (TX): American Heart Association; 2001.

[33] Ho KL, Anderson KM, Kannel WB, et al. Survival after the onset of congestive heart failure in Framingham heart study subjects. Circulation 1993;88(1):107–15.

[34] Falk JL, O'Brien JF, Shesser R. Heart failure. In: Marx JA, Hockberger RS, Walls RM, editors. Rosen's emergency medicine: concepts and clinical practice. 5th ed. St. Louis (MO): Mosby; 2002. p. 1113–9.

[35] Packer M. How should physicians view heart failure? The philosophical and physiological evolution of three conceptual models of the disease. Am J Cardiol 1993;71:3C–11C.

[36] Michalsen A, Konig G, Thimme W. Preventable causative factors leading to hospital admission with decompensated heart failure. Heart 1998;80:437–41.

[37] Yamasaki N, Kitaoka H, Matsumura Y, et al. Heart failure in the elderly. Intern Med 2003; 42(5):383–8.

[38] Cline CM, Bjorck-Linne AK, Israelsson BY, et al. Non-compliance and knowledge of prescribed medication in elderly patients with heart failure. Eur J Heart Fail 1999;1(2):145–9.

[39] Kalra PR, Collier T, Cowie MR, et al. Haemoglobin concentration and prognosis in new cases of heart failure. Lancet 2003;362(9379):211–2.

[40] Tresch DD, Jamali I. Cardiac disorders. In: Duthie EH, Katz PR, editors. Practice of geriatrics. 3rd ed. Philadelphia (PA): WB Saunders; 1998. p. 497.

[41] Tresch DD. Clinical manifestations, diagnostic assessment, and etiology of heart failure in elderly patients. Clin Geriatr Med 2000;16(3):445–56.

[42] Badgett RG, Lucey CR, Mulrow CD. Can the clinical examination diagnose left-sided heart failure in adults. JAMA 1997;277(21):1712–9.

[43] Ezekowitz JA, McAlister FA, Armstrong PW. Anemia is common in heart failure and is associated with poor outcomes: insights from a cohort of 12,065 patients with new-onset heart failure. Circulation 2003;107:223–5.

[44] Cohen HW, Madhavan S, Alderman MH. High and low serum potassium associated with cardiovascular events in diuretic-treated patients. J Hypertens 2001;19(7):1315–23.

[45] Goto T, Takase H, Toriyama T, et al. Circulating concentrations of cardiac proteins indicate the severity of congestive heart failure. Heart 2003;89(11):1303–7.

[46] Hunt SA, Baker DW, Chin MH, et al. ACC/AHA guidelines for the evaluation and management of chronic heart failure in the adult: executive summary a report of the ACC/AHA task force on practice guidelines. Circulation 2001;104(24):2996–3007.

[47] Maisel A, Hollander JE, Guss D, et al. Primary results of the rapid emergency department heart failure outpatient trial. A multicenter study of b-type natriuretic peptide levels, emergency department decision making, and outcomes in patients presenting with shortness of breath. J Am Coll Cardiol 2004;44(6):1328–33.

[48] McCullough PA, Nowak RM, McCord J, et al. B-type natriuretic peptide and clinical judgment in emergency diagnosis of heart failure: analysis from the breathing not properly multinational study. Circulation 2002;106(4):416–22.

[49] Maisel AS, McCord J, Nowak RM, et al. Bedside b-type natriuretic peptide in the emergency diagnosis of heart failure with reduced or preserved ejection fraction. Results from the breathing not properly multinational study. J Am Coll Cardiol 2003;41(11):2010–7.

[50] Maisel AS, Clopton P, Krishnaswamy P, et al. Impact of age, race, and sex on the ability of b-type natriuretic peptide to aid in the emergency diagnosis of heart failure: results from the breathing not properly multinational study. Am Heart J 2004;147(6):1078–84.

[51] Kollef MH. Ventilator-associated pneumonia. A multivariate analysis. JAMA 1993; 270(16):1965–70.

[52] Bersten AD, Holt AW, Vedig AE, et al. Treatment of severe cardiogenic pulmonary edema with continuous positive airway pressure delivered by face mask. N Engl J Med 1991; 325(26):1825–30.

[53] Sharon A, Shpirer I, Kaluski E, et al. High-dose intravenous isosorbide-dinitrate is safer and better than bi-pap ventilation combined with conventional treatment for severe pulmonary edema. J Am Coll Cardiol 2000;36(3):832–7.

[54] Howard PA, Dunn MI. Aggressive diuresis for severe heart failure in the elderly. Chest 2001;119(3):807–10.

[55] VMAC investigators. Intravenous nesiritide vs nitroglycerin for treatment of decompensated congestive heart failure: a randomized controlled trial. JAMA 2002;287(12):1531–40.

[56] Varriale P, David W, Chryssos BE. Hemodynamic response to intravenous enalaprilat in patients with severe congestive heart failure and mitral regurgitation. Clin Cardiol 2993;16:235–8.

[57] Sacchetti A, Ramoska E, Moakes ME, et al. Effect of ED management on ICU use in acute pulmonary edema. Am J Emerg Med 1999;17:571–4.

[58] Caldicott LD, Hawley K, Heppell R, et al. Intravenous enoximone or dobutamine for severe heart failure after acute myocardial infarction: a randomized double-blinded trial. Eur Heart J 1993;14(5):696–700.

[59] Ferroni C, Fraticelli A, Paciaroni E. Intermittent dobutamine therapy in patients with advanced congestive heart failure. Arch Gerontol Geriatr 1996;23(3):313–27.

[60] Rame JE, Sheffield MA, Dries DL, et al. Outcomes after emergency department discharge with a primary diagnosis of heart failure. Am Heart J 2001;142:714–9.

[61] Poses RM, Smith WR, McClish DK, et al. Physicians' survival predictions for patients with acute congestive heart failure. Arch Intern Med 1997;157(9):1001–7.

[62] American Heart Association. 2005 heart and stroke statistical update. Dallas (TX): Author; 2004.

[63] Bunch TJ, White RD, Gersh BJ, et al. Long-term outcomes of out-of-hospital cardiac arrest after successful early defibrillation. N Engl J Med 2003;348(26):2626–33.

[64] Longstreth WT, Cobb LA, Fahrenbruch CE, et al. Does age affect outcomes of out-of-hospital cardiopulmonary resuscitation. JAMA 1990;264(16):2109–10.

[65] Rogove HJ, Safar P, Sutton-Tyrrell K, et al. Old age does not negate good cerebral outcome after cardiopulmonary resuscitation: analysis from the brain resuscitation clinical trials. The brain resuscitation clinical trial I and II study groups. Crit Care Med 1995;23(1):18–25.

[66] Bunch TJ, White RD, Khan AH, et al. Impact of age on long-term survival and quality of life following out-of-hospital cardiac arrest. Crit Care Med 2004;32(4):963–7.

[67] Swor RA, Jackson RE, Tintinalli JE, et al. Does advanced age matter in outcomes after out-of-hospital cardiac arrest in community-dwelling adults. Acad Emerg Med 2000;7(7): 762–8.

[68] Kim C, Becker L, Eisenberg MS. Out-of-hospital cardiac arrest in octogenarians and nonagenarians. Arch Intern Med 2000;160(22):3439–43.

[69] Church TR, Hodges M, Bailey JJ, et al. Risk stratification applied to CAST registry data: combining 9 predictors. Cardiac arrhythmia suppression trial. J Electrocardiol 2002; 35(Suppl):117–22.

[70] Bikkina M, Larson MG, Levy D. Prognostic implications of asymptomatic ventricular arrhythmias: the Framingham heart study. Ann Intern Med 1992;117(12):990–6.

[71] Crispell KA. Common cardiovascular issues encountered in geriatric critical care. Crit Care Clin 2003;19:677–91.

[72] Aronow WS, Ahn C, Mercando AD, et al. Prevalence and association of ventricular tachycardia and complex ventricular arrhythmias with new coronary events in older men and women with and without cardiovascular disease. J Gerontol A Biol Sci Med Sci 2002; 57(3):M178–80.

[73] Hudson KG, Brady WJ, Chan TC, et al. Electrocardiographic manifestations: ventricular tachycardia. J Emerg Med 2003;25(3):303–14.

[74] Saliba WI, Natale A. Ventricular tachycardia syndromes. Med Clin North Am 2001;85(2): 267–304.

[75] Cummins RO, Field JM, Hazinski MF. ACLS provider manual. American Heart Association; 2001.

[76] Brugada P, Brugada J, Mont L, et al. A new approach to the differential diagnosis of a regular tachycardia with a wide QRS complex. Circulation 1991;83(5):1649–59.

[77] Griffith MJ, Garratt CJ, Mounsey P, et al. Ventricular tachycardia as default diagnosis in broad complex tachycardia. Lancet 1994;343(8894):386–8.

[78] Isenhour JL, Craig S, Gibbs M, et al. Wide-complex tachycardia: continued evaluation of diagnostic criteria. Acad Emerg Med 2000;7(7):769–73.

[79] Herbert ME, Votey SR, Morgan MT, et al. Failure to agree on the electrocardiographic diagnosis of ventricular tachycardia. Ann Emerg Med 1996;27(1):35–8.

[80] Sung RJ. Facilitating electrical cardioversion of persistant atrial fibrillation by antiarrhythmic drugs: update on clinical trial results. Card Electrophysiol Rev 2003;7(3):300–3.

[81] Opolski G, Stanislawska J, Gorecki A, et al. Amiodarone in restoration and maintenance of sinus rhythm in patients with chronic atrial fibrillation after unsuccessful direct-current cardioversion. Clin Cardiol 1997;20(4):337–40.

[82] Moss AJ, Hall WJ, Cannom DS, et al. Improved survival with an implanted defibrillator in patients with coronary disease at high risk for ventricular arrhythmia. N Engl J Med 1996; 335:2933–40.

[83] AVID investigators. A comparison of antiarrhythmic-drug therapy with implantable defibrillators in patients resuscitated from near fatal ventricular arrhythmias. The antiarrhythmics versus implantable defibrillators (AVID) investigators. N Engl J Med 1997;337(22): 1576–83.

[84] Zeltser D, Justo D, Halkin A, et al. Drug-induced atrioventricular block: prognosis after discontinuation of the culprit drug. J Am Coll Cardiol 2004;44(1):105–8.

[85] Hayden GE, Brady WJ, Pollack M, et al. Electrocardiographic manifestations: diagnosis of atrioventricular block in the emergency department. J Emerg Med 2004;26(1):95–106.

[86] Brady WJ, Swart G, DeBehnke DJ, et al. The efficacy of atropine in the treatment of hemodynamically unstable bradycardia and atrioventricular block: prehospital and emergency department considerations. Resuscitation 1999;41:47–55.

[87] Link MS, Estes NA 3rd, Griffin JJ, et al. Complications of dual chamber pacemaker implantation in the elderly. Pacemaker selection in the elderly (PACE) investigators. J Interv Card Electrophysiol 1998;2(2):175–9.

[88] Feinberg WM, Blackshear JL, Laupacis A, et al. Prevalence, age distribution, and gender of patients with atrial fibrillation. Analysis and implications. Arch Intern Med 1995;155(5): 469–73.

[89] Benjamin EJ, Levy D, Vaziri SM, et al. Independent risk factors for atrial fibrillation in a population-based cohort. The Framingham heart study. JAMA 1994;271(11):840–4.

[90] Fumagalli S, Boncinelli L, Bondi E, et al. Does advanced age affect the immediate and long-term results of direct-current external cardioversion of atrial fibrillation. J Am Geriatr Soc 2002;50(7):1192–7.

[91] Kilborn MJ, Rathore SS, Gersh BJ, et al. Amiodarone and mortality among elderly patients with acute myocardial infarction with atrial fibrillation. Am Heart J 2002;144(6): 1095–101.

[92] Vasishta S, Toor F, Johansen A, et al. Stroke prevention in atrial fibrillation: physicians' attitudes to anticoagulation in older people. Arch Gerontol Geriatr 2001;33(3):219–26.

[93] Man-Son-Hing M, Laupacis A. Anticoagulant-related bleeding in older persons with atrial fibrillation: physicians' fears often unfounded. Arch Intern Med 2003;163(13): 1580–6.

[94] Gullov AL, Koefoed BG, Peterson P. Bleeding during warfarin and aspirin therapy in patients with atrial fibrillation: the AFASAK 2 study. Atrial fibrillation aspirin and anticoagulation. Arch Intern Med 1999;159(12):1322–8.

[95] Fang MC, Chang Y, Hylek EM, et al. Advanced age, anticoagulation intensity, and risk for intracranial hemorrhage among patients taking warfarin for atrial fibrillation. Ann Intern Med 2004;141(10):745–52.

[96] Wolf PA, Abbott RD, Kannel WB. Atrial fibrillation as an independent risk factor for stroke: the Framingham study. Stroke 1991;22(8):983–8.

[97] Stollberger C, Chnupa P, Abzieher C, et al. Mortality and rate of stroke or embolism in atrial fibrillation during long-term follow-up in the embolism in left atrial thrombi (ELAT) study. Clin Cardiol 2004;27(1):40–6.

[98] Tsivgoulis G, Spengos K, Zakopoulos N, et al. Efficacy of anticoagulation for secondary stroke prevention in older people with non-valvular atrial fibrillation: a prospective case series study. Age Ageing 2005;34(1):35–40.

[99] Wyse DG, Waldo AL, DiMarco JP, et al. A comparison of rate control and rhythm control in patients with atrial fibrillation. N Engl J Med 2002;347:1825–33.

[100] Hagens VE, Ranchor AV, Van Sonderen E, et al. Effect of rate or rhythm control on quality of life in persistent atrial fibrillation. Results from the rate control versus electrical cardioversion (RACE) study. J Am Coll Cardiol 2004;43(2):241–7.

[101] Daily PO, Trueblood W, Stinson EB, et al. Management of acute aortic dissections. Ann Thorac Surg 1970;109:237–47.

[102] Von Kodolitsch Y, Schwartz AG, Nienaber CA. Clinical prediction of acute aortic dissection. Arch Intern Med 2000;160:2977–82.

[103] Hagan PG, Nienaber CA, Isselbacher EM, et al. The International Registry of Acute Aortic Dissection: new insights into an old disease. JAMA 2000;283:897–903.

[104] Spittell PC, Spittell JA, Joyce JW, et al. Clinical features and differential diagnosis of aortic dissection: experience with 236 cases (1980 – 1990). Mayo Clin Proc 1993;68:642–51.

[105] Mehta RH, O'Gara PT, Bossone E, et al. Acute type A aortic dissection in the elderly: clinical characteristics, management, and outcomes in the current era. J Am Coll Cardiol 2002; 40:685–92.

[106] Khan I, Nair C. Clinical, diagnostic, and management perspectives of aortic dissection. Chest 2002;122:311–28.

[107] Suzuki T, Mehta RH, Ince H, et al. Clinical profiles and outcomes of acute type B aortic dissection in the current era: lessons from the International Registry of Aortic Dissection (IRAD). Circulation 2003;108(Suppl 1):II312.

[108] Klompas M. Does this patient have an acute thoracic dissection. JAMA 2002;287(17): 2262–72.

[109] Spittell PC, Spittell JA Jr, Joyce JW, et al. Clinical features and differential diagnosis of aortic dissection: experience with 236 cases (1980 through 1990). Mayo Clin Proc 1993;68:642.

[110] Nienaber CA, von Kodolitsch Y, Nicolas V, et al. The diagnosis of thoracic aortic dissection by noninvasive imaging procedures. N Engl J Med 1993;328:1–9.

[111] Bansal RC, Chandrasekaran K, Ayala K, Smith DC. Frequency and explanation of false negative diagnosis of aortic dissection by aortography and transesophageal echocardiography. J Am Coll Cardiol 1995;25:1393–401.

[112] Mehta RH, Suzuki T, Hagan PG, et al. Predicting death in patients with acute type A aortic dissection. Circulation 2002;105:200–6.

[113] Kawahito K, Adachi H, Yamaguchi A, et al. Early and late surgical outcomes of acute type A aortic dissection in patients aged 75 years and older. Ann Thorc Surg 2000;70:1455–9.

[114] Melton LJ III, Bickerstaff LK, Hollier LH, et al. Changing incidence of abdominal aortic aneurysms: a population-based study. Am J Epidemiol 1984;120:379–86.

[115] Powell JT, Greenhalgh RM. Clinical practice: small abdominal aortic aneurysms. N Engl J Med 2003;348:1895–901.

[116] Lederle FA, Johnson GR, Wilson SE, et al. Prevalence and associations of abdominal aortic aneurysm detected through screening. Ann Intern Med 1997;126:441–9.

[117] Reed WW, Hallett JW Jr, Damiano MA, et al. Learning from the last ultrasound: a population-based study of patients with abdominal aortic aneurysm. Arch Intern Med 1997;157:2064–8.

[118] Nevitt MP, Ballard DJ, Hallett JW Jr. Prognosis of abdominal aortic aneurysms: a population-based study. N Engl J Med 1989;321:1009–14.

[119] Johansson G, Swedenborg J. Ruptured abdominal aortic aneurysms: a study of incidence and mortality. Br J Surg 1986;73(2):101–3.

[120] Rutledge R, Oller D, Meyer A, et al. A statewide, population-based, time-series analysis of the outcome of ruptured abdominal aortic aneurysm. Ann Surg 1996;223(5):492–505.

[121] Bengtsson H, Bergqvist D. Ruptured abdominal aneurysm: a population-based study. J Vasc Surg 1993;18(1):74–80.

[122] Lederle FA, Simel DL. Does this patient have abdominal aortic aneurysm? JAMA 1999; 281:77–82.

[123] LaRoy LL, Cormier PJ, Matalon TA, et al. Imaging of abdominal aortic aneurysms. AJR Am J Roentgenol 1989;152:785–92.

[124] Shuman WP, Hastrup W Jr, Kohler TR, et al. Suspected leaking abdominal aortic aneurysm: use of sonography in the emergency room. Radiology 1988;168:117–9.

[125] Weinbaum FI, Dubner S, Turner JW, Pardes JG. The accuracy of computed tomography in the diagnosis of retroperitoneal blood in the presence of abdominal aortic aneurysm. J Vasc Surg 1987;6:11–6.

[126] Sullivan CA, Rohrer MJ, Cutler BS. Clinical management of the symptomatic but unruptured abdominal aortic aneurysm. J Vasc Surg 1990;11:799–803.

[127] Brown MJ, Sutton AJ, Bell PR, et al. A meta analysis of 50 years of ruptured abdominal aortic aneurysm repair. Br J Surg 2002;89(6):714–30.

[128] Evans SM, Adam DJ, Brittendon J, et al. Long term survival following repair of ruptured abdominal aortic aneurysm in patients over 75 years of age. Br J Surg 1999;86(5):696–701.

[129] Mohler ER, Fairman RM. Management of abdominal aortic aneurysm. In: Up to date. Version 12.3. Accessed via the Web on 11/23/2004.

[130] Donaldson MC, Rosenberg JM, Bucknam CA. Factors affecting survival after ruptured abdominal aortic aneurysm. J Vasc Surg 1985;2:564–70.

**ELSEVIER
SAUNDERS**

Emerg Med Clin N Am
24 (2006) 371–388

EMERGENCY
MEDICINE
CLINICS OF
NORTH AMERICA

Abdominal Pain in the Elderly

Joseph P. Martinez, MD*,
Amal Mattu, MD, FAAEM, FACEP

*Division of Emergency Medicine, University of Maryland School of Medicine,
110 South Paca Street, Sixth Floor, Suite 200, Baltimore, MD 21201, USA*

High risk for and subtle presentations of serious pathologic conditions in the elderly patient who has abdominal pain require careful, timely evaluations and aggressive management. The elderly patient who has abdominal pain consumes more time and resources than any other emergency department (ED) patient presentation [1]. Their length of stay is 20% longer than younger patients who have the same complaint, they require admission nearly half the time, and they require surgical intervention one third of the time [2]. In contrast to many other patient presentations, the elderly patient who has abdominal pain requires the ED physician to do more than determine "sick or not sick" and make a disposition of admission versus discharge. Failure to identify an acute surgical condition in the emergency department can lead to increased mortality even if the patient is admitted for observation [2]. Of those elderly patients who have abdominal pain and are discharged home, nearly one third returns to the ED with continued symptoms.

The population of the United States is continuing to age. Twelve percent of the population is older than the age of 65 years, and this number is expected to increase to 20% by the year 2030. The fastest growing subset is the group of people over the age of 85 years. There is likely to be an increase in the number of elderly patients who present to the emergency department with abdominal pain.

Challenges to diagnosis

Several variables create complexities in securing a diagnosis in this age group. These include the physiologic changes that accompany aging, difficulties with taking an adequate history, medications that cause or confound

---

* Corresponding author.
E-mail address: jmartine@umaryland.edu (J.P. Martinez).

pathology, lack of expected vital sign changes and physical findings, significant comorbidities, and seemingly normal laboratory values in the face of surgical disease.

Physiologic changes

Although the actual number of T cells does not decline with age, their function does [3]. This renders the elderly person less able to fight infection. Moreover, they have alteration in their physical barriers to infection, such as skin and mucous membrane strength and integrity. Altered pain perception is well documented in elderly patients. A 1960 study demonstrated a prolongation in time necessary to sense a painful stimulus and to perceive it as painful [4]. Painless cardiac ischemia and infarction have long been recognized in elderly patients [5]. More recent studies now extend this decreased pain perception to intra-abdominal conditions [6,7]. This decreased sensitivity may be one factor why elderly patients present to EDs later in their disease course with resultant poorer prognosis.

History taking

Several factors contribute to the difficulty that may be encountered in taking an adequate history from an elderly patient. Decreased hearing or memory may exacerbate the problem. Stoicism commonly is encountered, coupled with the fear of losing independence should a serious condition be found. Acute or chronic alteration in mental status is encountered frequently.

Medications

Medication use may mask or create pathology. More elderly patients are taking nonsteroidal anti-inflammatory drugs (NSAIDs) than ever before, which may increase their risk for peptic ulcer disease. Steroid medications are useful for various conditions found in elderly patients, such as rheumatoid arthritis and temporal arteritis, but they also may increase the risk for ulcer formation. In addition, they may block the expected inflammatory response to peritonitis, leading to less abdominal tenderness. Anticholinergic medications may induce abdominal pain through urinary retention or ileus. Several other common medications, including digoxin, colchicine, and metformin, can produce abdominal pain. Beta blockers may blunt the expected tachycardia often seen with serious intra-abdominal pathology. Acetaminophen and NSAIDs may reduce the likelihood of fever, whereas corticosteroids may alter the serum leukocyte count and blunt the inflammatory response. Chronic narcotic use may blunt the pain that normally accompanies an abdominal catastrophe. Antibiotic use may cause abdominal pain, vomiting, and diarrhea. This is important to keep in mind when evaluating the elderly patient who has a long list of medications.

Physical examination

Evaluation of vital signs is the first step of a physical examination. This too may be fraught with uncertainty in the elderly patient. Despite serious intra-abdominal pathology, elderly patients are often normothermic or even hypothermic [8]. As noted earlier, the expected tachycardia may be blunted by medications or intrinsic conduction system abnormalities. Normal appearing blood pressure may reflect significant hypotension for a patient who has chronic hypertension. Tachypnea should be noted, and although it may reflect the expected response to pain, it also may be a compensatory mechanism for progressive acidosis caused by sepsis or ischemic bowel.

Physical examination should not be limited to the abdomen. General appearance is important, as is overall volume status. Conjunctivae should be examined for pallor. The cardiopulmonary examination is crucial. It may suggest a diagnosis by showing signs of pneumonia, congestive heart failure, pericarditis, or pulmonary emboli. The presence of atrial fibrillation is of particular significance, because it increases the risk for mesenteric ischemia. Examination of the extremities may reveal the presence of peripheral emboli or stigmata of vascular disease. Neurologic findings of previous cerebrovascular accident also may be a clue to underlying vascular disease.

The abdomen should be assessed fully, taking special note of surgical scarring, distention, organomegaly, ecchymosis, masses, or bruits. Abdominal musculature is often thin in elderly patients, leading to less guarding and rigidity even in the presence of frank peritonitis. A detailed search for hernias should be conducted, because they may be the cause of bowel obstruction and strangulation. Although the rectal examination does not assist in limiting the differential diagnosis, it may reveal the presence of gross or occult blood and may be the only way to discover prostatitis as a source of pain.

Comorbidities

Diabetes may blunt the normal response to serious abdominal pathology, including acute cholecystitis and acute appendicitis, making these surgical conditions more difficult to identify. Patients who have known gastrointestinal malignancies may have their abdominal pain written off as cancer pain, when in fact they may have a perforated viscous or other surgical process. The higher prevalence of vascular disease in elderly patients means that vascular catastrophes, such as leaking abdominal aortic aneurysm, mesenteric ischemia, and mesenteric venous thrombosis, all of which are difficult to diagnose in a timely fashion, are more likely to be the cause of abdominal pain in an older patient.

Laboratory values

It is prudent for the clinician to have a low threshold for obtaining laboratory studies in elderly patients who have abdominal pain. The clinician should not be swayed by normal laboratory values, however, nor be confused by abnormalities that do not fit the clinical picture. Laboratory values are often normal despite the presence of surgical disease. Over-reliance on the leukocyte count is another common pitfall. Up to one quarter of patients who have appendicitis may not develop leukocytosis [9]. The same is often found in other surgical conditions. Hyperamylasemia is nonspecific, and although elevations may indicate pancreatitis, they also may be seen in more life-threatening entities, such as mesenteric ischemia. The presence of blood in the urine may be seen in patients who have nephrolithiasis or urinary tract infection, but it also may be found in cases of appendicitis, diverticulitis, or even ruptured abdominal aortic aneurysm (AAA). An electrocardiogram should be obtained early in the work-up of elderly patients who have abdominal pain.

Imaging studies

A discussion of plain radiographs and other imaging modalities deserves special consideration, because their role has changed with advances in technology, availability, and operator skills.

Plain radiographs

The general usefulness of plain radiographs is limited mainly to evaluation for free intra-peritoneal air, signs of obstruction, or the rare case of foreign body ingestion or insertion. Although neither cost effective nor diagnostically helpful as a general screening tool in the elderly patient who has abdominal pain, there are several clues to serious disease that may be found on plain radiographs [10]. Suggestion of cecal or sigmoid volvulus may be noted. Signs of biliary tract disease such as emphysematous cholecystitis may be seen. A calcified aneurysmal aorta may be noted. Despite these more subtle abnormalities, the presence of free intra-peritoneal air or bowel obstruction remain the most useful radiographic findings.

Ultrasound

As more and more emergency physicians (EPs) gain familiarity and skill with bedside ultrasound, more uses are found for it. Long used to evaluate the abdomen in trauma, EPs are now becoming more comfortable with other applications. In the geriatric patient who has abdominal pain, it is useful for diagnosing AAA. Although ultrasound cannot determine whether the AAA is leaking or not, in an unstable patient who has abdominal pain and who is found to have an AAA, emergent surgical exploration is mandated. Ultrasound is also the imaging modality of choice for biliary and pelvic disease. Ultrasound may be limited by body habitus, bowel gas, and operator dependence.

Computerized tomography

Advances in computerized tomography (CT) technology have been wide-spread in recent years. The advent of multidetector row CT scanners has led to improved image quality in shorter acquisition times with less motion artifact. In addition, reformatting the images allows for CT angiography to be performed with image quality near that of conventional angiography [11].

A 2004 study examined the ability of CT to alter decision making in elderly patients who have abdominal pain [12]. Results of CT scans altered the diagnosis in 45% of cases. It also changed the admission decision in one quarter of patients, the need for antibiotics in one fifth, and the need for surgery in 12% of cases. In addition, CT scanning doubled the diagnostic certainty of the attending EP from 36% before CT to 77% after CT.

CT is highly sensitive for diagnosing perforation, AAA, appendicitis, and other common entities. Although not the gold standard for diagnosing mesenteric ischemia, it is more useful than angiography in cases of suspected mesenteric venous thrombosis.

Angiography

Angiography is most helpful in cases in which the suspicion for acute mesenteric ischemia is high. Though invasive, potentially nephrotoxic, and not always easy to obtain, it should be sought on an emergent basis in such cases. Even in cases in which mesenteric ischemia is identified by CT, preoperative angiography should be pursued for diagnostic and therapeutic reasons.

Specific conditions

Bowel obstruction

Elderly patients may present with small bowel obstruction (SBO) or large bowel obstruction (LBO). The etiology is different depending on the site. Hernias and adhesions from prior surgeries are the most common causes of SBO. Large bowel obstructions are usually caused by cancer, diverticulitis, or volvulus. In addition, although gallstone disease accounts for only 2% of cases of bowel obstruction in the general population, it may lead to almost one quarter of cases of intestinal obstruction in elderly patients, usually women [13]. It predominantly causes SBO but may in rare cases lead to colonic obstruction.

Small bowel obstruction

The symptoms of SBO are similar in the elderly population to those in the general population. Abdominal pain, distention, and vomiting commonly are seen, accompanied by constipation. Early in the course, however, these symptoms may be absent. Diarrhea may be present because of hyperperistalsis distal to the obstruction. This may account for the high rate of misdiagnosis of SBO: it remains the second most common condition (behind appendicitis) to be inappropriately discharged home [2]. The mortality rate for SBO in the geriatric population remains high at 14% to 35%. Although plain radiographs may suggest SBO (Fig. 1), abdominal CT is much more sensitive and may reveal the cause of the obstruction. When patients who have nonspecific SBO are admitted to medical services for conservative treatment, there is evidence that surgical therapy, if it becomes necessary, may be delayed [14]. This leads to increased morbidity and mortality.

Large bowel obstruction

LBO is less common than SBO. Proportionally more cases of LBO are seen in elderly patients, because the two most common causes (diverticulitis and cancer) increase with age. The classic description is that of a patient who has abdominal pain, severe constipation or obstipation, and intractable vomiting. Nearly one fifth of elderly patients have diarrhea, however, and only half report constipation or vomiting [15]. A difficult diagnosis, LBO often is discovered late in its course. This contributes to the mortality rate of nearly 40%. All patients who have LBO should be questioned carefully about symptoms of weight loss, change in bowel habits or stool caliber, and fatigue, because these may be signs of colorectal cancer (Figs. 2 and 3).

Volvulus causes only 15% of cases of LBO but is more likely to require emergent surgical intervention [10]. Symptomatology depends on the site of the volvulus. Sigmoid volvulus accounts for nearly 80% of cases and tends

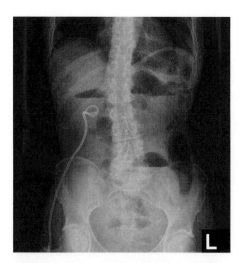

Fig. 1. Plain radiograph shows multiple air–fluid levels consistent with partial small bowel obstruction. Incidental finding is nephrostomy tube in right kidney.

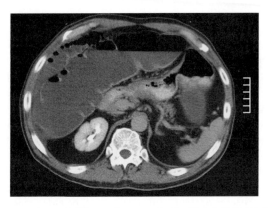

Fig. 2. Axial, contrast-enhanced CT scan shows markedly dilated, fluid-filled large bowel consistent with obstruction.

to present with more gradual onset of pain. Vomiting is seen in only one third of patients and constipation in half to three quarters. Cecal volvulus typically presents with acute onset of pain, nausea, and vomiting. On plain films, cecal volvulus usually shows a dilated loop of bowel with a kidney bean appearance in the left upper quadrant [16]. Virtually all cases of cecal volvulus require operative repair, whereas selected cases of sigmoid volvulus can be nonoperatively managed by decompressing the bowel with a rectal tube placed by way of a sigmoidoscope.

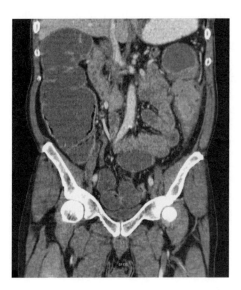

Fig. 3. Coronal reformatting of CT scan in Fig. 2 reveals the cause of obstruction to be a mass in the descending colon.

Biliary tract disease

Biliary disease remains the leading reason for acute abdominal surgery in the elderly population [17]. When cholecystectomy is performed emergently, the mortality rate is nearly fourfold that of the same procedure performed electively [18]. Cholelithiasis increases with age, and the severity of gallstone disease is much higher in the elderly population. The prevalence of gallbladder perforation, gangrene, emphysematous cholecystitis, ascending cholangitis, gallstone ileus, choledocholithiasis, and gallstone-induced pancreatitis are all higher [19].

Elderly patients who have cholecystitis tend to have right upper quadrant or epigastric pain with tenderness over the gallbladder. Other signs may be absent. Unlike younger patients, more than half of elderly patients who have acute cholecystitis have no nausea or vomiting and half also lack fever. Even with gallbladder empyema, gangrene, or frank perforation, one third still may be afebrile [20]. Laboratory studies also may be unreliable. Leukocytosis is absent in 30% to 40%, and a significant percentage have normal liver function tests. A recent study found no decrease in the accuracy of ultrasound or the sonographic Murphy's sign in elderly patients, even when they were premedicated with opioid analgesia [21]. Elderly patients have an increased likelihood of acalculous cholecystitis, however, which is not appreciated as readily on ultrasound [22]. A negative ultrasound combined with a high clinical suspicion for cholecystitis should prompt a radionuclide (HIDA) scan.

The incidence of complications caused by biliary disease is increased markedly in elderly patients. When the diagnosis of biliary disease is made, broad spectrum antibiotics, specifically covering gram-negative and anaerobic organisms, therefore should be started and prompt surgical evaluation initiated. Delayed surgical treatment in this population is associated with increased morbidity and mortality [23].

Choledocholithiasis is also more common, and with it, ascending cholangitis. Acute suppurative cholangitis rarely is seen before the seventh decade of life and mandates prompt decompression. Disseminated intravascular coagulation is common in both of these entities, and coagulation profiles should be monitored closely.

Pancreatitis

Pancreatitis remains the most common nonsurgical abdominal condition in the elderly population [24]. The incidence of pancreatitis increases 200-fold after the age of 65 years. Similar to most other abdominal conditions, the mortality rate in elderly patients is much higher, approaching 40% after the age of 70 years [25]. The presentation in elderly patients is varied. It may present classically with a boring pain radiating to the back, associated with nausea, vomiting, and dehydration. It also may be a hypermetabolic state resembling systemic inflammatory response syndrome. Unfortunately as many as 10% of cases of pancreatitis in elderly patients may present initially with hypotension and altered mental status [26]. This mandates maintaining a high index of suspicion for this condition. The astute clinician is not too quick to assume that mild elevations of amylase are pancreatitis without considering more lethal entities such as mesenteric ischemia. Elderly patients, especially those older than 80 years, are at higher risk for necrotizing pancreatitis, which places them in jeopardy of rapid deterioration [27]. The threshold for performing a CT scan in cases of pancreatitis in the elderly population should be low, especially if there are signs of impending sepsis.

Peptic ulcer disease

In a frequently quoted study from the 1960s, 35% of endoscopically proven peptic ulcer disease (PUD) was painless in patients older than age 60 years, compared with 8% of those younger than 60 years [28]. An acute abdomen is the first presentation of PUD in 50% of elderly patients, commonly because of perforation [26]. Other complications of PUD include hemorrhage, gastric outlet obstruction, and penetration into an adjacent viscus.

Perforation may present atypically in the elderly patient. Less than half of patients have the classic acute onset of abdominal pain. Rigidity is absent in nearly 80% [29]. Free intraperitoneal air on plain radiographs is absent in 40% of patients who have perforation [30]. When it is present (Figs. 4 and 5), it is often best visualized on a lateral film, which frequently is not obtained. The mortality of perforation in the general population is approximately 10%, whereas in the geriatric population it is 30% and increases

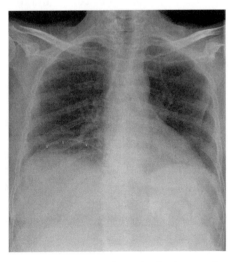

Fig. 4. Erect radiograph of patient ultimately determined to have perforated peptic ulcer shows free intraperitoneal air silhouetting the right side of the diaphragm (marked with small "x"s).

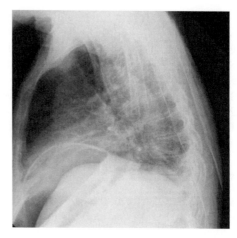

Fig. 5. Lateral radiograph of patient from Fig. 4 better demonstrates the presence of free intra-peritoneal air.

eightfold if the diagnosis is delayed by 24 hours [31]. In a well-publicized randomized, controlled trial showing identical mortality rates for conservative treatment of perforated peptic ulcer versus surgical treatment, the group of patients older than age 70 years was less likely to respond to conservative treatment [32].

Hemorrhagic complications of PUD are also more common in elderly patients. Nearly one fifth of cases of hemorrhage in elderly patients have shown no prior symptoms of peptic ulcer. When elderly patients do bleed from PUD, they are more likely than younger patients to require blood transfusions, to need surgery to control bleeding, and to re-bleed [33]. Early signs of bleeding such as tachycardia are often absent for reasons mentioned previously.

Diverticular disease

Diverticular disease increases in prevalence with age. The incidence is approximately 50% in patients older than age 70 years and 80% after age 85 years [34]. Diverticular disease typically manifests as lower gastrointestinal bleeding or diverticulitis. Diverticulitis in turn may result in abscess formation, bowel obstruction, free perforation, or fistula, and may be a cause of overwhelming sepsis. Free perforation is seen more commonly in elderly or immunocompromised populations. It carries a significant mortality rate, 25% in some studies [35].

Diverticulosis is the most common etiology of lower gastrointestinal bleeding in the geriatric population and may be massive. Nearly 15% of all people who have diverticular disease experience at least one episode of significant bleeding. Though it typically resolves spontaneously, 25% of patients re-bleed and some progress to hemorrhagic shock [36].

More people who have diverticular disease develop clinical diverticulitis than hemorrhage. Unfortunately it is misdiagnosed 50% of the time [37]. The classic findings of nausea, distention, fever, palpable left lower quadrant mass, and leukocytosis are frequently absent. As with many other conditions in this population, leukocytosis may be lacking in a large number of cases. Irritation of the bladder or ureter by the inflamed diverticulum may induce pyuria or hematuria and result in the erroneous diagnosis of nephrolithiasis or urinary tract infection. A palpable mass in women often leads to suspicion of gynecologic malignancy and provokes unnecessary worry of cancer. Right-sided diverticulitis may provoke unnecessary operations for presumed appendicitis. Liberal use of abdominal and pelvic CT scan usually can distinguish between these entities. Early diverticulitis and early appendicitis may be missed by CT scan.

Appendicitis

Appendicitis used to be thought of as a disease of the young. Although it certainly is more common in younger patients, it is the third most common indication for abdominal surgery in the elderly population [38]. In addition, the mortality rate in the general population is less than 1%, whereas in the geriatric population it ranges from 4% to 8% [39]. Despite the lower incidence of appendicitis in this population, elderly patients account for half of all deaths from appendicitis [40]. The incidence of perforation is much higher in elderly patients, nearly 70% in some studies [41].

A recent study was performed comparing appendicitis in elderly patients over 10 years at one institution to the previous 10 years [42]. Despite improved technology, knowledge of the disease, and awareness, the admitting diagnosis was still incorrect in 54% of cases. Half of all cases had perforated by the time of surgery, and delays to surgery of more than 24 hours occurred in one quarter of those initially misdiagnosed. This delay was associated with a perforation rate of nearly 75%.

Some of the challenges to diagnosing appendicitis include delayed presentation to care by the patient and atypical symptoms. Up to one fifth of elderly patients who have appendicitis present after 3 days of symptoms and another 5% to 10% after 1 week of symptoms [43]. In the study cited previously, it was noted that CT scans were obtained in less than half of cases in which symptoms had been present for greater than 48 hours.

Atypical symptoms are another confounding issue. Less than one third of elderly patients have fever, anorexia, right lower quadrant pain, and leukocytosis. Again, nearly half of patients are afebrile, half demonstrate no rebound or involuntary guarding, and nearly one quarter have no right lower quadrant tenderness at all [30,42]. It must be emphasized again that although appendicitis is not uncommon in this population, the typical presentation is. Liberal use of CT scanning is encouraged for any patient in this age group who still possesses an appendix. Early surgical consultation should be obtained in suspicious or equivocal cases, because delays in diagnosis lead to increased risk for perforation, with resultant increases in morbidity and mortality. Many studies have demonstrated decreased morbidity and mortality with rapid diagnostic laparotomy rather than watchful waiting [44–46].

Vascular catastrophes

Ruptured abdominal aortic aneurysm

Ruptured AAA remains the thirteenth leading cause of death in the United States [47]. The mortality is extremely high. One study demonstrated a mortality rate of 70%, even with an average ED time of only 12 minutes before surgery [48]. Although the diagnosis is fairly straightforward in the elderly patient who has abdominal pain, hypovolemic shock, and a pulsatile abdominal mass, this is the exception rather than the rule. Hypotension is absent in nearly 65% of cases, presumably because of tamponade in the left retroperitoneal space [49]. This affords the EP an opportunity to diagnose the condition before catastrophic rupture. Unfortunately atypical presentations are common, and the misdiagnosis rate is as high as 30% to 50% [50,51].

The most common misdiagnosis is that of renal colic [50,51]. Patients who have ruptured AAA often have back pain radiating toward the groin associated with microscopic hematuria caused by irritation of the ureter by the AAA. As a general rule, any elderly patient presenting with symptoms of new onset nephrolithiasis should have an evaluation of their aorta to detect AAA. This can be accomplished by ultrasound or noncontrast CT scan, which is often used to diagnose renal colic. Similarly, when diagnosing musculoskeletal back pain in elderly patients, the clinician should have a low threshold for imaging the aorta. Other conditions that are mimicked by ruptured AAA include diverticulitis (palpable left lower quadrant mass), lower gastrointestinal (GI) bleed (from aortoenteric fistula), and acute coronary syndrome (if the patient presents with syncope). Any patient who has previous aneurysm repair and who presents with GI bleeding must be considered to have an aortoenteric fistula until proven otherwise. The already high mortality rate of this condition increases further with any delay in diagnosis. The diagnosis of AAA should be considered in any patient who has syncope or hypotension in combination with abdominal or back pain.

Treatment decisions should be based on the stability of the patient. Early consultation with a vascular surgeon in suspected cases of AAA is essential. An unstable patient in whom AAA is diagnosed by history (known AAA), physical (pulsatile abdominal mass), or testing (bedside ultrasound) should be transported emergently to the operating room without delay [48]. Bedside ultrasound has been remarkably effective in making the diagnosis, even in the hands of inexperienced operators [52,53]. In stable patients, CT with contrast remains the test of choice because of its high sensitivity for detection of aneurysm and presence of rupture (Fig. 6). If renal function or

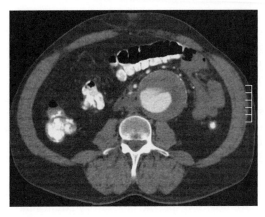

Fig. 6. Axial, contrast-enhanced CT scan demonstrates 7×7-cm non-ruptured AAA with thrombus lining its wall.

allergy precludes the use of intravenous contrast, unenhanced CT still can visualize acute hemorrhage [54,55].

Volume resuscitation in patients who are perfusing peripheral tissues adequately and who exhibit normal mentation should be deferred. Increasing blood pressure may lead to loss of the retroperitoneal tamponade with subsequent exsanguination [56]. At least 10 units of blood should be available for the operating room, because transfusion needs are usually substantial [48]. Advanced age is not a contraindication for repair. Mortality rates do not differ significantly with age, and AAA rupture is uniformly fatal without surgical treatment [57].

Mesenteric ischemia

Acute mesenteric ischemia (AMI) is one of the most difficult diagnoses to make. It requires a high index of suspicion, coupled with the willingness to image suspected cases aggressively.

Mesenteric ischemia encompasses four distinct entities: superior mesenteric artery (SMA) embolus, SMA thrombosis, mesenteric venous thrombosis (MVT), and nonocclusive mesenteric ischemia (NOMI). Embolus of the SMA accounts for most cases [58]. It presents as severe abdominal pain out of proportion to physical examination and may be associated with vomiting and diarrhea. Typically the patient has risk factors for embolic disease, such as atrial fibrillation, valvular disease, ventricular aneurysm, or postinfarction ventricular thrombi. Although atrial fibrillation is the most common cause, it is present in less than 50% of cases [59]. Patients who have SMA thrombosis typically have a long history of pain after meals (intestinal angina) and may report "food fear" and subsequent weight loss [60]. They often have known atherosclerotic disease, and their acute event occurs when an atherosclerotic plaque ruptures in the SMA. The acute presentation is then similar to that of SMA embolus. MVT conversely tends to be less acute, and presentation may be delayed days to weeks [61]. It is highly associated with an underlying hypercoagulable state. Half of patients have a personal or family history of deep venous thrombosis or pulmonary embolus [62]. Hypoperfusion secondary to sepsis, severe dehydration, or congestive heart failure predispose to NOMI. Although less common than embolic disease, the mortality of NOMI is exceedingly high [63].

The diagnosis of AMI is exceedingly difficult. Symptoms are often nonspecific, and the classic triad of abdominal pain, gut emptying, and underlying cardiac disease is found in the minority of cases. When present, vomiting and diarrhea may lead to the erroneous diagnosis of gastroenteritis. The physical examination is usually unhelpful. Abdominal tenderness, peritoneal signs, and bloody stools are absent early in the course until transmural necrosis develops. No specific laboratory studies have been found to date. A leukocytosis is generally present, as is some degree of metabolic acidosis and elevated lactate [64,65]. As noted previously, hyperamylasemia frequently is seen and should not sway the clinician to the diagnosis of pancreatitis.

Plain films are generally unhelpful. Mortality is actually much lower if plain radiographs are normal, presumably because the abnormalities that are visible on plain films are typically late findings [66]. As CT technology continues to improve, it will probably assume a larger role in the diagnosis of AMI, especially with the increasing quality of CT angiography. CT is the test of choice for MVT, because it often shows the thrombus itself [67]. For now, angiography remains the gold standard. The early, aggressive use of angiography is the only factor that has been shown to reduce overall mortality from mesenteric ischemia [68–70]. It should be considered in any at-risk patient who presents with acute abdominal pain and a paucity of physical findings. Despite the risks associated with angiography, it should not be delayed in these patients while obtaining other, less valuable tests or while waiting for peritoneal signs to develop.

Treatment of AMI is primarily surgical, although there have been studies investigating intra-arterial thrombolytics, vasodilators, or angioplasty [71–73]. Even in those cases in which AMI is diagnosed by another modality, angiography generally should be pursued, because it is needed in conjunction with surgical embolectomy to address the associated vasospasm [74].

Extra-abdominal causes

Elderly patients who have abdominal pain often have causes for their pain located outside of the abdominal cavity. The most important is acute myocardial infarction (MI). Elderly patients who have acute MI frequently lack chest pain. Nearly one third of women older than age 65 years have abdominal pain as their presenting symptom of acute MI [75]. Abdominal pain also may accompany other cardiac causes, such as decompensated heart failure, pericarditis, and endocarditis.

Pulmonary etiologies, including lower lobe pneumonias or pulmonary emboli, also may cause abdominal pain. Pleural effusions, empyemas, or pneumothoraces can mimic intra-abdominal conditions. Endocrine conditions, such as diabetic ketoacidosis, hypercalcemia, or adrenal crisis, may lead to nonspecific abdominal pain. Herpes zoster, porphyria, medication effects, and gynecologic or genitourinary conditions are additional etiologies to consider.

Disposition

Given the likelihood of atypical presentations, unreliability of physical examination findings, and lack of sensitivity of laboratory testing, the elderly patient who has abdominal pain should be approached systematically, keeping the differential diagnosis broad and searching for potentially life-threatening etiologies. The EP should not be swayed by aspects of the history that do not follow classic teachings, normal vital signs, laboratory values that are seemingly normal, or laboratory abnormalities that do not explain the patient's presentation. Liberal use of imaging and early surgical consultation is encouraged. The importance of serial examinations and even serial laboratory studies cannot be overemphasized.

Even after a thorough work-up has been pursued in the ED, the clinician should realize that certain entities may not become obvious until the disease course has progressed further. The EP should have a low threshold for admission to the hospital or to an ED observation unit for further monitoring.

Those patients who are selected for discharge home should have a repeat abdominal examination documented, have improvement in their clinical course noted, in most cases have a normal imaging study, and be able to tolerate oral nutrition. They also should have a reliable caretaker and a timely follow-up evaluation. Finally, the clinician should avoid labeling undifferentiated abdominal pain with a more benign diagnosis, such as gastroenteritis. Patients should be informed that the cause of their symptoms is unclear, and they should be given specific instructions regarding signs and symptoms to monitor themselves for or to seek further medical attention.

Summary

The population of the United States continues to age. As such, all physicians will be seeing more geriatric patients. Abdominal pain remains one of the most common and potentially serious complaints that EPs encounter. Vascular catastrophes should be considered early in the course of all elderly patients who have abdominal pain, because the window for successful intervention is small. A thorough work-up is essential and a broad differential should be kept in mind. The astute clinician should always be mindful that elderly patients may have delayed presentations of serious illnesses, and their signs and symptoms of disease may be atypical. Early imaging, surgical consultation, and hospital admission in equivocal cases should always be considered.

References

[1] Baum SA, Rubenstein Z. Old people in the emergency room: age-related differences in emergency department use and care. J Am Geriatr Soc 1987;35:398–404.
[2] Brewer RJ, Golden GT, Hitsch DC, et al. Abdominal pain: an analysis of 1,000 consecutive cases in a university hospital emergency room. Am J Surg 1976;131:219–24.
[3] Evans R. Physiology of aging. In: Sanders AB, editor. Emergency care of the elder person. St. Louis: Beverly Cracom Publications; 1996. p. 11–28.
[4] Sherman ED, Robillard E. Sensitivity to pain in the aged. Can Med Assoc J 1960;83:944–7.
[5] Bayer AJ, Chadha JS, Farag RR, et al. Changing presentation of myocardial infarction with increasing old age. J Am Geriatr Soc 1986;34:263–6.
[6] Cooper GS, Shlaes DM, Salata RA. Intraabdominal infection: differences in presentation and outcome between younger patients and the elderly. Clin Infect Dis 1994;19:146–8.
[7] Clinch D, Banerjee AK, Ostick G. Absence of abdominal pain in elderly patients with peptic ulcer. Age Ageing 1988;13:120–3.
[8] Fenyo G. Diagnostic problems of acute abdominal diseases in the aged. Acta Chir Scand 1974;140:396–405.
[9] Horratas MC, Guyton DP, Wu D. A reappraisal of appendicitis in the elderly. Am J Surg 1990;160:291–3.
[10] Hendrickson M, Naparst TR. Abdominal surgical emergencies in the elderly. Emerg Med Clin N Am 2003;21:937–69.
[11] Chow LC, Chan FP, Li KC. A comprehensive approach to MR imaging of mesenteric ischemia. Abdom Imaging 2002;27:507–16.
[12] Esses D, Birnbaum A, Bijur P, et al. Ability of CT to alter decision making in elderly patients with acute abdominal pain. Am J Emerg Med 2004;22(4):270–2.
[13] Sanson TG, O'Keefe KP. Evaluation of abdominal pain in the elderly. Emerg Med Clin N Am 1996;14(3):615–27.
[14] Schwab DP, Blackhurst DW, Sticca RP. Operative acute small bowel obstruction: admitting service impacts outcome. Am Surg 2001;67(11):1034–8.
[15] Greenlee HB, Pienkos EJ, Vanderbilt PC, et al. Acute large bowel obstruction. Arch Surg 1974;108:470–6.
[16] Prince LA. Abdominal radiography. In: Johnson GA, Cohen H, Wojtowycz AR, editors. Atlas of emergency radiology. Philadelphia: WB Saunders; 2001. p. 53–83.
[17] Rosenthal RA, Anderson DK. Surgery in the elderly: observations on the pathophysiology and treatment of cholelithiasis. Exp Gerontol 1993;28:458–72.
[18] Glenn F. Surgical management of acute cholecystitis in patients 65 years of age and older. Ann Surg 1981;193:56–9.
[19] Bedirli A. Factors effecting the complications in the natural history of acute cholecystitis. Hepatogastroenterology 2001;48(41):1275–8.
[20] Morrow DJ, Thompson J, Wilson SE. Acute cholecystitis in the elderly. Arch Surg 1978;113:1149–52.
[21] Nelson BP, Senecal EL, Ptak T, et al. Opioid analgesia in the elderly: is the diagnosis of gallbladder pathology hindered. Ann Emerg Med 2004;44(S4):S89.
[22] Shuman WP. Low sensitivity of sonography and cholescintigraphy in acalculous cholecystitis. Am J Roentgenol 1984;142(3):531–4.
[23] Madden JW, Croker JR, Beynon GPJ. Septicemia in the elderly. Postgrad Med 1981;57:502–6.
[24] Martin SP, Ulrich CD II. Pancreatic disease in the elderly. Clin Geriatr Med 1999;15:579–605.

[25] Hoffman E, Perez E. Acute pancreatitis in the upper age groups. Gastroenterology 1959;36: 675–85.

[26] Caesar R. Dangerous complaints: the acute geriatric abdomen. Emerg Med Rep 1994;15: 191–202.

[27] Paajanen H. AP in patients over 80 years. Eur J Surg 1996;162(6):471–5.

[28] Leverat M. Peptic ulcer disease in patients over 60: experience in 287 cases. Am J Dig Dis 1966;11:279–85.

[29] Fenyo G. Acute abdominal disease in the elderly: experience from two series in Stockholm. Am J Surg 1982;143:751–4.

[30] McNamara RM. Acute abdominal pain. In: Sanders AB, editor. Emergency care of the elder person. St. Louis: Beverly Cracom Publications; 1996. p. 219–43.

[31] Wakayama T. Risk factors influencing the short-term results of gastroduodenal perforation. Surg Today 1994;24(8):681–7.

[32] Crofts TJ, Park KG, Steele RJ. A randomized trial of nonoperative treatment for perforated peptic ulcer. N Engl J Med 1989;320(15):970–3.

[33] Borum ML. Peptic-ulcer disease in the elderly. Clin Geriatr Med 1999;15:457–71.

[34] Ferzoco LB. Acute diverticulitis [review]. N Engl J Med 1998;338(21):1521–6.

[35] Krukowski ZH, Matheson NA. Emergency surgery for diverticular disease complicated by generalized and faecal peritonitis: a review. Br J Surg 1984;71:921–7.

[36] Henneman PL. Gastrointestinal bleeding. In: Marx JA, Hockberger RS, Walls RM, et al, editors. Rosen's emergency medicine: concepts and clinical practice. 5th edition. St. Louis: Mosby Inc; 2002. p. 194–200.

[37] Ponka JL, Welborn JK, Brush BE. Acute abdominal pain in aged patients: an analysis of 200 cases. J Am Geriatr Soc 1963;11:993–1007.

[38] Kauvar DR. The geriatric acute abdomen. Clin Geriatr Med 1993;9:547–58.

[39] Gupta H, Dupuy D. Abdominal emergencies: has anything changed? Surg Clin N Am 1997; 77:1245–64.

[40] Shoji BT, Becker JM. Colorectal disease in the elderly patient. Surg Clin N Am 1994;74: 293–316.

[41] Yamini D, Vargas H, Bongard F, et al. Perforated appendicitis: is it truly a surgical urgency? Am Surg 1998;64:970–5.

[42] Storm-Dickerson TL, Horratas MC. What have we learned over the past 20 years about appendicitis in the elderly? Am J Surg 2003;185:198–201.

[43] Freund HR, Rubinstein E. Appendicitis in the aged: is it really different? Am Surg 1984;50:573–6.

[44] Graham A, Henley C. Laparoscopic evaluation of acute abdominal pain. J Laparoendosc Surg 1991;1:165–8.

[45] Forde KA. The role of laparoscopy in the evaluation of the acute abdomen in critically ill patients. Surg Endosc 1992;6:219–21.

[46] Koruda MJ. Appendicitis: laparoscopic strategy in diagnosis and treatment. N Carol Med J 1992;53:196–8.

[47] Gillum RF. Epidemiology of aortic aneurysm in the United States. J Clin Epidemiol 1995;48: 1289–98.

[48] Johansen K, Kohler TR, Nicholls SC, et al. Ruptured abdominal aortic aneurysm: the Harborview experience. J Vasc Surg 1991;13:240–5.

[49] Rutherford RB, McCroskey BL. Ruptured abdominal aneurysm: special considerations. Surg Clin North Am 1989;69:859–68.

[50] Marston WA, Ahlquist R, Johnson G Jr, et al. Misdiagnosis of ruptured abdominal aortic aneurysms. J Vasc Surg 1992;16:17–22.

[51] Salkin MS. Abdominal aortic aneurysm: avoiding failure to diagnose. ED Legal Letter 1997; 8:67–78.

[52] Kuhn M, Bonnin RL, Davey MJ, et al. Emergency department ultrasound scanning for abdominal aortic aneurysm: accessible, accurate, and advantageous. Ann Emerg Med 2000;36: 213–9.

[53] Shuman WP, Hastrup W, Kohler TR, et al. Suspected leaking abdominal aortic aneurysm: use of sonography in the emergency room. Radiology 1988;168:117–9.

[54] Siegel CL, Cohan RH. CT of abdominal aortic aneurysms. Am J Roentgenol 1994;163: 17–29.

[55] Weinbaum FI, Dubner S, Turner JW, et al. The accuracy of computed tomography in the diagnosis of retroperitoneal blood in the presence of abdominal aortic aneurysm. J Vasc Surg 1987;6:11–6.

[56] Ernst CB. Abdominal aortic aneurysm. N Engl J Med 1993;328:1167–72.

[57] Barry MC. An "all comers" policy for ruptured abdominal aortic aneurysms: how can results be improved? Eur J Surg 1998;164(4):263–70.

[58] McKinsey JF, Gewertz BL. Acute mesenteric ischemia. Surg Clin N Am 1997;77(2):307–18.

[59] Park WM, Gloviczki P, Cherry KJ Jr, et al. Contemporary management of acute mesenteric ischemia: factors associated with survival. J Vasc Surg 2002;35(3):445–52.

[60] Kazmers A. Operative management of chronic mesenteric ischemia. Ann Vasc Surg 1998;12: 299–308.

[61] Sack J, Aldrete JS. Primary mesenteric venous thrombosis. Surg Gynecol Obstet 1982;154: 205–8.

[62] Rhee RY, Gloviczki P, Mendonca CT, et al. Mesenteric venous thrombosis: still a lethal disease in the 1990s. J Vasc Surg 1994;20:688–97.

[63] Bassiouny HS. Nonocclusive mesenteric ischemia. Surg Clin North Am 1997;77(2):319–26.

[64] Meyer T, Klein P, Schweiger H, et al. How can the prognosis of acute mesenteric artery ischemia be improved? Results of a retrospective analysis (German). Zentrablatt Fur Chirurgie 1998;123:230–4.

[65] Glenister KM, Corke CF. Infarcted intestine: a diagnostic void. ANZ J Surg 2004;74:260–5.

[66] Ritz JP, Runkel N, Berger G, et al. Prognosefactoren des mesenterialinfarktes. Zentralbl Chir 1997;122:332–8.

[67] Bradbury MS, Kavanaugh PV, Chen MY, et al. Noninvasive assessment of portomesenteric venous thrombosis: current concepts and imaging strategies. J Comput Assist Tomogr 2002; 26(3):392–404.

[68] Boley SJ, Sprayregen S, Siegelman SS, et al. Initial results from an aggressive roentgenologic and surgical approach to acute mesenteric ischemia. Surgery 1977;82:848–55.

[69] Clark RA, Gallant TE. Acute mesenteric ischemia: angiographic spectrum. AJR Am J Roentgenol 1984;142:555–62.

[70] Lobo Martinez E, Carvajosa E, Sacco O, et al. Embolectomy in mesenteric ischemia. Rev Esp Enferm Dig 1993;83:351–4.

[71] Boley SJ, Feinstein FR, Sammartano R, et al. New concepts in the management of emboli of the superior mesenteric artery. Surg Gynecol Obstet 1981;153:561–9.

[72] Savassi-Rocha PR, Veloso LF. Treatment of superior mesenteric artery embolism with a fibrinolytic agent: case report and literature review. Hepatogastroenterology 2002; 49(47):1307–10.

[73] Rivitz SM, Geller SC, Hahn C, et al. Treatment of acute mesenteric venous thrombosis with transjugular intramesenteric urokinase infusion. J Vasc Interv Radiol 1995;6:219–23.

[74] Boley SJ, Regan JA, Tunick PA, et al. Persistent vasoconstriction—a major factor in nonocclusive mesenteric ischemia. Curr Top Surg Res 1971;3:425–33.

[75] Lusiani I, Perrone A, Pesavento R, et al. Prevalence, clinical features, and acute course of atypical myocardial infarction. Angiology 1994;45:49–55.

ELSEVIER
SAUNDERS

Emerg Med Clin N Am
24 (2006) 389–412

EMERGENCY
MEDICINE
CLINICS OF
NORTH AMERICA

Atraumatic Joint and Limb Pain in the Elderly

Lori Harrington, MD, Jeffrey I. Schneider, MD*

*Department of Emergency Medicine, Boston Medical Center,
Dowling 1 South, 1 Boston Medical Center Place, Boston, MA 02118, USA*

Here we address some of the more common etiologies of atraumatic joint and limb pain.

Gout

Gout, a rheumatologic disorder characterized by the deposition of mono-sodium urate crystals in the joints, is the most common form of crystalline arthopathy, and has been estimated to effect 2.1 million persons in the United States [1]. Although it is often considered to be solely a disease of middle-aged men, gout does affect women and the elderly. Population studies have demonstrated an annual incidence of 3.2 per 1000 in men compared with 0.5 per 1000 in women [2], although the overall prevalence in the general population ranges from 0.7% to 1.4% in men and 0.5% to 0.6% in women [3]. However, in people over 65 years old, this prevalence increases to 4.4% to 5.2% in men and 1.8% to 2.0% in women. Among those patients with onset of gout after the age of 60, the distribution of disease is almost equal between men and women. In patients with onset after age 80, women predominate [3].

Pathophysiology

Crucial in the pathogenesis of gout is an elevation of uric acid levels in the body. Although only a minority of individuals with elevated serum uric acid levels go on to develop the disease, hyperuricemia is clearly associated with an increased risk of developing gout [4]. Although the exact mechanism is poorly understood, hyperuricemia (a result of overproduction in 10–20% of cases and underexcretion in 80–90% of cases [5]) results in the generation

---

* Corresponding author.
E-mail address: jeffrey.schneider@bmc.org (J.I. Schneider).

doi:10.1016/j.emc.2006.01.004
emed.theclinics.com

of uric acid salts that are deposited in the synovium of joints. These uric acid crystals bind immunoglobulins and other protein molecules that activate proinflammatory cytokines and chemotactic factors stimulating the influx of neutrophils into the synovial fluid. These phagocytic cells engulf the crystal–protein complexes, causing release of intracellular lysosomal enzymes, further propagating the release of collagenase, and other proteolytic enzymes into the joint [1]. Clinically, the physician recognizes this as inflammation of a joint.

Clinical presentation

Asymptomatic, long-standing hyperuricemia is generally present before the first clinical manifestation of acute gouty arthritis. Initially, monoarticular in 85% to 90% of patients, the first flare of gouty arthritis involves the first metatarsophalangeal (MTP) joint in approximately 50% to 60% of cases [3]. Classically, the patient complains of sudden onset of severe pain with associated signs of inflammation. Examination will demonstrate a warm, erythematous, and extremely tender joint. Generally self limited, with resolution expected in from 2 to 3 weeks, examination and laboratory studies may reveal an uncomfortable, febrile patient with a fever, leukocytosis, and elevated sedimentation rate. Although most commonly affecting the MTP joint, gouty arthritis also frequently affects the ankles, knees, elbows, and wrists.

After resolution of the flare, the patient may be asymptomatic for months or years and have no physical signs or symptoms. If untreated, most individuals will have a recurrence of the acute arthritis, which can lead to chronic arthritis involving multiple joints. Before the institution of urate-lowering drugs, as many as 20% to 40% of untreated patients developed chronic tophaceous gouty arthritis [5]. This refers to the deposition of urate crystal–protein complexes and associated inflammation *outside* the synovial fluid. The deposition classically occurs in periarticular tissues such as tendons, ligaments, cartilage, bone, and bursae. Tophi are often seen in periarticular areas of feet, fingers, and knees, and in and around olecranon, and prepatellar bursae, as well as on the ear and nose.

As with many other disease entities, elderly patients often present in a manner other than with the "classic" presentation. Instead of a red, warm, swollen MTP joint, the elderly may initially have symptoms more consistent with chronic tophaceous gout [6]. Gouty attacks in the older patient tend to be polyarticular, sometimes mimicking rheumatoid arthritis, with a more subacute onset and a more indolent course. Furthermore, the elderly more often have disease affecting the joints of the fingers. This is believed to be a result of osteoarthritic changes, placing individuals at increased risk for crystal deposition in these joints [7]. Older adults also tend to present with tophi earlier in their course in such atypical locations as the digital pulp, occasionally even before arthritis develops [8].

As with other disease processes involving the inflammatory cascade, the elderly may exhibit systemic symptoms such as fever, change in mental status, and decreased ability to perform activities of daily living. This may occur in the absence of complaints related to joint pathology and inflammation. Risk factors associated with the onset of gout are also different in the elderly. Although middle-age men with the disease are often afflicted with obesity, hyperlipidemia, high alcohol intake, and family history of gout, the elderly patient may have renal disease (and a subsequent decline in glomerular filtration), medication use such as low dose aspirin and diuretic use, and lympho- and myeloproliferative disorders [5].

The association of gout with diuretic use and renal insufficiency in the elderly is especially prominent. Specifically, diuretic use has been reported in over 75% of patients with elderly onset gout, with a frequency of 95% to 100% in women [9]. A retrospective cohort study documented an almost twofold increase in the risk of initiating antigout therapy in patients within 2 years of starting thiazide diuretics for hypertension compared with non-thiazide therapy [10].

Confirmation of clinically suspected gout requires arthrocentesis. The presence of needle-shaped, negatively birefringent crystals under polarized light is pathognomonic for the disorder. Although most sensitive if performed in the acutely inflamed joint, previously inflamed joints may still show evidence of monosodium urate crystals [11]. In addition to crystal examination, synovial fluid analysis should include cell count with differential, Gram stain, and culture. Typically, synovial fluid in acute gout will have a white blood count of 5000 to 75,000/mm^3 with a predominance of neutrophils [12]. Interestingly, serum uric acid levels may be normal during an acute attack, and plain radiography, while sometimes helpful, is generally not definitive [5]. Characteristically, one may see preservation of normal bone density until later in the disease, after numerous gouty flares. Other characteristic lesions include well-marginated para-articular erosions with overhanging edges or margins and punctate bone sclerosis due to intraosseous deposition of tophi [1].

Treatment

The goal of therapy is twofold: treating the pain of an acute attack, and reducing the likelihood of recurrence to avoid chronic disease. Treatment of acute inflammation from gout generally includes nonsteroidal anti-inflammatory drugs (NSAIDs), colchicine, narcotics, and\or corticosteroids. Early initiation of therapy is essential for optimal results. Although NSAIDs are generally the drug of choice in acute gouty arthritis, the clinician would be wise to consider the side effects of this class of medication, particularly in the elderly. For example, the incidence of peptic ulcer disease, gastritis, renal insufficiency, and fluid retention are all increased in the geriatric population [12]. Consequently, only short-term use of these drugs is recommended.

In young, healthy patients with recent onset of symptoms, colchicine can be a very effective treatment in up to 75% of cases. However, its use is limited by side effects and narrow therapeutic window [13], and it should be avoided in patients with renal or hepatic insufficiency. For theses reasons, it is often considered a second line therapy in the elderly. Corticosteroids, given intra-articularly or orally, or adrenocorticotropic hormone (ACTH) intra-muscularly or subcutaneously are another option to treat acute gout. Intra-articular steroids have come into favor because of the low risk of systemic side effects. Short courses of oral steroids are generally considered safe and side effects such as renal failure, fluid retention, ulcer disease, hyperten-sion, and hyperglycemia are rarely seen or short-lived [5], and are recom-mended when NSAIDs are contraindicated. Oral corticosteroids are particularly helpful in elderly patients who present with polyarticular disease in which intraarticular therapy is not practical. Parenteral ACTH has been shown to be effective in resolution of acute gouty arthritis in complicated patients with multiple medical problems for which NSAIDs or colchicine were contraindicated. However, there is no evidence to suggest that ACTH is superior to corticosteroids [14].

The second consideration in treatment of gout is to prevent further at-tacks that may lead to chronic arthritis. Prophylactic doses of colchicine may be used, if tolerated, and have shown to clearly diminish the rate of re-current attacks, irrespective of the serum urate concentration [13]. However, recurrent gouty attacks can also be prevented by lowering serum urate levels. One retrospective study of 267 patients with acute gout demonstrated a reduction in the frequency or prevention of future gouty attacks with the reduction of serum urate levels to 6 mg/dL [15]. This reduction in blood uric acid levels may be accomplished by either increasing excretion (with medi-cations such as probenecid), or by decreasing production (with medications such as allopurinol). Allopurinol is considered the drug of choice in the elderly, although dosing must be based on creatinine clearance [8].

Pseudogout

Pseudogout, like gout, is characterized by deposition of crystals into joints. As its name suggests, pseudogout often presents similarly to gout, and the two are frequently confused. The pathogenesis of pseudogout can be traced to the deposition of calcium pyrophosphate dihydrate (CPPD) crystals in articular cartilage, and is often referred to as CPPD deposition disease. This phenomenon, when visualized as intraarticular calcifications on plain radiography, is known as chondrocalcinosis. As with gout, the presence of crystals in the joints stimulates the influx of pro-inflammatory proteins and cells into the synovium leading to an inflammatory arthritis. Unlike gout, however, in which elevated serum urate levels lead to supersat-uration and deposition in joints, the CPPD crystals can invade a joint with-out a serum abnormality [12]. Several metabolic diseases associated with

CPPD disease include hyperparathyroidism, hypothyroidism, hypomagnesemia, hypophosphatemia, and hemachromatosis [7]. These disorders are seen in less than 5% of cases of pseudogout, making the majority of cases idiopathic [12].

Clinical presentation

CPPD disease can present in a variety of different manners. The three most common presentations include: (1) an acute attack of monoarthritis or polyarthritis mimicking gout, septic arthritis, or rheumatoid arthritis; (2) a chronic arthropathy mimicking osteoarthritis; or (3) an asymptomatic process that is discovered as an incidental radiologic finding. Frequently, however, acute pseudogout is characterized by an acute monoarthritis. The disease tends to occur in the elderly, in an equal distribution of females and males, with an average age at presentation of 65 years [16]. Although any joint may be afflicted, CPPD disease most commonly affects the knee and wrist joints, followed by the shoulder and the ankle. More than one joint is involved in about 10% of acute cases [7]. Although a flare may occur at any time, one study demonstrated that approximately 10% of patients manifested acute pseudogout after surgery, whereas 25% occurred during a severe intercurrent illness [16].

Chondrocalcinosis, while a common finding in older individuals, is uncommon in those younger than 40 years old. The incidence of this finding in the general population is estimated to be 10% to 15% in those aged 65 to 75, and over 40% in those over age 80 [7]. Chronic pyrophosphate arthropathy is typically seen in elderly women (older than 75 years) [16], who present with complaints of chronic pain, stiffness, and restricted movement of joints, particularly knees and wrists, with signs of synovitis on exam. The age-related increase in the diagnosis of chondrocalcinosis and osteoarthritis has led some to question if there may be a relationship between these two entities. In some patients, calcium crystal deposition can be quite indistinguishable from osteoarthritis—especially radiographically [7].

The diagnosis of CPPD disease is dependent on clinical presentation, findings of synovial fluid analysis, and radiographic films. Arthrocentesis of an acutely inflamed joint shows CPPD crystals that are pleiomorphic and weakly positively birefringent crystals under polarizing light. Generally, synovial fluid white blooc cell (WBC) counts will be 10,000 to 20,000/mm^3, but higher counts may be seen, and have been reported up to 80,000/mm^3 [16]. Plain radiographs commonly show calcification in the knee menisci, triangular ligaments of the wrists, and other cartilages [12]. Chondrocalcinosis may be punctate or linear, and occurs in fibrocartilage and hyaline cartilage [17]. As mentioned previously, pyrophosphate arthropathy can look indistinguishable from osteoarthritis on plain radiographs. Serum calcium, phosphate, urate, iron, and free thyroxin levels should be evaluated, given the small association of the disease with metabolic and endocrine disorders [16].

Treatment

Treatment of CPPD disease focuses on treatment of the pain and inflammation of acute attacks. Treatment modalities are similar to those for gout. NSAIDs and oral or intraarticular corticosteroids may be used for acute pain and inflammation. Aspiration of joint fluid can be helpful in significantly relieving pain and discomfort and increasing the mobility of affected joints. Colchicine, although shown to be helpful, is rarely necessary, as other less toxic modalities tend to be quite successful, and is only indicated in resistant cases [7]. Management of chronic pyrophosphate arthropathy is similar to that of osteoarthritis—pain control with NSAIDs, physical therapy, and intra- and periarticular steroid injection. End-stage disease may necessitate joint replacement.

Septic arthritis

Bacterial arthritis occurs in 2 to 10 per 100,000/year in the general population, 28 to 38 per 100,000/year in patients with rheumatoid arthritis [18], and 40 to 68 per 100,000/year in patients with prosthetic joints [19] It is the most rapidly destructive joint disease, and is most commonly a result of hematogenous seeding of joints from bacteremia. Less frequently, it is the result of joint surgery, direct inoculation by steroid injection, joint aspiration, animal or human bite, or other penetrating wound, or by direct extension from contiguous osteomyelitis. Reports of intraarticular steroid injection causing a septic joint have been reported as low as 18 cases in 250,000 [20]. The synovium is extremely vascular, and has no limiting basement membrane, allowing for relatively easy invasion of pathogens into the joint space [21].

Although numerous bacteria have been isolated from septic joints, the most common pathogen is *Staphylococcus aureus* [18]. This is followed by streptococci species, Gram negatives, including *Haemophilus influenza*, *Escherichia coli*, and Pseudomonas, and *Neisseria gonorrhea* [22]. In the United States, disseminated gonococcal infection is the most common cause of bacterial arthritis in young, healthy, sexually active adults, and occurs in 1% to 3% of untreated gonorrhea [23]. As a result, septic arthritis is generally divided into two categories in the literature—that resulting from gonococcal infection, and that which is nongonococcal in etiology. Interestingly, in Europe, disseminated gonococcal infection is rarely seen [18].

Nongonococcal septic arthritis is generally monoarticular, and most commonly affects the knee, but may also affect the shoulder, hip, wrist, elbow, and interphalangeal joints. More frequently an affliction of the elderly, the classic presentation includes the abrupt onset of a single, warm, edematous, painful joint. As mentioned above, the knee accounts for about 50% of infections, and up to 10% to 20% of infections may be polyarticular, with two or three joints involved. In addition, as many as 78% of patients may present with fever [24].

host factors that may predispose a patient to recurrent infections or
on of a joint space. Hosts with impaired defense mechanisms such
une deficiencies including HIV and diabetes, those with chronic con-
s such as liver failure or cancer, and intravenous drug users are at
r risk for infection [24]. Patients with defects in complement are at
ticularly high risk for disseminated gonococcal infection. Other host
rs including previous trauma, previous arthritis, or the presence of
sthetic joint increases the ability of a pathogen to seed a joint. Kaan-
et al [19] performed a prospective study to analyze those patients at in-
sed risk for septic arthritis and found that patients over the age of 80,
e with rheumatoid arthritis, diabetes mellitus, skin infection, and those
hip or knee prosthesis were significantly more likely to develop septic
ritis.

eatment

The case-fatality rate of septic arthritis is estimated to be 10% to 25%,
d as many as 50% of the surviving patients suffer a permanent loss of
int function as a result of the infection [19]. Therefore, septic arthritis is
onsidered a medical emergency requiring aggressive and early interven-
ion. Optimal therapy includes systemic antibiotics and surgical drainage.
Patients should be admitted to the hospital for parenteral broad-spectrum
antibiotics pending results of aspirate or drainage. A young, healthy, sexually active individual, should be treated with penicillin or cetriaxone/
ceftizoxime/cefotaxime for suspected disseminated gonococcal infection,
whereas, an elderly patient with suspected nongonococcal infection should
be treated more broadly for the most common causes of infection, namely
S aureus, streptococcal species, and Gram negatives. Empiric treatment generally includes a beta-lactam in combination with an aminoglycoside, or
a quinolone [18].

As discussed previously, culture-positive aspirates can prove difficult to
produce. As a result, response to treatment may be used as an indicator
of appropriate therapy. For example, gonococcal arthritis can be expected
to improve rapidly—typically within 24 to 48 hours of treatment. Although
no definitive studies on optimal antibiotic treatment length have been performed, 2 to 4 weeks of parenteral antibiotics followed by oral antibiotics
to complete a 4- to 6-week course is generally considered acceptable [26].
Drainage can be provided by repeated needle aspiration or with open surgical drainage if no clinical improvement, or if there is difficulty in attaining
repeated needle aspiration. Over 95% of patients with gonococcal arthritis
recover completely, while less than 50% of patients with staphylococcal infections recover without residual damage [24].

Special consideration should be given to the treatment of joint infections
in those with prostheses. In addition to antibiotics, therapy usually requires
open drainage and prosthesis removal because of the ability of the bacteria

Conversely, disseminated gonococcal infecti
in younger, healthier adults who frequently prese
pearing illness compared with that seen in nong(
coccal septic arthritis, although not unheard of, i:
cause of an infected joint in the elderly. The symp
gratory polyarthralgias, tenosynovitis, rash, and
may result in multiple tendons of multiple joints b(
taneously, while the rash is characterized by numer(
ing 3 to 4 days. These may appear as pustules, v(
macules, or papules. Disseminated gonococcal infe(
without a rash, but with a purulent arthritis that can
more commonly, asymmetric and polyarticular. Only
tients with disseminated gonococcal infection present
swollen, tender joint [24]. The difference in presentatio(
poorly understood, but is thought to be due to the varied
ent strains of gonorrhea or perhaps to presentation at dif(
same disease process [21].

Bacteriologic diagnosis

Definitive diagnosis of septic arthritis requires arthrocent(
fication of organisms by Gram stain or culture. Typically
analysis from a septic joint shows grossly purulent materi(
150,000 WBCs with a predominance of neutrophils. Although
agnosis is by identification of the organism, synovial fluid Gram
itive in only 50% of cases of nongonococcal arthritis and
gonococcal arthritis. Relatedly, synovial fluid cultures are p(
time with nongonococcal infection and only 50% of time with (
infection. Therefore, presumptive diagnosis of gonococcal arthri(
required if cultures are negative in the setting of a very high clini(
cion and positive urogenital cultures for gonorrhea. Genitourinary
are positive in 80% of patients with disseminated gonococcal infect(
Blood cultures are positive in 50% to 70% of patients with nongon(
arthritis [22]. The difficulty in recovering a positive Gram stain or cu(
suspected cases of disseminated gonococcal infection is likely due to t(
ficult in vitro growth requirements needed for *N. gonorrhea*. In a liter(
review by Swan et al [25], the sensitivity for culture was estimated to be
to 95% and 50% to 75% for Gram stain, in patients with nongonoco(
arthritis who had not been treated. These estimates decrease when includ(
patients who are treated with antibiotics before the joint aspiration. Becat(
of the high morbidity and mortality associated with septic arthritis, and le(
than ideal diagnostic testing, high clinical suspicion is essential when diag(
nosing septic arthritis.

It is important to remember that a relatively small number of individuals
who develop bacteremia subsequently develop septic arthritis. There are

to attach to the prosthetic material and the subsequent difficulty in eradicating these infections. Increased adverse outcomes have been seen in the elderly, in patients with preexisting joint disease, and in those joints containing synthetic material [27]. In these individuals, urgent orthopedic evaluation is warranted.

Osteoarthritis

Osteoarthritis, also known as degenerative joint disease, is the most common type of arthritis diagnosed in the elderly population. Estimates from the Rochester, Minnesota, community indicate an incidence of 600 to 1500 newly diagnosed cases of symptomatic hip or knee arthritis per 100,000 persons older than age 60 [12]. Men and women are affected equally, but symptoms occur earlier in women and appear more severe. In the Framingham Osteoarthritis Study, the prevalence of radiographically evident osteoarthritis was slightly higher in women than in men (although this difference was not statistically significant). However, symptomatic knee osteoarthritis was significantly higher in women than in men (11.4% compared with 6.8%). Furthermore, this study also revealed that the prevalence of osteoarthritis increases with age among persons over age 65, and about 40% of patients over the age of 80 had symptomatic knee osteoarthritis [28]. Other longitudinal studies have suggested that 4% of women per year experience progressive knee osteoarthritis, while 1% per year have the new onset of symptomatic knee arthritis [29].

The precise etiology of osteoarthritis is poorly understood. Although experience tells us that degenerative changes are the predominant factor leading to osteoarthritis, other key elements are yet to be completely elucidated. Part of the pathogenesis is thought to be related to abnormal function of chondrocytes. Normally, these cells are continuously replacing and remodeling articular cartilage. Interruption of this proccess, or an alteration in their conventional function is believed to contribute to osteoarthritis. Specifically, an aberration in aging chondrocytes that results in decreased function and responsiveness to stimuli results in a loss of tissue maintenance, loss of cartilage, and further leads to an increase in cartilage degradation and injury to articular bone surfaces. As a result, osteophyte and subchondral cyst formation ensues [30]. Risk factors for the development of osteoarthritis include age, joint immobilization, previous joint injury, joint instability, obesity, peripheral neuropathy, and prolonged joint stress from occupation or athletic activity. Maintenance of appropriate body weight may be the single most important preventative and controllable factor [31].

Clinical presentation

Those who are afflicted with osteoarthritis often seek health care because of joint pain. Typically polyarticular and symmetric in nature, the disease most often affects the distal interphalangeal joints, proximal interphalangeal joints, base of the thumb, knees, cervical and lumbar spine, and the first MTP joint [12]. More uncommon, osteoarthritis affecting the hip or acromioclavicular joints can cause severe limitations in ambulation and strength or range of motion of the upper extremity [32]. The pain of osteoarthritis is usually exacerbated by mild to moderate activity or joint use. As the disease progresses, prolonged joint stiffness and enlargement may become evident.

Diagnosis

The diagnosis of osteoarthritis is often a clinical one—based on a history of atraumatic joint pain in an elderly patient, which is worse with use and improves with rest [30]. Examination of the affected joint should be meticulous so as to differentiate this disorder from other disorders of the joints, including tendonitis, bursitis, or tenosynovitis. The joint is generally not erythematous, and there is no effusion present. Later in the disease, the clinician may elicit crepitus, as well as joint enlargement. Radiographs can help to confirm the diagnosis by demonstrating joint space narrowing, subchondral cysts, increased density of subchondral bone, or osteophytes. However, the absence of these radiographic abnormalities does not preclude the diagnosis. Synovial fluid analysis classically reveals few inflammatory cells. Generally, the aspirate of an osteoarthritic joint shows less than 2000 white cells/mm^3 with a predominance of mononucleated forms [33].

Treatment

As no treatment modality has been shown to affect the natural history of the disease, the clinician's therapy should be aimed at alleviating pain while improving function and quality of life [34]. Although NSAIDs are again a hallmark of conventional treatment, their side effect profile must be acknowledged, particularly in the elderly. Nephrotoxicity, gastritis and gastrointestinal bleeding, fluid retention in those with cardiomyopathy, and new literature suggesting a possible link to cardiovascular disease should temper the physician's eagerness to prescribe this class of medication. However, the short-term use of NSAIDs, if appropriately monitored, does safely provide many patients with relief of their pain. However, no study has demonstrated an advantage of NSAIDs over acetaminophen in the management of osteoarthritic pain, and some with acute pain may gain relief with intraarticular glucocorticoid injections [12]. Narcotic analgesics may be required during flares of disease, but again, should be used carefully in a geriatric population.

Finally, physical therapy and rehabilitation can play a crucial role in the treatment of those with osteoarthritis. Strengthening and stretching exercises, education and teaching of the use of assist devices to aid in ambulation, dressing, reaching, and bathing can maintain or restore a patient's ability to function independently. Aggressive physical and occupational therapy are critical in the management of patients with functional limitations [34]. Joint replacement is reserved for those who have intractable pain or whose ability to perform the necessary functions of daily living is severely impaired and recalcitrant to other therapeutic interventions [35].

Rheumatoid arthritis

Rheumatoid arthritis (RA) is a progressive, autoimmune arthritis characterized by a symmetric, peripheral polyarthritis. Epidemiologic studies have shown the overall prevalence of RA is about 1% in the Caucasian population [36], while the average annual incidence has been reported to be 34 to 42 per 100,000. The disease primarily affects the elderly and females—the incidence increases fourfold for those over age 50, and is two to three times more common in women [37]. One population study reported that RA was present in 2% of persons age 60 and older [38].

Diagnosis

The diagnosis of rheumatoid arthritis is based on the integration of clinical findings, radiologic findings, and laboratory tests. The American College of Rheumatology has published criteria for the diagnosis of rheumatoid arthritis. Patients must demonstrate: (1) morning stiffness in and around joints lasting at least 1 hour before maximal improvement; (2) soft tissue swelling of three or more joint areas; (3) swelling of the proximal interphalangeal, metacarpophalangeal, or wrist joints; (4) symmetric swelling; (5) rheumatoid nodules; (6) the presence of rheumatoid factor; and (7) radiographic erosions or periarticular osteopenia in hand or wrist joints. To fulfill the criteria, patients must demonstrate at least four of the above (criteria 1 through 4 must have been present for at least 6 weeks) [39].

Clinically, patients present with arthritis commonly affecting the hand, fingers, and wrist joints. The predominant symptoms are pain, stiffness, and swelling of peripheral joints. The disease is classically symmetric, providing one manner by which to separate from other arthritides such as gout or septic arthritis [40]. Although rheumatoid factor is present in the serum of 70% to 80% of patients with RA, it is neither sensitive nor specific, and can also be seen in those with lupus, Sjogren's syndrome, and even in some healthy individuals [41].

Treatment

As RA is a progressive and potentially debilitating disease, treatment focuses on pain management, delay or prevention of sequelae of the disease process, and promotion and maintenance of long-term function. In addition, recent advances in the understanding of the pathogenesis of RA have allowed for targeting of specific immune modulators that are believed to play a critical role in the development of the disease. Although the initiation of these medications is likely beyond the scope and expertise of the emergency physician, one should have a fundamental understanding of their role in the management of RA. In addition to the NSAIDs and corticosteroids that have classically been used to manage the disease, therapies include methotrexate, hydroxychloroquine, sulfasalazine, or newer specific anticytokine medications such as etanercept, infliximab, or anakinra [42]. Frequent reevaluation is necessary to determine maximal management and to avoid toxic side effects. In combination with pharmacologic therapy, physical and occupational therapy can improve motion and restore function. Reconstructive or prosthetic surgery is recommended in patients with end-stage joint disease causing intractable pain or intolerable functional limitation.

Polymyalgia rheumatica and giant cell arteritis

Polymyalgia rheumatica (PMR), originally described by Bruce in 1888, and coined "senile rheumatic gout" [43], and temporal arteritis are related conditions that involve an arthritis of the proximal joints, and nearly exclusively affect an older population. PMR and temporal arteritis, also referred to as giant cell arteritis (GCA), are thought to represent a spectrum of disease, but their true relationship is still not completely understood [44]. Although several studies have examined the prevalence of PMR, the lack of a "gold standard" definition has hampered accurate measurement. Several epidemiologic studies have suggested that the incidence of PMR increases with age, from 19.8 per 100,000/year in the 50 to 59 age group to 112 per 100,000/year in the 70 to 79 age group [45]. In a sample of women in the eighth decade of life, the incidence was as high as 168/100,000/year [46]. Relatedly, another study reported the incidence of giant cell arteritis in a Swedish population to be 28.6 per 100,000/year in those over age 50 [47]. This number also tends to increase with age, reaching a peak in those who are between 70 and 90. In addition, afflicted women outnumber men two to one [46,48,49].

Clinical presentation

Although no universally accepted, formal diagnostic criteria exist, PMR is characterized by pain and morning stiffness in the neck, shoulder girdle, and pelvic girdle, and often includes constitutional symptoms such as malaise, fatigue, anorexia, and fever. It rarely affects those less than 50 years old, and sedimentation rates are typically greater than 40 mm/h [45,50]. The muscle stiffness of PMR tends to ease through the day, and muscle strength is not impaired, but instead hindered by pain. Shoulder discomfort is the presenting finding in the majority of patients (70–95%), with the hip and neck being less frequently involved (50–70% of patients) [43]. The presentation of symmetric arthritis in an elderly female can easily result in it being mistakenly classified as rheumatoid arthritis [44]. Physical examination, however, will demonstrate a lack of synovitis, swelling, or warmth that are often seen with other arthritides. In addition, unlike RA, PMR is not a progressive disease process.

The clinical syndrome of giant cell arteritis is one of tenderness of the superficial temporal arteries, and partial occlusion of these vessels, which may result in severe headaches and can cause jaw claudication. In the most severe cases, ischemic optic neuropathy occurs due to occlusion of branches of the ophthalmic artery, presenting as sudden, painless visual loss—the most feared complication of GCA [51]. The American College of Rheumatology describes GCA as a disease affecting those over age 50 who have onset of new headache, temporal artery tenderness or decreased artery pulse, elevated erythrocyte sedimentation rate (ESR) greater than or equal to 50 mm/h, and arterial biopsy showing necrotizing arteritis, characterized by a predominance of mononuclear or multinucleated giant cell infiltrates The presence of three or more of the above criteria is associated with a sensitivity of 93.5% and specificity of 91.2% for the disease [52]. Several have reported on the relationship between GCA and PMR, indicating that PMR is seen in as many as 50% of those with biopsy-proven GCA [44,53]. Conversely, Salvarani [46] reported that 13% to 17% of patients with a diagnosis of PMR also had symptoms of GCA.

Treatment

Corticosteroids are the treatment of choice for both PMR and GCA. An initial dose of 10 to 20 mg of prednisone per day is often adequate to treat PMR, while GCA often requires initial doses of 40 to 60 mg per day. For those with impending visual loss, high-dose intravenous therapy is recommended [43]. As a general rule, the relief of arthritic symptoms is rapid (24–48 hours). A lack of improvement should cause one to question the original diagnosis [54]. Very slow tapering of the steroid treatment is necessary after response to avoid relapse of symptoms [43]. Most studies indicate that between one third and one half of patients can stop steroids after 2 years; however, relapses are more likely during the initial 18 months of treatment and within 1 year of withdrawal of steroids [51]. Again, the clinician must remember the side effects and complications associated with long-term steroid use in this elderly population.

Although the above is not an exhaustive description of the atraumatic arthritides that affect the elderly, it should serve as an introduction to several of the more common disease entities that the emergency physician encounters. Other such illnesses not discussed include systemic lupus erythematosus, mixed connective tissue disorders, fibromyalgia, and spondyloarthopathies, including reactive arthritis, psoriatic arthritis, and ankylosing spondylitis.

Cervical radicular limb pain

As one ages, degenerative changes in the cervical and lumbar spine predispose individuals to nerve root compression and adjacent inflammation.

The pain and neurologic sequelae can dramatically affect patients—particularly the elderly, who might have marginal reserve to overcome such limitations in movement, strength, and sensation. It has been reported that neck and back pain are common in the elderly, with one study indicating a 15% 1-month prevalence rate for back pain and 11% for neck pain [55].

Pathophysiology

Initially described by Parkinson in 1817, cervical radiculopathy identifies a constellation of signs and symptoms that are associated with altered function of cervical spine nerve roots. This may manifest itself as pain in the neck region as well as discomfort in a radicular distribution in one or both upper extremities. Additionally, the pain can occur in combination with sensory, motor, or reflex changes [56].

Although there are a number of disease processes that might affect the cervical spine and exiting nerve roots (vertebral fracture or dislocation, compression by tumor or abscess, vertebral collapse, spondylolisthesis, and trauma to cervical roots), cervical disc herniation and cervical spondylosis are the most common etiologies causing radicular symptoms of the upper extremities [57]. A 1969 study reported that 97% of patients with radiculopathy had radiographic evidence of foraminal stenosis [58]. Age-related alterations in the chemical structure of the nucleus pulposis and annulus fibrosus result in a disturbance of the normal architecture of the cervical spine. Specifically, there is a loss of height between the vertebral bodies as the discs bulge posteriorly into the spinal canal. As the vertebral bodies become closer to each other, there is infolding of the ligamentum flavum and facet joint capsule. The formation of osteophytes as part of a normal aging process, in combination with the posteriorly protruded disc material and redundant soft tissue, results in a reduction in the spinal canal and foraminal dimensions. This, in turn, may result in extrinsic compression of the nerve root or spinal cord [59]. The nerve roots of the cervical spine exit at nearly a horizontal orientation, in close proximity to the bone and disc—factors that are critical to the pathogenesis of nerve root compression and radiculopathy [57]. Specifically, the boundaries of the neuroforaminae include the uncovertebral joint anteromedially, facet joints, and articular processes posterolaterally, and pedicles of superior and inferior bodies both superiorly and inferiorly.

Although cervical radiculopathy is the most common reason for atraumatic limb pain, the clinician must remember to consider other etiologies for the upper extremity pain, weakness, or sensory deficits. Peripheral nerves are prone to compression and subsequent irritation at many points along their route from the spinal cord to the hand. Bony prominences, tendon sheaths, muscles, and vascular structures can all provide a substrate for nerve impingement and dysfunction. Although not discussed in detail here, carpel tunnel syndrome, pronator syndrome, and thoracic outlet syndrome are all examples of such disease entities [57,60,61].

History and physical examination

Although the clinical presentation of radiculopathies differ somewhat between individuals, the majority initially present with some combination of pain, weakness, and sensory loss. Henderson et al examined 736 patients who were diagnosed with cervical radiculopathy and reported that 99.4% had arm pain, 85.2% had sensory deficits, 79.7% had neck pain, 71.2% had reflex abnormalities, 68% had motor deficits, and 52.5% had scapular pain [62]. Radhakrishnan et al. performed an epidemiologic survey and reported similar results [56].

Although the variability in precise clinical presentation can make diagnosis difficult, patterns of signs and symptoms do allow for physicians to recognize some of the more common characteristics of particular nerve root dysfunction. Neurocompression at the C2–C3 level (which affects the exiting C3 root), is uncommon and results in pain and numbness in the head and nape of the neck that can be very difficult to separate from other syndromes such as tension headache. In addition, there is no specific motor weakness that is characteristic of this radiculopathy. Compression of the C4 root results in pain along the base of the neck with radiation to the shoulder and posteriorly to the scapula. C5 nerve root compression can cause numbness over the top of the shoulder and down the lateral arm. Patients experience pain throughout the shoulder, which is easily confused with that resulting from an injury to the shoulder joint. They may have weakness of the deltoid, limiting their ability to raise the arm on the affected side [57].

Compression of the C6 nerve root, which is more commonly encountered than those above, results in pain across the neck to the shoulder, down the arm along the biceps, into the radial aspect of the forearm, and to the back of the hand between or into the thumb and index finger. On examination, patients exhibit weakness of the biceps and wrist extensors and a decreased brachioradialis reflex. C7 radiculopathy, also common, causes pain across the posterior shoulder and arm through the posterolateral forearm with radiation toward the index finger. Examination of these patients often reveals weakness of the triceps, finger extensors, wrist flexors, and the pronator teres, along with a decrease in the triceps reflex. Sensory changes may be reported in the index finger and thumb. Finally, patients with significant C8 nerve root compression exhibit a decrease in sensation which primarily involves the fourth and fifth fingers, but which may extend proximally. Motor symptoms may include a decrease in fine motor control of the fingers, as small muscles of the hand such as the interossei are primarily affected [57].

In an attempt to alleviate the pain and neurologic symptoms of a cervical radiculopathy, patients may assume positions that increase the physical space in the neuroforaminae and decrease the tension on nerve roots. One such position, referred to as the "shoulder abduction sign," involves the patient raising their arm over their head and resting the hand or wrist on top of the head [63], or they may tilt their head to the contralateral side.

In contrast, the Spurling maneuver in which the lateral rotation of the head is toward the symptomatic side, may exacerbate the pain [64]. Provocative testing using these movements may be useful in discriminating between cervical radicular pain and muscular or joint pain from shoulder pathology.

Lumbar radiculopathy

As with cervical radiculopathy, lumbar radiculopathy can debilitate the young and old alike. In an analogous manner to cervical disease, age-related degeneration of vertebral architecture is thought to play a role in the pathophysiology of symptoms. In addition, studies have demonstrated that the low back pain can be experimentally reproduced with the injection of hypertonic saline into the supraspinous, intraspinous, and longitudinal ligaments, ligamenta flava, and facet-joint capsules [65]. Nerve fibers that innervate these structures, as well as the annulus fibrosus, are afferent branches of the posterior primary rami [66]. The efferent branches of these nerves innervate the paraspinal musculature, and by a poorly understood mechanism, trigger the muscle spasm that is often part of the low back pain syndrome [67].

The lifetime prevalence of low back pain has been estimated to be as high as 60% to 90%, with an annual incidence of 5% [68]. Men and women are believed to be similarly affected, with more women reporting symptoms after age 60 [69]. Lumbar pain and radiculopathy can result from a number of disease processes. As one might expect, treatment options vary widely, and include conservative therapies such as bed rest, oral medications, lumbar corsets, and physical therapy. Failing these, some studies have demonstrated that nerve root injections with anesthetics and corticosteroids may obviate the need for surgical intervention [70]. Although many will improve with these less aggressive treatments, some patients will require surgery [71].

Of those with acute low back pain, a relatively small number (approximately 1%) experience true sciatica—defined as pain in the distribution of a lumbar nerve root, often accompanied by neurosensory and motor deficits. In addition to epidemiologic studies reporting an association between low back pain and factors such as occupation and certain psychologic profiles, several physiologic factors that increase in frequency with aging have been implicated in the pathogenesis of low back pain and sciatica. These include isthmic spondylolisthesis, osteoarthritis, disc disease, osteoporosis, and spinal stenosis [67]. Intervertebral disc herniations are the most common cause of lumbar radiculopathy, and 10% to 15% of these patients will eventually require surgical intervention [72]. When these conditions cause irritation and inflammation of nerve roots, limb pain and weakness can ensue. An inability to ambulate, increased susceptibility to falls, and difficulty caring for oneself may become serious concerns for the elderly patient.

In the elderly in particular, however, the clinician would be wise to consider etiologies other than musculoskeletal disorders as the cause of back or leg pain. For example, aortic aneurysm, pancreatitis, pancreatic tumor, kidney diseases, and sickle cell disease have all been known to mimic more benign causes of back and leg pain [73].

Spinal stenosis

Stenosis of the spine is defined as narrowing of the spinal canal, which may result in pain, radicular symptoms, and lower extremity claudication. Initially described by Henk Verbiest in 1954 [74], it is becoming a more frequently recognized etiology of low back pain, particularly in the elderly [75]. Formerly a diagnosis made by myelography, the advent of axial imaging with CT and MRI has allowed physicians to document the presence and extent of canal stenosis with relative ease.

Stenosis of the lumbar spine can be classified as that resulting from congenital–developmental abnormalities, and that which is a consequence of degenerative changes of the spine. Most commonly occurring between the third and fourth and fourth and fifth vertebrae of the lumbar spine, symptoms of degenerative stenosis usually do not develop until one reaches 60 years old (some argue that it is nearly exclusively a disease of those older than 50 years) [76,77]. As our population ages and average lifespans increase, the prevalence of diseases such as lumbar spinal stenosis also should be expected to increase. Alterations in the normal architecture of an aging spine, including changes in the zygapophyseal joints, ligamentum flavum, intervertebral discs, epidural venous structures, laminae, and pedicles, can result in impingement on the spinal canal and irritation and inflammation of exiting nerve roots [78].

Natural history

Lumbar spinal stenosis generally presents as either back or leg pain, which is exacerbated by standing and walking (especially on flat surfaces or downhill—positions in which the spine is extended), and relieved by sitting or lying with the hips flexed (resulting in flexion of the lumbar spine). Physical examination may demonstrate mild weakness of the lower extremities, but localizing symptoms and findings are generally not present, and provocative testing with straight leg testing is not revealing. Treatment options are varied, and include conservative therapy such as bed rest, analgesics, and back support, but may also involve more aggressive measures such as surgical decompression or caudal epidural blocks.

Although there are no prospective, randomized, controlled trials of various treatment modalities in lumbar spinal stenosis (one can imagine that it would be difficult to deny a patient who is in severe pain a particular therapy), there have been several short, observational prospective studies. Johnsson et al [79] presented a series of 32 patients, observed over 49 months, in which 15% improved, 70% remained unchanged, and 14%

deteriorated at 4 years. The Maine Lumbar Study reported on 67 surgically treated and 52 conservatively treated patients who were observed for a 4-year period. Their results indicated that patient satisfaction after 4 years of treatment was higher in those treated surgically (63–42%). The benefit of surgery, however, was noted to decline over time, whereas the symptoms of nonsurgically treated patients improved modestly and remained stable over 4 years [80]. In one slightly larger investigation, 100 patients, were followed for 10 years. In this study, 19 patients with severe symptoms were treated surgically, and 50 patients with moderate symptoms were treated nonoperatively. The remaining 31 patients were randomized between the two treatment arms. Of those who initially did not have surgery, 29% had to undergo delayed surgical intervention because of deterioration [81]. None of these studies, however, addressed the elderly as a separate population.

Although there is clearly some percentage of patients who will fail conservative therapy, no studies have been able to identify predictors that would allow the clinician to identify those who will need an operation to alleviate their symptoms. Furthermore, those who initially favor a nonsurgical approach will still benefit from the operation if it becomes necessary. Thus, many argue that all patients should be offered a trial of nonoperative therapy initially [82]. Finally, most agree that the only true indications for surgical intervention are intractable pain after the failure of conservative measures, and the presence of bowel or bladder dysfunction, or progressive neurologic deficit in a radicular distribution [82].

In a geriatric population, in which the side effects of narcotic analgesia may be intolerable, or patient comorbidities or preference may preclude surgery, some have suggested that epidural blocks might provide a valuable alternative. A relatively small study involving epidural injections of Xylocaine and Depo-Medrol in elderly patients (average age 76) with MRI-documented lumbar spinal stenosis demonstrated significant pain relief and very few complications [73]. Although this study only followed patients for 10 months after therapy, it suggests that local injection provides adequate pain relief in a patient population that might not tolerate other treatment modalities. Not surprisingly, a 1996 study reported an increase in mortality and complications in spinal stenosis surgery in patients who were older [83]. There are, however, no randomized controlled studies comparing conservative and invasive therapies in the geriatric population, and the encouraging results of the above study have not been reproduced in some additional studies involving all age groups [84].

Gait disturbances

Disturbances of gait are extremely common in the elderly, and lead to significant morbidity and mortality. One population based study suggested that 15% of people over 60 years old had some abnormality of gait [85], while another examining a cohort of 79 year olds reported that 25% used some form of mechanical aid for ambulation [86]. Accidental deaths, many of which are the result of falls, are a significant cause of death and disability in the elderly. A loss of balance or misstep can lead to head injuries, orthopedic injuries such as hip fractures, and a fear of falling, which may severely restrict an elder's ability to care for himself and live independently. A 1981 study reported that half of elders surveyed reported that their fear of falling limited their activity [87].

As one ages, a number of physiologic changes occur that significantly impact gait and balance. To begin, the amount of sway while erect has been shown to intensify with increasing age [88]. As one becomes older, the reliance on proprioception to prevent falls increases, while the efficiency of the motor and sensory systems that relay the information necessary for one to comprehend the position of their limbs in space becomes less efficient and accurate [89]. Disease processes that affect the neurologic system are particularly critical to the integration of numerous sensory and motor pathways that are critical for balance and ambulation. For example, cervical myelopathy, Parkinson's disease, stroke and resulting hemiparesis, and normal pressure hydrocephalus can significantly impact the gait of elders.

Myelopathy

Myelopathy, often the result of cervical spondylosis, is a common cause of gait instability in the geriatric patient. Degenerative osteophytes in the cervical spine impinge on the spinal canal and spinal cord, causing the typical clinical findings of spasticity and hyperreflexia of the legs, dorsal column signs, and urinary urgency. The gait of these individuals is usually stiff-legged with reduced toe clearance. Although imaging may reveal characteristic osteophytes, neck pain and radicular symptoms of the upper extremities are not universally present [89].

Parkinson's Disease

Parkinson's Disease affects approximately 1.8% of the population over age 65 [90]. The gait of afflicted individuals can be described as one of flexed posture, lessened arm swing, and a difficulty with the initiation of movement and turning. This may be so severe that a patient may remain still until given a small push allowing the legs to move forward [91]. In addition, there is often a decrease in balance as the disease progresses. Although medical therapy may improve the gait, the disturbance of balance may not recover.

Stroke

An alteration of gait is the presenting complaint in those who have experienced a cerebrovascular accident in more patients than one might initially expect. Although a large stroke resulting in hemiparesis may be clinically obvious, those that result in a loss of proprioception or sensation in the feet or legs may be more subtle. In one series, 16% of those with an abnormal gait had evidence of cerebral infarcts on CT scan, but no history of hemiparesis or major motor deficit from a stroke [92]. Persistent falling to one side, difficulty in initiating movement, shuffling gait, poor standing balance, and difficulty raising feet off of the ground during ambulation should alert the clinician to the possibility of stroke. Imaging of the brain with CT or MRI may reveal infarcts in the basal ganglia, cerebellum, or periventricular white matter [89].

Normal pressure hydrocephalus

Initially described in 1965, normal pressure hydrocephalus (NPH) is a syndrome of "slowness and paucity of thought and action, unsteadiness of gait, and unwitting urinary incontinence" in the setting of a cerebrospinal fluid pressure of less than 180 mmHg [93]. The gait of afflicted patients can be described as that of shuffling feet, reduced speed, unsteady turning, and poor balance [94,95]. Improvement after the removal of 49 to 50 mL of cerebrospinal fluid may be both diagnostic and therapeutic [96]; however, the magnitude of improvement can differ substantially [94]. In addition, the gait abnormalities of NPH may precede dementia by months, or even years [97].

Although the above are some of the more common etiologies of unstable gait, the complete list is exceptionally long. In the elderly in particular, the clinician would be wise to also consider infectious diseases such as neurosyphillis, metabolic disorders such as uremia or hepatic failure, medications such as benzodiazepines and neuroleptics, spinal cord lesions such as cervical tumors and posterior column degeneration, peripheral neuropathies, vitamin B12 deficiency, and mechanical conditions such as osteoarthritis, which may result in an antalgic gait. In as many as 20% of elderly patients with abnormal gait, no specific etiology is identified [98].

In summary, the geriatric patient may present with a wide range of complaints related to atraumatic joint and limb pain. The emergency physician may be the first clinician to evaluate these complaints, and early diagnosis and treatment may prevent further morbidity. Finally, therapy should be tailored to the patient, with careful consideration of both the medical and social impacts of the disease and treating medications.

References

[1] Monu MB, Pope TL. Gout: a clinical and radiologic review. Radiol Clin North Am 2004; 42(1):169–84.
[2] Abbott RD, Brand FN, Kannel WB, et al. Gout and coronary artery disease: the Framingham Study. J Clin Epidemiol 1988;41(3):237–42.
[3] Agudelo CA, Wise CM. Geriatric rheumatology: crystal-associated arthritis in the elderly. Rheum Dis Clin North Am 2004;26(3):527–46.
[4] Terkeltaub RA. Gout. N Engl J Med 2003;349(17):1647–55.

[5] Fam AG. Gout in the elderly: clinical presentation and treatment. Drugs Aging 1998;13(3): 229–43.

[6] Campell SM. Gout: how presentation, diagnosis, and treatment differ in the elderly. Geriatrics 1988;43(11):71–7.

[7] Doherty M, Dieppe P. Crystal deposition disease in the elderly. Rheum Dis Clin North Am 1986;12(1):97–111.

[8] Gonzalez EB, Miller SB, Agudelo CA. Optimal management of gout in older patients. Drugs Aging 1994;4(2):128–34.

[9] MacFarlane DG, Dieppe PA. Diuretic-induced gout in elderly women. Br J Rheumatol 1985;24(2):155–7.

[10] Gurwitz JH, Kalish SC, Bohn RL, et al. Thiazide diuretics and the initiation of antigout therapy. J Clin Epidemiol 1997;50(8):953–9.

[11] Agudelo CA, Weinberger A, Schumacher HR, et al. Definitive diagnosis of gout by identification of urate crystals in asymptomatic metatarsophalangeal joints. Arthritis Rheum 1979;22(5):559–60.

[12] Michet CJ Jr, Evans JM, Fleming KC, et al. Common rheumatologic disease in elderly patients. Mayo Clin Proc 1995;70(12):1205–14.

[13] Emmerson BT. The management of gout. N Engl J Med 1996;334(7):445–51.

[14] Ritter J, Kerr LD, Valeriano-Marcet J, et al. ACTH revisted: effective treatment for acute crystal induced synovitis in patients with multiple medical problems. J Rheumatol 1994; 21(4):696–9.

[15] Shoji A, Yamanaka H, Kamatani N. A retrospective study of the relationship between serum urate level and recurrent attacks of gouty arthritis: evidence for reduction of recurrent gouty arthritis with antihyperuricemic therapy. Arthritis Rheum 2004;51(3):321–5.

[16] Bonafede RP. Evaluating CPPD crystal deposition, an important disease of aging. Geriatrics 1988;43(11):59–68.

[17] Sagarin MJ. Pseudogout. J Emerg Med 2000;18(3):373–4.

[18] Goldenberg DL. Septic arthritis. Lancet 1998;351(9097):197–202.

[19] Kaandorp CJ, Van Schaardenburg D, Krijnen P, et al. Risk factors for septic arthritis in patients with joint disease: a prospective study. Arthritis Rheum 1995;38(12):1819–25.

[20] Hollander JL. Intrasynovial corticosteroid therapy in arthritis. Md State Med J 1970;19(3): 62–6.

[21] Shirtliff ME, Mader JT. Acute septic arthritis. Clin Microbiol Rev 2002;15(4):527–44.

[22] Ryan MJ, Kavanaugh R, Wall PG, et al. Bacterial joint infection England and Wales: analysis of bacterial isolates over a four year period. Br J Rheumatol 1997;36(3):370–3.

[23] Dubost JJ, Soubrier M, DeChamps C, et al. No changes in the distribution of organisms responsible for septic arthritis over a 20 year period. Ann Rheum Dis 2002;61(3):267–9.

[24] Goldenberg DL, Reed JI. Bacterial arthritis. N Engl J Med 1985;312(12):764–71.

[25] Swan A, Amer H, Dieppe P. The value of synovial fluid assays in the diagnosis of joint disease: a literature survey. Ann Rheum Dis 2002;61(6):493–8.

[26] Gupta MN, Sturrock RD, Field M. Prospective comparative study of patients with culture proven and high suspicion of adult onset septic arthritis. Ann Rheum Dis 2003;62(4):327–31.

[27] Kaandorp CJ, Krijnen P, Moens HJB, et al. The outcome of bacterial arthritis: a prospective community-based study. Arthritis Rheum 1997;40(5):884–92.

[28] Felson DT, Naimark A, Anderson J, et al. The prevalence of knee osteoarthritis in the elderly: the Framingham Osteoarthritis Study. Arthritis Rheum 1987;30(8):914–8.

[29] Felson DT, Zhang Y, Hannan MT, et al. The incidence and natural history of knee osteoarthritis in the elderly: the Framingham Osteoarthritis Study. Arthritis Rheum 1995;38(10): 1500–5.

[30] Hinton R, Moody RL, Davis AW, et al. Osteoarthritis: diagnosis and therapeutic considerations. Am Fam Physician 2002;65(5):841–8.

[31] Felson DT, Zhang Y, Hannan MT, et al. Risk factors for incident radiographic knee osteoarthritis in the elderly: the Framingham Study. Arthritis Rheum 1997;40(4):728–33.

[32] Buttaci CJ, Stitik TP, Yonclas PP, et al. Osteoarthritis of the acromioclavicular joint: a review of anatomy, biomechanics, diagnosis, and treatment. Am J Phys Med Rehabil 2004; 83(10):791–7.

[33] Siva C, Velazquez C, Mody A, et al. Diagnosing acute monoarthritis in adults: a practical approach for the family physician. Am Fam Phycician 2003;68(1):83–90.

[34] American College of Rheumatology Subcommittee on Osteoarthritis Guidelines. Recommendations for the medical management of osteoarthritis of the hip and knee: 2000 update. Arthritis Rheum 2000;43(9):1905–15.

[35] Hawker GA, Wright JG, Badley EM, et al. Perceptions of, and willingness to consider, total joint arthroplasty in a population-based cohort of individuals with disabling hip and knee arthritis. Arthritis Rheum 2004;51(4):635–41.

[36] Spector TD. Rheumatoid arthritis. Rheum Dis Clin North Am 1990;16(3):513–37.

[37] Chan KA, Felson DT, Yood RA, et al. Incidence of rheumatoid arthritis in central Massachusetts. Arthritis Rheum 1993;36(12):1691–6.

[38] Rasch EK, Hirsch R, Paulose-Ram R, et al. Prevalence of rheumatoid arthritis in persons 60 years of age and older in the United States: effect of different methods of case classification. Arthritis Rheum 2003;48(4):917–26.

[39] Arnett FC, Edworthy SM, Bloch DA, et al. The American Rheumatism Association 1987 revised criteria for the classification of rheumatoid arthritis. Arthritis Rheum 1988;31(3): 315–24.

[40] Lee DM, Weinblatt ME. Rheumatoid arthritis. Lancet 2001;358(9285):903–11.

[41] Shmerling RH, Delbanco TL. The rheumatoid factor: an analysis of clinical utility. Am J Med 1991;91:528–34.

[42] American College of Rheumatology Subcommittee on Rheumatoid Arthritis Guidelines. Guidelines for the management of rheumatoid arthritis: 2002 update. Arthritis Rheum 2002;46(2):328–46.

[43] Salvarini C, Cantini F, Boiardi L, et al. Medical progress: polymyalgia rheumatic and giant cell arteritis. N Engl J Med 2002;347(4):261–71.

[44] Cantini F, Niccoli L, Storri L, et al. Are polymyalgia rheumatica and giant cell arteritis the same disease? Semin Arthritis Rheum 2004;33(5):294–301.

[45] Chuang TY, Hunder GG, Ilstrup DM, et al. Polymyalgia rheumatica: a 10-year epidemiologic and clinical study. Ann Intern Med 1982;97(5):672–80.

[46] Salvarani C, Gabriel SE, O'Fallon WM, et al. Epidemiology of polymyalgia rheumatica in Olmsted County, Minnesota, 1970–1991. Arthritis Rheum 1995;38(3):369–73.

[47] Bengtsson BA, Malmvall BE. The epidemiology of giant cell arteritis including temporal arteritis and polymyalgia rheumatica. Incidences of different clinical presentations and eye complications. Arthritis Rheum 1981;24(7):899–904.

[48] Salvarani C, Crowson CS, O'Fallon WM, et al. Reappraisal of the epidemiology of giant cell arteritis in Olmstead County, Minnesota, over a fifty-year period. Arthritis Rheum 2004; 51(2):264–8.

[49] Boesen P, Sorensen SF. Giant cell arteritis, temporal arteritis, and polymyalgia rheumatica in a Danish county. A prospective investigation, 1982–1985. Arthritis Rheum 1987;30(3) 294–9.

[50] Healey LA. Long-term follow-up of polymyalgia rheumatica: evidence for synovitis. Sem Arthritis Rheum 1984;13(4):322–7.

[51] Swannell AJ. Fortnightly review: polymyalgia rheumatica and temporal arteritis: diagnosis and management. BMJ 1997;314(7090):1329–32.

[52] Hunder GG, Bloch DA, Michel BA, et al. The American College of Rheumatology 1990 criteria for the classification of giant cell arteritis. Arthritis Rheum 1990;33(8):1122–8.

[53] Gonzalez-Gay MA. Giant cell arteritis and polymyalgia rheumatica: two different but often overlapping conditions. Sem Arthritis Rheum 2004;33(5):289–93.

[54] Brooks RC, McGee SR. Diagnostic dilemmas in polymyalgia rheumatica. Arch Intern Med 1997;157(2):162–8.

[55] Hartvigsen JDC, Christensen K, Frederiksen H. Back and neck pain exhibit many common features in old age: a population-based study of 4,486 Danish twins 70–102 years of age. Spine 2004;29(5):576–80.

[56] Radhakrishnan K, Litchy WJ, O'Fallon WM, et al. Epidemiology of cervical radiculopathy: a population-based study from Rochester, Minnestoa, 1976 through 1990. Brain 1994;117: 325–35.

[57] Ahlgren BD, Garfin SR. Cervical radiculopathy. Orthop Clin North Am 1996;27(2):253–63.

[58] Wilkinson HA, LeMay ML, Ferris EJ. Clinical-radiographic correlations in cervical spondylosis. J Neurosurg 1969;30(3):213–8.

[59] Rao R. Neck pain, cervical radiculopathy, and cervical myelopathy: pathophysiology, natural history, and clinical evaluation. J Bone Joint Surg Am 2002;84-A(10):1872–81.

[60] Younger DS. Entrapment neuropathies. Primary Care Clin Office Pract 2004;31(1):52–65.

[61] Viera AJ. Management of carpel tunnel sundrome. Am Fam Physician 2003;68(2):265–72.

[62] Henderson CM, Hennessy RG, Shuey HM Jr, et al. Posterior-lateral foraminotomy as an exclusive operative technique for cervical radiculopathy: a review of 846 consecutively operated cases. Neruosurgery 1983;13:504–12.

[63] Davidson RI, Dunn EJ, Metzmaker JN. The shoulder abduction test in the diagnosis of radicular pain in cervical extradural compressive monoradiculopathies. Spine 1981;6(5): 441–6.

[64] Levitz CL, Reily PJ, Torg JS. The pathomechanics of chronic, recurrent cervical nerve toor neurapraxia. The chronic burner syndrome. Am J Sports Med 1997;25(1):73–6.

[65] Hirsch C, Ingelmark B-E, Miller M. The anatomical basis for low back pain: studies on the presence of sensory nerve endings in ligamentous, capsular, and intervertebral disc structures in the human lumbar spine. Acta Orthp Scand 1963;33:1–17.

[66] Wyke B. Receptor systems in lumbrosacral tissues in relation to the production of low back pain. In: White AA, Gordon SL, editors. American Academy of Orthopaedic Surgeons Symposium on idiopathic low back pain. St. Louis (MO): C.V. Mosby; 1982. p. 97–107.

[67] Frymoyer JW. Back pain and sciatica. N Engl J Med 1988;318(5):291–300.

[68] Frymoyer JW, Pope MH, Clements JH, et al. Risk factors in low-back pain: an epidemiological survey. J Bone Joint Surg 1983;65-A(2):213–8.

[69] Biering-Sørensen F. Physical measurements as risk indicators for low-back trouble over a one year period. Spine 1984;9(2):106–19.

[70] Riew KD, Yin Y, Gilula L, et al. The effect of nerve-root injections on the need for operative treatment o flumbar radicular pain: a prosective, randomized, controlled, double-blind study. J Bone Joint Surg Am 2000;82-A(11):1589–93.

[71] Vad VB, Bhat AL, Lutz GE, et al. Transforaminal epidural steroid injections in lumbosacral radiculopathy: a prospective randomized study. Spine 2002;27(1):11–5.

[72] Bush K, Cowan N, Katz DE, et al. The natural history of sciatica with associated disc pathology: a prospective study with clinical and independent radiologic follow-up. Spine 1992; 17(10):1205–12.

[73] Ciocon JO, Galindo-Ciocon D, Amaranath L, et al. Caudal epidural blocks for elderly patients with lumbar canal stenosis. J Am Geriatr Soc 1994;42(6):593–6.

[74] Verbiest H. A radicular syndrome from developmental narrowing of the lumbar vertebral canal. J Bone Joint Surg 1954;36:230–7.

[75] Taylor VM, Deyo RA, Cherkin DC, et al. Low back pain hospitalization. Recent United States trends and regional variations. Spine 1994;19(11):1207–12.

[76] Hall S, Bartleson J, Onofrio BM, et al. Lumbar spinal stenosis. Clinical features, diagnostic procedures, and results of surgical treatment in 68 patients. Ann Intern Med 1985;103(2): 271–5.

[77] Clinchot DM, Kaplan PE, Lamb JF. Lumbar spinal stenosis in an elderly patient. J Gerontol 1998;53A(1):M72–5.

[78] Spengler DM. Degenerative stenosis of the lumbar spine. J Bone Joint Surg 1987;69-A(2): 305–8.

[79] Johnsson KE, Rosen I, Uden A. The natural course of lumbar spinal stenosis. Clin Orthop 1992;279:82–6.
[80] Atlas SJ, Keller RB, Robson D, et al. Surgical and nonsurgical management of lumbar spinal stenosis: four year outcomes from the Maine Lumbar Spine Study. Spine 2000;25(5):556–62.
[81] Amundsen T, Weber H, Nordal HJ, et al. Lumbar spinal stenosis: conservative or surgical management? A prospective 10-year study. Spine 2000;25(11):1424–35.
[82] Sengupta DK, Herkowitz HN. Lumbar spinal stenosis: treatment strategies and indications for surgery. Orthop Clin North Am 2003;34(2):281–95.
[83] Ciol MA, Deyo RA, Howell E, et al. An assessment of surgery for spinal stenosis: time trends, geographic variations, complications, and reoperations. J Am Geriatr Soc 1996; 44(3):285–90.
[84] Cuckler JM, Bernini PA, Wiesel SW, et al. The use of epidural steroids in the treatment of lumbar radicular pain. A prospective, randomized, double-blind study. J Bone Joint Surg Am 1985;67(1):63–6.
[85] Newman G, Dovenmuehle RH, Busse EW. Alterations in neurologic status with age. J Am Geriatr Soc 1960;8:915–7.
[86] Lundgren-Lindquist B, Aniansson A, Rundgren Å. Functional studies in 79-year-olds: walking performance and climbing capacity. Scand J Rehabil Med 1983;15(3):125–31.
[87] Imms FJ, Edholm OG. Studies of gait and mobility in the elderly. Age Ageing 1980;10(3): 147–56.
[88] Sheldon JH. The effect of age on the control of sway. Gerontol Clin (Basel) 1963;5:129–38.
[89] Desforges JF. Geriatrics: gait disorders in the elderly. N Engl J Med 1990;322(20):1441–6.
[90] Ben-Shlomo Y. How far are we in understanding the cause of Parkinson's disease? J Neurol Neurosurg Psychiatry 1999;61(1):4–16.
[91] Cunha UV. Differential diagnosis of gait disorders in the elderly. Geriatrics 1988;43(8):33–8.
[92] Sudarsky L, Ronthal M. Gait disorders among elderly patients: a survey study of 50 patients. Arch Neurol 1983;40(12):740–3.
[93] Adans RD, Fisher CM, Hakim S, et al. Symptomatic occult hydrocephalus with "normal" cerebrospinal-fluid pressure: a treatable syndrome. N Engl J Med 1965;273:117–26.
[94] Alexander NB. Gait disorders in older adults. J Am Geriatr Soc 1996;44(4):434–51.
[95] Sudarsky L, Simon S. Gait disorders in late-life hydrocephalus. Arch Neurol 1987;44(3): 263–7.
[96] Wikkelsø C, Andersson H, Blomstrand C, et al. The clinical effect of lumbar puncture in normal pressure hydrocephalus. J Neurol Neurosurg Psychiatry 1982;45(1):64–9.
[97] Fisher CM. Hydrocephalus as a cause of disturbances of gait in the elderly. Neurology 1982; 32(12):1358–63.
[98] Koller WC, Glatt SL, Fox JH. Senile gait: a distinct neurologic entity. Clin Geriatr Med 1985;1(3):661–9.

ELSEVIER
SAUNDERS

Emerg Med Clin N Am
24 (2006) 413–432

EMERGENCY
MEDICINE
CLINICS OF
NORTH AMERICA

Trauma and Falls in the Elderly

Miriam T. Aschkenasy, MD, MPH*, Todd C. Rothenhaus, MD, FACEP

*Department of Emergency Medicine, Boston Medical Center, Dowling 1 South,
One Boston Medical Center Place, Boston, MA 02115, USA*

The United States' population is living longer than ever before. The average American life span has increased by almost 30 years in the past century, from 47 years in the early 1900s to 76 years in 2000. It is predicted that the number of people over the age of 85 will likely double by the year 2020, and that by 2050 people over age 64 will make up over 20% of the US population compared with 12% today [1].

Trauma is the fifth leading cause of death in patients over the age of 65 [2]. The elderly sustain a disproportionate share of fractures and serious injury, accounting for approximately 28% of deaths due to trauma while representing only 12% of the overall trauma population [3].

Trauma in the elderly poses special challenges. Physiologic changes impact morbidity and mortality. Geriatric patients have different injury patterns that impact care [4]. Older victims of trauma may have significant comorbid medical conditions and may be taking medications that can complicate injury and resuscitation.

Until the early 1980s, trauma research traditionally focused on the pediatric and young adult population, and few studies focused specifically on the elderly [5]. Since that time, a plethora of studies have been performed on geriatric trauma. Unfortunately, most have been retrospective trauma registry reviews. Few prospective and even fewer randomized controlled trials have been performed. Much of the literature on geriatric trauma remains to be written [6].

Although it is clear that morbidity and mortality from major trauma in the geriatric population is high, the vast majority of patients survive to hospital discharge, and a significant percentage return to their previous levels of function and activities of daily living [7–9].

* Corresponding author.
E-mail address: maschkemd@hotmail.com (M.T. Aschkenasy).

0733-8627/06/$ - see front matter © 2006 Elsevier Inc. All rights reserved.
doi:10.1016/j.emc.2006.01.005   *emed.theclinics.com*

Every day, throughout the United States, patients are overtriaged to trauma canters, and undertriaged to local hospitals. The role of emergency physicians is paramount to the treatment of elderly victims of trauma. It is incumbent on all emergency physicians, regardless of venue, to take a consistent and thorough approach to the management of geriatric trauma patients. By identifying occult instability, resuscitating and stabilizing the victim, identifying important injuries and relevant comorbidities, and making an appropriate hospital disposition of transfer, emergency physicians can have a tremendous impact on the morbidity and mortality of geriatric trauma patients.

This article reviews the current literature on the management of elderly patients with trauma. We begin with a discussion of the physiologic changes of aging, and the impact of comorbidities and medications, that particularly influence management and outcome. We then turn to mechanisms of injury distinctive to geriatric trauma. We then discuss aspects particular to the resuscitation of geriatric trauma victims, focusing on pitfalls in evaluation and injury patterns unique to the geriatric patient. We also include a discussion of the evaluation and management of falls in the elderly, including assessment of fall risk.

The physiology of aging

It is clear that the effects of aging do not begin abruptly at 65 years of age. In a study of nearly 200,000 trauma patients, it was determined that mortality from severe trauma begins to increase at the age of 40 years [10]. For each 1-year increase in age over 65, the odds of dying after trauma increases by over 6% [11].

Aging can be defined as the normal, predictable, and irreversible changes of various organ systems over the passage of time that ultimately lead to death. Physiologic changes that occur with age affect patients in a number of ways, but generally results in a loss of functional reserve in most organ systems.

The effects of aging should not be confused with coexisting disease. Although distinguishing the effects of aging from the effects of disease may be difficult, the presence of comorbidity impacts the morbidity and mortality from trauma independent of the normal process of aging [2,12]. For example, it is clear that the bones of elderly patients are less able to withstand the mechanical forces of trauma, and that injuries occur with the transmission of less kinetic energy than in younger patients. This effect acts synergistically with the disease of osteoporosis, making the incidence of fractures in patients with osteoporosis significantly higher than in age-matched patients without the disease, and the incidence of fractures in elderly patients higher than in children or younger adults.

Cardiac functional reserve is diminished with age. Older patients have a lower cardiac output, decreased cardiac reserve, and are less likely to be able to tolerate hemodynamic stress as well as younger patients. Aging of the electrical conducting system, or pharmacologic activity of beta-blockers or calcium blockers, result in a decrease heart rate response to catecholamines. It is well known that elderly patients can have a blunted inotropic and chronotropic response to trauma. Compensatory tachycardia, seen almost universally in young patients in response to hypovolemia or shock, is frequently absent. The less vigilant clinician can miss significant hemorrhage or easily underestimate severity of illness [13–19].

Superimposed on the normal effects of age on the heart may be the presence of heart failure, which may further diminish cardiac output; heart block, which can further blunt the rate response to stress; and coronary artery disease, which may manifest as demand ischemia during the stress of trauma. The risk of an acute cardiac event must be considered in every case of trauma in the elderly. An ECG is mandatory early in the workup.

Pulmonary changes with age include a loss of elasticity in the chest wall and lungs, leading to decreased mechanical compliance and an increase in baseline work of breathing. Alveolar loss and decreased diffusion capacity result in an age-dependent decline in arterial oxygen tension. As a result, a patient 80 years of age can be expected to have a baseline PaO_2 of between 78 and 92 mmHg. Mucociliary clearance declines with age leading to a concomitant decrease in the ability to clear the bronchial tree. Vital capacity, forced expiratory volume, and functional reserve are also compromised with age and need to be considered in management of ventilation [13].

Coexisting hepatic disease seems to impact mortality in trauma patients significantly [11]. Patients with end-stage liver disease and cirrhosis have a much higher mortality from the risk of bleeding and uncontrolled hemorrhage. Patients with end-stage renal disease also carry a high mortality after trauma. The number of functioning nephrons decreases with age, leading to a age-related decline in creatinine clearance that is nearly always underappreciated in elderly patients, as muscle mass (the primary source of creatinine) also decreases significantly with age. Decision making regarding contrast in diagnostic studied should take into account that a "normal creatinine" in an elderly patient may actually reflect a significant reduction in renal function.

A number of changes occur to the aging brain including an approximately 200-g decrease in brain weight, with a concomitant decrease in brain size. Stretching of the bridging vessels over the surface of the brain results in increased susceptibility to tearing under shear forces. In addition, there seems to be a significant, age-related decline in cerebrovascular autoregulation that may partially explain the worse outcomes seen in elderly patients with head injury [20].

The effects of aging on skin are multifactorial and result in a decrease in nearly all skin functions, most importantly reduced defenses against microorganisms and loss of temperature autoregulation. Age-related changes in wound healing occur across all four phases of wound healing: hemostasis, inflammation, proliferation, and resolution [21].

Glucose tolerance declines significantly with age [2]. As hyperglycemia has been associated with worse outcome in patients with traumatic brain injury, glycemic control has become an important goal in critically ill trauma patients. Identification of diabetes mellitus and hyperglycemia (and well as hypoglycemia) should occur early during resuscitation. Finger stick glucose should be considered mandatory during initial evaluation [22].

Pre-existing medications

A number of medications have been strongly associated with trauma in the elderly, including psychotropic medications (ie, antidepressants, neuroleptics, and sedatives) and antihypertensive (ie, beta-blockers, calcium blockers, diuretics, and in particular, multiple) medications. Less commonly implicated have been antiepileptic and glaucoma agents. Over 80% of patients evaluated after accidental fall are found to be on medications easily implicated in contributing to the fall [23]. The presence of four or more chronic medications seems to correlate well with an increasing risk of falls.

Critical to the emergency department (ED) management of trauma victims are medications that can impact outcome and management of the victim. Beta-blockers, as we have noted, may decrease the patient's compensatory hemodynamic response to hemorrhage or volume loss. Antihypertensive medications in general may make resuscitation more difficult. Consideration of antihypertensive overdose or other therapeutic misadventure should be considered in patients without a source of hemorrhage and persistent hypotension. However, hypotension should never be attributed to blood pressure medications until hemorrhage and ischemia have been ruled out. Most importantly, *the patient with a history of hypertension and a normal blood pressure is unstable until proven otherwise.*

Chronic therapy with oral warfarin (Coumadin), as well as other anticoagulants, aspirin, and newer antiplatelet agents has become commonplace. Use of warfarin is indicated in a number of medical conditions including venous thromboembolism, atrial fibrillation, stroke, and valve replacement [24]. The frequency of warfarin use increases with age. Unfortunately, the risk of major bleeding complications from warfarin use also increases with age (as well as increased international normalized ratio [INR]). Warfarin appears to worsen outcome from severe head injury, but has a less dramatic impact on mortality in patients without head injury [11,25–29]. Similarly, aspirin and clopidogrel (Plavix) seem to increase the risk of death in patients who sustain intracranial injury, although there is also a significant association with concomitant comorbid disease in patients prescribed antiplatelet agents [30].

Treatment options for patients taking warfarin who sustain injury need to be individualized and balanced between the need for warfarin therapy (ie, mechanical valve and risk of embolic stroke) and the need for immediate reversal (life-threatening hemorrhage, intracranial bleeding), nonurgent reversal (preoperative), simple withdrawal of warfarin (subsequent risk of falls), or no change in therapy. For patients requiring immediate reversal in the ED, published guidelines suggest the administration of prothrombin complex concentrate, supplemented with 10 mg of vitamin K via slow intravenous (IV) infusion [31,32]. If prothrombin complex concentrate is unavailable, fresh frozen plasma is indicated. Repeat treatment may be necessary, depending on the result of subsequent INR measurements. For nonemergent reversal of warfarin, administering a single (1–2.5 mg) oral or parenteral dose of vitamin K may be considered, but should generally be made in conjunction with the patient's primary care or admitting physician [31,32].

Desmopressin, a synthetic vasopressin analog, has been shown to have hemostatic properties in patients taking aspirin. However, no controlled trials in trauma patients have been performed. Patients taking aspirin that suffer severe head injury can be treated with Desmopressin 15 μg/mL. However the efficacy of this may be limited [33]. The impact of preinjury warfarin or antiplatelet agents on considerations for neuroimaging is discussed below.

Mechanism of injury

In a study of prehospital data of trauma patients over age 70 presenting to the ED, the majority of injuries where due to falls (60.7%), followed by motor vehicle accidents (21.5%). Interestingly, the frequency of motor vehicle accidents declined for patients aged 90 years or older (3.4%). A small number of patients in the study had a suspected medical etiology as the reason for the trauma. The most common bodily site of injury was the head and face followed by the extremities [34]. Alcohol and other drugs may actually play an important role in contributing to geriatric trauma, especially falls and to a lesser extent motor vehicle collisions [35].

Falls

Numerous studies confirm that the most common reason for trauma in the elderly is due to falls [7,8,36–43]. Low-level falls (falls from a standing height) are the most common reason for injury in geriatric patients. Complications resulting from falls are the leading cause of death from injury in men and women older that age 65. The incidence of falls increases with age over 64 years and varies according to living status. Approximately 30% to 40% of community-dwelling seniors will sustain a significant fall in their lifetime. Approximately 50% of individuals living in a long-term care facility will sustain a fall, and this percentage climbs to 60% if there has been a fall within the previous year [8,36–39].

Injuries sustained by geriatric patients from falls tend to be more severe than the injuries sustained by younger patients from similar falls. Injuries to the head, pelvis, and lower extremities are extremely common. Although elderly patients account for less than 15% of trauma admissions due to falls, they account for half of deaths due to falls. Overall mortality is about 11% [44]. High-level falls (>15 feet) in the elderly are less common, but carry a mortality approaching 25% [45]. Increased morbidity is associated with increased disability, hospital admissions, and inpatient length of stay.

Major risk factors for falls include; older age, female gender, history of a previous fall, lower extremity weakness, balance difficulties, psychotropic drug use, and arthritis. Cognitive impairment "discovered" after injury may actually predate the index visit, and may contribute to the risk of falls [43]. Table 1 lists contributing factors to injuries in elderly patients. Particular etiologies to consider include vision impairment, medications, chronic medical conditions such as Parkinson's disease or osteoarthritis, environmental hazards, acute medical conditions such as syncope, transient ischemic attacks, neoplastic malignancies, metabolic derangements, infection, and anemia. Multiple risk factors for falls significantly increases the risk for subsequent falls. In one study, patients with four or more established risks for falls had a 78% risk of subsequent fall, compared with 27% in patients with zero or one risk factor [8].

When evaluating a geriatric patient who has fallen, all aspects of the incident should be reviewed. Complications of prolonged immobility such as rhabdomyolisis, dehydration, and infection need to be considered. Was the fall due to an environmental factor (rug, stairs, uneven ground, and so forth), acute or chronic medical conditions, trauma, or substance abuse? Can the patient function on the same level as before the fall? Can the patient ambulate, take care of their personal needs and manage at home?

Table 1
Contributing factors to injuries in elderly patients.

Chronic medical conditions	Environmental factors	Acute medical conditions	Other
• Osteoarthritis	• Rugs	• Syncope	• Older age
• Osteoporosis	• Lighting	• Dysrhythmias	• Female gender
• CVA	• Stairs	• CVA, TIA	• Alcohol and
• Ischemic heart	• Bathtubs/showers	• Acute MI	drug use
disease	• Footwear	• Seizure	• Elder abuse
• Anemia	• Uneven ground	• Acute renal failure	
• DM	• Weather	• Infection	
• HTN	• Walking aids	• Hypoglycemia	
• Gait and balance		• AAA	
disturbances		• New medications	
• Visual impairment		• Dehydration	
• Depression		• Acute fractures	
• Polypharmacy		• Self inflicted injury	
• Parkinson's disease			
• Dementia			

Abbreviations: AAA, abdominal aortic aneurysm; CVA, cerebral vascular accident; DM, diabetes mellitus; HTN, hypertension; MI, myocardial infarct; TIA, transient ischemic attack.

Adapted from Sattin RW. Falls among older persons a public health perspective. Annu Rev Public Health 1992;13:489–508.

Fear of falling can inhibit social and functional status. Consider what additional resources or assistance are necessary to assure a safe discharge. This assessment can be difficult and time consuming. Involvement of family members, primary care physician, visiting nurse, or social worker can help in certain situations. Geriatrics consultation or case management in the ED can help address the issues involved in the safe discharge of geriatric trauma patients from the ED. Transfer to a skilled nursing or rehab facility may be appropriate.

Motor vehicle collisions

Although a significant amount of research has been done on falls in the elderly, there is only a modest amount of published research on elderly patients involved in motor vehicle crashes. The pathophysiology of aging and the presence of acute and chronic medical conditions that affect vision, reflexes, balance and cognition, and place elderly persons at high risk for involvement in motor vehicle crashes.

It is reasonable to expect that motor vehicle trauma involving elderly patients will continue to climb over the coming decades as the US population ages. Elderly patients have an increased severity of injuries from motor vehicle collisions when compared with nonelderly. However, the pattern of injury for geriatric patients in motor vehicular trauma appears quite similar to the pattern of injury for younger patients, except for an increased incidence (11%) of sternal fractures from seatbelts in patients over 65 years of age, compared with an incidence of 1.5% in the under 65 age category [46].

Pedestrians struck by automobiles

Pedestrians injured by automobiles represent some of the most seriously injured patients in trauma. The elderly are at particular risk for being struck as pedestrians, and make up a significant percentage of pedestrians who have been struck by a motor vehicle [46,47]. Slow ambulation, impaired reflexes, misjudgment, and visual, auditory, and gait impairment appear to be involved, as elderly patients are frequently struck within marked crosswalks or walk directly into the path of an oncoming vehicle.

Sklar and colleagues specifically looked at elderly pedestrians who had been struck by a motor vehicle and found a significantly increased mortality rate. Fatal injuries tended to be from severe head injury or major vascular damage, with the majority of deaths occurring at the scene or in the ED. Once hospitalized, patients died from complications of prolonged ventilation and infection [47]. Patients struck by cars sustain twice as many lower extremity injuries as their younger counterparts. Recent data reveals that age plays a tremendous role in severity of injury in pedestrians struck. Injuries to the brain, spine, and thorax, as well as skeletal injuries increase dramatically with age, although injuries to the abdomen do not. Mortality is greater than 25% in patients struck as pedestrians over the age of 65 [48].

Burns

Elderly patients constitute approximately 13% of all patients admitted to burn units. Total body surface area burned, mortality, and hospital length of stay are all higher in the elderly [49–51]. Physiologic changes associated with aging, acute and chronic medical conditions, and social isolation are factors that increase the morbidity and mortality from burns in the geriatric population.

In a study of life expectancy and living status of elderly patients surviving burn injury, overall in hospital mortality approached 50%, and mortality was 100% in patients over the age of 60 who had sustained a body surface area burn of 50% or greater [49]. As with other forms of trauma, burn treatment in the elderly is complicated by coexisting disease and impaired functional reserve. Despite increased morbidity and mortality associated with burns in the elderly population, no data is available suggesting changes in initial burn treatment protocols other than taking into consideration underlying medical conditions that may require additional care. However, liberal transfer to a burn unit is recommended, especially in patients with significant coexisting medical condition [52].

Accidental hypothermia

Geriatric patients are at an increased risk for accidental hypothermia [53–55]. Acute and chronic medical conditions predispose the elderly to hypothermia, especially when ambient temperatures are low. Dementia can result in a patient getting lost in cold weather with inadequate protective clothing. Financial limitations may lead to insufficient heating of the home, and ultimately to homelessness.

Older patients have a lower basal metabolic rate, and can have problems maintaining core body temperature when the ambient air temperature drops. Medical conditions that predispose to hypothermia include hypoglycemia, hypothyroidism, hypopituitarism, hypoaldosteronism, sepsis, and substance abuse [56]. Acute medical etiologies for hypothermia should be considered. A cerebrovascular accident or fall can result in an elderly patient remaining in a cold house or room for a prolonged period of time. Frequently, it may be difficult to determine on initial evaluation if the patient fell and then became hypothermic, or had some precipitating event that made them hypothermic resulting in a fall.

Initial treatment of the hypothermic geriatric patient follows the same guidelines for hypothermia in general. There is little direct research on the treatment of older hypothermic patients. Several studies examining cardiopulmonary bypass for severe hypothermia list age over 64 as a relative contraindication to bypass, but these studies excluded older patients without explanation.

Geriatric patients presenting to the ED with mild to moderate hypothermia are not uncommon. We recommend a low threshold to admit to observe these patients for complications such as renal failure, infection, dehydration, pulmonary edema, cardiac stress, compartment syndrome, pancreatitis, coagulopathy, electrolyte abnormalities, and rhabdomyolisis. With little or no data on how to specifically treat the older patient with hypothermia it is important to be mindful of baseline medical problems that could complicate therapy and to address any acute medical issues that may have led to the episode. Most cases of accidental hypothermia are preventable. Taking the time to address behavioral and social issues may prevent repeat presentation to the ED.

Elder abuse and neglect

Like all forms of abuse and neglect, elder abuse is prevalent, insidious, and underreported. This issue is difficult to study, and there is very little data available on incidence, outcome, morbidity, or mortality. According to the National Elder Abuse Incidence Study, nearly 450,000 persons over age 60 experienced some form of domestic abuse, although only 16% of these cases are reported [57]. Risk factors for abuse include female gender, age >80, and physical and mental frailty. Risk factors pertaining to the perpetrator include being related to the victim (often an adult child), age younger then the injured, financial dependence on the victim, substance abuse, and prior history of violence.

Evaluation of all geriatric injury victims in the ED should include an assessment for signs and symptoms of abuse. Bruises in multiple stages of healing, unexplained fractures, untreated injuries, sign of neglect such as dehydration, malnutrition, and bedsores are important clues to the possibility of abuse or neglect, and should trigger further inquiry as to whether elder patients are victims of violence or other forms of abuse. When a clinician suspects abuse (or a patient reports abuse), it is the duty of the physician to protect the patient, treat injuries, and report the case to the proper authorities such as the police or elder services. Reporting laws exist, but differ from state to state. The reader is referred to a complete review of elder abuse elsewhere in this volume.

Management of the geriatric trauma victim

Prehospital care

It is a difficult task for the emergency physician to determine if the geriatric patient will be safe returning to the home environment. Information gathered by Emergency Medical Services (EMS) is invaluable to ED providers in assessing the elderly trauma victim. Particular attention should be paid to the social environment and home situation. The elderly may be reluctant or unable to provide accurate information regarding their home life, and deny inability to care for themselves. Even a loss of driving privileges or independent living means a loss if autonomy.

A number of questions should be asked of prehospital providers. Does the patient live alone? Does it appear that the patient is unable to care for him or herself? Does it appear as if the patient has been on the ground for a prolonged period of time? Is there evidence of substance abuse? What medications are present and does it appear that the patient has been compliant? Is there a cane or wheelchair that the patient uses? Is the home a fall hazard (rugs, stairs, poor lighting) or a safe place for the elderly patient to live? Concerns expressed by prehospital providers over the safety of a patient living individually should be highly respected, and essentially seal a decision to admit the patient, transfer the patient to a skilled facility, or trigger prompt follow up for a comprehensive geriatric assessment.

Triage

Studies show that patients who sustain serious injury are best managed in a trauma center. Development of a statewide trauma system led to improved survival for geriatric trauma patients [58]. Standard triage criteria for trauma patients include age > 55 as an important, although not absolute, determinant of trauma center disposition in injured patients [52]. At least one study advocates trauma team activation for all patients over age 75 [59]. Some argue that triage of isolated injuries (ie, hip fractures) to trauma centers overburdens the trauma system, while others support the concept of a team approach to all geriatric trauma [60]. Once admitted to a trauma center, trauma surgeons direct the patient's care, where management of coexisting medical issues and comprehensive evaluation of potential medical etiologies for the injury may be inconsistent [61]. Currently, many seriously injured patients, and most patients with less serious injury, will not be taken to a trauma center.

Injury scoring systems, including the injury severity score (ISS) have been examined in an attempt to better triage patients with major trauma. Studies in geriatric patients have been mixed. A case–control study of major trauma in geriatric patients found that the currently employed ISS, if age adjusted, performs adequately as an indicator of outcome for the older trauma patient [62]. In another study, ISS was evaluated in elderly patients and not found to accurately predict survival [63]. This was thought to be due in part to the fact that ISS does not consider the impact of pre-existing disease. The validity of the ISS for geriatric patients involved in motor vehicle collisions is still at issue. McCoy and colleagues [46] suggested a weighted scoring system, but this is yet to be developed and validated.

Initial resuscitation

The initial resuscitation of the geriatric trauma victim should be guided by standard protocols, always keeping in mind that standard hemodynamic parameters, especially heart rate, are inadequate to determine the stability of geriatric patients. Patients who appear stable should undergo aggressive testing to uncover occult instability or injury. Arterial blood gases should be considered mandatory because they may reveal an increased base deficit, or an elevated serum lactate concentration, which are harbingers of occult hypovolemia or impending shock. *While an increased base deficit is clearly a marker of serious illness, a normal base deficit does not rule out serious injury or risk of death in elderly patients* [64]. Patients who exhibit any evidence of impaired perfusion should undergo aggressive monitoring and resuscitation, as this has clearly been shown to improve outcome [19,65]. In the absence of a pulmonary artery catheter, a central venous catheter and serial arterial blood gases (looking at the base deficit) or serum lactate levels are suggested to guide therapy [66]. Noninvasive hemodynamic monitoring using bioimpedance technology has been gaining acceptance as a substitute for pulmonary artery catheterization, and has been shown in the elderly trauma patients to be reliable [67]. A second determination of either serum lactate or base deficit, drawn between 30 to 45 minutes after arrival, should be strongly considered in all geriatric patients who remain in the ED. Persistently high results should alert the clinician to ongoing hemorrhage, inadequate resuscitation, or other complications such as compartment syndrome. The elderly are at increased risk for the development of hypothermia during resuscitation, and diligence should be exercised in maintaining core temperature using external warming devices [68].

Evaluation of the initial ABCs in geriatric trauma patients include a number of important considerations. The elderly have decreased airway reflexes, and expeditious and deliberate management of the airway should be considered to prevent aspiration. Because the ventilatory response to hypoxia and hypercarbia are blunted in the elderly, occult respiratory insufficiency is common. Analysis of pH and arterial carbon dioxide tension is essential.

Anatomically, the geriatric airway can be difficult to manage. Mouth opening may be impaired. Coupled with the need to maintain in-line stabilization of the spine, kyphosis, or impaired mobility in a cleared cervical spine, laryngosopy may be difficult. Pharmacologic therapy for rapid sequence intubation in the geriatric patient also merits special consideration. Doses of nearly all sedatives, including barbiturates, benzodiazepines, and etomidate, should be reduced in the elderly to avoid hypotension. Doses of lidocaine and opiates, frequently used as premedication before intubation of patients suffering head injury, should also be reduced. Priming or administration of a defasciculating dose of a nondepolarizing neuromuscular blocker may abolish respirations prematurely, resulting in apnea with inadequate relaxation. Doses of neuromuscular blocking agents should not be reduced [17].

Patterns of injury

Elderly trauma patients clearly have different patterns of injury. Such knowledge should aid the clinician in diagnosing injuries, and determining severity of illness.

Central nervous system

Multiple investigators have recommended liberal use of computed tomography for elderly people. Case reports and case series have shown that intracranial hemorrhage can result in elderly patients who sustain minor head trauma (no loss of consciousness) and who are neurologically intact on arrival to the ED [69]. This incidence, while small, is further increased if the patient is taking warfarin and perhaps other anticoagulants or antiplatelet agents [70,71]. In a subgroup analysis of the NEXUS derivation study, 12.5% of patients over 65 were found to have significant intracranial injury, versus 7.9% of patients under 65. Furthermore, elderly patients sustaining minor head injury had a high risk of significant intracranial injury despite no evidence of significant skull fracture, neurologic deficit, or altered level of consciousness [72]. Liberal use of CT is warranted in this population until better clinical decision rules are available.

Spine

Elderly patient undergoing radiography of the cervical spine after trauma have at least twice the likelihood of cervical spine fracture than younger patients [73]. Interestingly, elderly patients who fall from low heights are at significantly increased risk of injury between the occiput and C-2, while patients in motor vehicle collisions and high falls are more likely to injure lower cervical vertebrae. Injuries to the cervical spine at multiple levels are common [74].

In the Canadian C-spine rule, age greater than 65 was used as exclusion criteria, essentially mandating cervical spine imaging in all geriatric trauma patients [75]. In contrast, the NEXUS clinical decision rule *has* been validated in a cohort of geriatric patients. The NEXUS investigators estimate that application of the decision rule could reduce the need for cervical spine imaging by 14%. Of note, 15% of injured geriatric patients were considered intoxicated at time of evaluation [73].

Given the high incidence of injuries to the atlantoaxial (C1–C2) complex, a quite justifiable strategy is to CT the cervical spine of all elderly patients requiring CT of the head. Some centers have advocated CT of C1–C2 in all patients undergoing head CT for trauma, regardless of indications for imaging the cervical spine. As CT of the cervical spine has recently been found to be far superior to plain radiography for detecting fractures, and CT of the brain is likely be indicated in nearly all elderly patients with trauma, CT should probably be considered the primary imaging modality of the cervical spine in most elderly patients, especially those over the age of 75 [74].

Cervical spondylosis predisposes to a syndrome of spinal cord injury in the absence of bony abnormality not uncommon in geriatric trauma patients. Mechanism for this phenomenon has been attributed to narrowing of the spinal canal, making the spinal cord more susceptible to compression when the neck is hyperextended, resulting in either a central cord or

Brown-Séquard like syndrome [76]. Cases of spinal cord injury without bony injury frequently mandate emergent MRI to rule out acute disc herniation requiring decompression and to further delineate other causes of cord injury.

Rib fractures and other thoracic injuries

Rib fractures are both an important injury in and of themselves, and a marker of injury severity in the multiply injured geriatric patient. Elderly patients with rib fractures have nearly twice the mortality as younger victims, despite a lower ISS and higher Glasgow coma scale (GCS). In addition, mortality rises significantly with the number of rib fractures, from 12% in patients sustaining one to two fractures, to nearly 40% in patients with seven or more fractures. Pulmonary complications including respiratory failure, pneumonia, and pleural effusion are more common in the elderly. Even the presence of a single rib fracture in the elderly carries significant morbidity and mortality [77,78].

Abdominal trauma

The abdomen is one region that is injured at a rate surprisingly similar to that of younger persons. The spleen is smaller in size from involution and apparently less prone to injury. Unfortunately, when solid organ injury is present, nonoperative management of spleen or liver injury has been challenging. Extreme age was once considered an absolute contraindication to nonoperative management of blunt solid organ injury. However, recent data suggest that age alone is not a contraindication to nonoperative management, and an expanded number of patients can now safely be observed [79].

Abdominal examination is traditionally considered less reliable in elderly patients, as evidenced by the lack of sensitivity for surgical disease in nontraumatic conditions [2]. Liberal use of abdominal CT after trauma should be considered in all geriatric trauma patients.

Musculoskeletal system

Fractures of the hip are the second most common (after wrist) fractures in elderly patients who sustain injures after a fall [23]. Patients sustaining isolated hip fracture have similar injury severity scores, and a similar incidence of severe complications, as the trauma population in general [60]. Despite this, most patients with isolated hip fracture in the United States are seen primarily by an emergency physician and admitted to either an orthopedist or to the patient's primary care physician. Although this practice has recently been questioned, it remains to be investigated whether outcome can be improved by triage of patients with isolated hip fractures directly to trauma centers, transfer of patients from community hospital EDs to trauma centers, or by the development of specialized hip fracture care centers [80].

A common presentation in the elderly is the persistence of hip pain despite negative radiographs. Such patients have a significant incidence of occult fracture. In a study of patients presenting to the ED with hip pain and negative plain films, 4.4% were diagnosed with fracture [81]. Over 90% of patients were over 65 years of age. MRI is superior to CT for the detection of fracture, and is more likely to reveal pathology not seen on CT. Fractures of the acetabulum can also easily missed on plain radiographs, particularly after falls. Periprosthetic fractures are relatively rare, but carry a high rate of complications including infection and nonunion [3].

Vertebral fractures in elderly patients are common, even after minor or unapparent trauma. The prevalence of vertebral fractures in the general population increases dramatically with age. Patients present with pain at the level of fracture, and may or may not complain of radicular symptoms. Three types of fractures are common: anterior wedge, biconcave, and crush deformities. All elderly patients who present with back pain should undergo radiographs to evaluate for fracture. Even in the presence of negative radiographs, fracture may still be present. MRI or delayed bone scanning may be employed [82].

Fractures of the pelvis carry tremendous morbidity in elderly patients. In one study of elderly ED patients, pubic rami fractures were the most common (56%), followed by acetabular fractures (19%) and ischium fractures (11%). Multiple fractures were present in over half of patients, and mortality was nearly four times higher than in nongeriatric patients [83]. In studies of major trauma patients, pelvic fractures in the elderly patients are more likely to hemorrhage and undergo angiography [84]. Elderly patients are far more likely to suffer lateral compression fractures, as opposed to anterior compression fractures, are more likely to require transfusion, and are far more likely to die. Mortality in patients suffering pelvic fracture has been reported between 12% and 21% [84,85].

Spontaneous osteoporotic fractures of the pelvis, also known as sacral insufficiency fractures, are a rare and infrequently diagnosed cause of low back, hip, and leg pain. Patients may present after minimal or minor trauma with symptoms suggestive of cauda equina syndrome and marked sacral tenderness. Plain radiographs are frequently normal. CT or MRI of the lumbosacral spine may be required to make the diagnosis [86,87].

Disposition, aftercare care, and outcome

Nearly all geriatric patients who sustain multiple injuries will need to be admitted. Geriatric patients involved in serious trauma have high admission rates to intensive care and correspondingly high morbidity and mortality rates [88]. Most deaths occur in the first 24 hours of admission and survivors suffer a significant decline in function [63,64,88]. Geriatric trauma patients have longer hospital stays, incur higher overall hospital charges, and require longer periods of rehabilitation [18,89,90]. These patients also have a higher rate of complications, leading to worse outcomes [91]. Functional outcome after blunt trauma is predictably worse with increasing age, but outcomes between patients 65 to 97 years and patients over 80 years are remarkably similar [92]. Recovery from injury can be prolonged, but with aggressive management over 90% of patients survive and many can return home [93]. Prolonged intensive care unit stay is not associated with an unfavorable long-term outcome [94].

Although no prospective randomized trial examining the outcome of transfer versus no transfer for geriatric trauma patients has been performed, evidence strongly suggests that multiply injured geriatric trauma patients are likely best served in a trauma center [95,96]. Patients requiring general surgical or neurosurgical intensive care or burn care should be transferred once best attempts to stabilize the victim have occurred. Patients requiring repeat operation or particular orthopedic or other surgical expertise should also be considered for transfer. Lengthy attempts at defining all injuries in the initial receiving hospital are not warranted if they will not significantly change management or will delay transfer for definitive care of more life-threatening injuries. Unfortunately, studies done by referring hospitals are frequently repeated at the receiving facility, increasing the costs of care [97].

Selected patients sustaining isolated injures (usually after falls) may be considered candidates for discharge from the ED. Patients who presenting after a fall who report recurrent falls, have an abnormal mental status, or exhibit gait instability upon evaluation are poor candidates for discharge, and require a falls assessment by a geriatric specialist or team [98]. Patients with lower extremity injuries are particularly high risk. Interestingly, assist devices such as canes and walkers have not been shown to reduce the risk of falls [98].

Comprehensive geriatric assessment has become the "gold standard" of care for at risk elderly, and has been shown to reduce the rate of hospital admission, reduce repeat ED visits, and improve outcomes in patients discharged from the ED [99]. A clinical prediction rule developed to assess fall risk in the elderly has shown that mental impairment (confusion, disorientation, or agitation), toileting difficulties, vision problems, and difficulty with transfer or mobility accurately predict falls in hospitalized patients [100]. Presence of these in the ED likely puts the patient at substantial risk for subsequent falls.

Summary

As the US population ages the geriatric population grows. Trauma in the elderly is responsible for a significant number of visits to EDs and will continue to increase. Knowledge of the physiologic changes associated with aging, the impact of coexistent acute and chronic medical conditions, and an understanding of the unique patterns of injury in geriatric trauma patients is critical to maximizing outcome.

Older patients tend to injure themselves most often after falls. Even falls from standing can result in significant fractures and head injury. Geriatric trauma victims demand aggressive management, a high index of suspicion for occult instability, and a low threshold for laboratory and radiographic investigation to delineate injuries.

Ultimately, trauma in the elderly should be addressed not just in the ED and hospital, but also from a public health perspective with emphasis on services and prevention. Research that addresses the different presentations, injury patterns, predictors of morbidity and mortality, and public health research on prevention will help further enlighten emergency physicians on how to best treat geriatric trauma patients to help them maintain high functional status. Much research remains to be done [101].

References

[1] Day J. Population projections of the united states by age, sex, race, and hispanic origin: 1995 to 2050. Washington (DC): US Bureau of the Census, Current Population Reports, P25-1130, US Government Printing Office; 1996.

[2] McMahon DJ, Schwab CW, Kauder D. Comorbidity and the elderly trauma patient. World J Surg 1996;20:1113–20.

[3] Koval KJ, Meek R, Schemitsch E, et al. An AOA critical issue. Geriatric trauma: young ideas. J Bone Joint Surg Am 2003;85-A:1380–8.

[4] Eliastam M. Elderly patients in the emergency department. Ann Emerg Med 1998;18: 1222–9.

[5] Champion HR, Copes WS, Buyer D, et al. Major trauma in geriatric patients. Am J Public Health 1989;79(9):1278–82.

[6] Jacobs DG. Special considerations in geriatric injury. Curr Opin Crit Care 2003;9(6):535–9.

[7] Currie CT, Lawson PM, Robertson CE, et al. Elderly patients discharged from accident and emergency departments—their dependency and support. Arch Emerg Med 1984;1: 205–13.

[8] Tinetti ME, Speechley M, Ginter SF. Risk factors for falls among elderly persons living in the community. N Engl J Med 1988;319:1701–7.

[9] Mosenthal AC, Livingston DH, Lavery RF, et al. The effect of age on functional outcome in mild traumatic brain injury: 6-month report of a prospective multicenter trial. J Trauma 2004;56:1042–8.

[10] Morris JA Jr, MacKenzie EJ, Damiano AM, et al. Mortality in trauma patients: the interaction between host factors and severity. J Trauma 1990;30:1476–82.

[11] Grossman MD, Miller D, Scaff DW, et al. When is an elder old? Effect of preexisting conditions on mortality in geriatric trauma. J Trauma 2002;52:242–6.

[12] Milzman DP, Boulanger BR, Rodriguez A, et al. Pre-existing disease in trauma patients: a predictor of fate independent of age and injury severity score. J Trauma 1992;32:236–43.

[13] Wright AS, Schurr MJ. Geriatric trauma: review and recommendations. Wis Med J 2001; 100(2):57–9.

[14] Schwab CW, Kauder DR. Trauma in the geriatric patient. Arch Surg 1992;127:701–6.

[15] Mandavia D, Newton K. Geriatric trauma. Emerg Clin North Am 1998;16:257–74.

[16] Levy DB, Hanion DP, Townsend RN. Geriatric trauma. Clin Geriatr Med 1993;9:601–21.

[17] Milzman DP, Rothenhaus TC. Resuscitation of the geriatric patient. Emerg Clin North Am 1996;14:233–45.

[18] DeMaria EJ. Evaluation and treatment of the elderly trauma victim. Clin Geriatr Med 1993;9(2):461–71.
[19] Scalea TM, Simon HM, Ducan AO, et al. Geriatric blunt multiple trauma: improved survival with early invasive monitoring. J Trauma 1992;30:129–34.
[20] Czosnyka M, Balestreri M, Steiner L, et al. Age, intracranial pressure, autoregulation, and outcome after brain trauma. J Neurosurg 2005;102:450–4.
[21] Gosain A, DiPietro LA. Aging and wound healing. World J Surg 2004;28:321–6.
[22] Jeremitsky E, Omert LA, Dunham CM, et al. The impact of hyperglycemia on patients with severe brain injury. J Trauma 2005;58(1):47–50.
[23] Nordell E, Jarnlo GB, Jetsen C, et al. Accidental falls and related fractures in 65–74 year olds: a retrospective study of 332 patients. Acta Orthop Scand 2000;71:175–9.
[24] Hirsh J, Fuster V, Ansell J, et al. American Heart Association/American College of Cardiology Foundation guide to warfarin therapy. Circulation 2003;107:1692–711.
[25] Kirsch MJ, Vrabec GA, Marley RA, et al. Preinjury warfarin and geriatric orthopedic trauma patients: a case-matched study. J Trauma 2004;57:1230–3.
[26] Lavoie A, Ratte S, Clas D, et al. Preinjury warfarin use among elderly patients with closed head injuries in a trauma center. J Trauma 2004;56:802–7.
[27] Mina AA, Bair HA, Howells GA, et al. Complications of preinjury warfarin use in the trauma patient. J Trauma 2003;54:842–7.
[28] Wojcik R, Cipolle MD, Seislove E, et al. Preinjury warfarin does not impact outcome in trauma patients. J Trauma 2001;51:1147–51.
[29] Kennedy DM, Cipolle MD, Pasquale MD, et al. Impact of preinjury warfarin use in elderly trauma patients. J Trauma 2000;48:451–3.
[30] Ohm C, Mina A, Howells G, et al. Effects of antiplatelet agents on outcomes for elderly patients with traumatic intracranial hemorrhage. J Trauma 2005;58:518–22.
[31] Ansell J, Hirsh J, Dalen J, et al. Managing oral anticoagulant therapy. Chest 2001;119: 22S–38S.
[32] Baker RI, Coughlin PB, Gallus AS, et al. Warfarin reversal: consensus guidelines, on behalf of the Australasian Society of Thrombosis and Haemostasis. Med J Aust 2004;181: 492–7.
[33] Pleym H, Stenseth R, Wahba A, et al. Prophylactic treatment with desmopressin does not reduce postoperative bleeding after coronary surgery in patients treated with aspirin before surgery. Anesth Analg 2004;98:578–84.
[34] Spaite DW, Criss EA, Valenzuela TD, et al. Geriatric injury: an analysis of pre-hospital demographics, mechanisms, and patterns. Ann Emerg Med 1990;19:1418–21.
[35] Zautcke JL, Coker SB Jr, Morris RW, et al. Geriatric trauma in the state of Illinois: substance use and injury patterns. Am J Emerg Med 2002;20(1):14–7.
[36] Graafmans WC, Ooms ME, Hofstee HM, et al. Falls in the elderly: a prospective study of risk factors and risk profiles. Am J Epidemiol 1996;143:1129–36.
[37] Campbell AJ, Borrie MJ, Spears GF. Risk factors for falls in community-based prospective study of people 70 years and older. J Gerontol 1989;44(4):M112–7.
[38] Thapa PB, Brockman KG, Gideon P, et al. Injurious falls in nonambulatory nursing home residents: a comparative study of circumstances, incidence, and risk factors. J Am Geriatr Soc 1996;44:273–8.
[39] Nevitt MC, Cummings SR, Hudes ES. Risk factors for injurious falls: a prospective study. J Gerontol 1991;46:M164–70.
[40] Kiel DP. Overview of falls in the elderly. Up to date online; 2004 (www.uptodate.com accessed November 4, 2004).
[41] Hogue C. Injury in late life: part I. Epidemioogy. J Am Geriatr Soc 1982;30(3):183–90.
[42] Sattin RW. Falls among older persons: a public health perspective. Annu Rev Public Health 1992;13:489–508.
[43] Aharon-Peretz J, Kliot D, Amyel-Zvi E, et al. Neurobehavioral consequences of closed head injury in the elderly. Brain Inj 1997;11:871–5.

[44] Mosenthal AC, Livingston DH, Elcavage J, et al. Falls: epidemiology and strategies for prevention. J Trauma 1995;38:753–6.

[45] Demetriades D, Murray J, Brown C, et al. High-level falls: type and severity of injuries and survival outcome according to age. J Trauma 2005;58:342–5.

[46] McCoy GF, Johnstone RA, Duthie RB. Injury to the elderly in road traffic accidents. J Trauma 1989;29(4):494–7.

[47] Sklar DP, Demarest GB, McFeeley P. Increased pedestrian mortality among the elderly. Am J Emerg Med 1989;7(4):387–90.

[48] Demetriades D, Murray J, Martin M, et al. Pedestrians injured by automobiles: relationship of age to injury type and severity. J Am Coll Surg 2004;199:382–7.

[49] Manktelow A, Meyer AA, Herzog SR, et al. Analysis of life expectancy and living status of elderly patients surviving burn injury. J Trauma 1989;29(2):203–7.

[50] Anous MM, Heimbach DM. Causes of death and predictors in burned patients more then 60 years of age. J Trauma 1986;26:135–9.

[51] Linn BS. Age differences in the severity and outcome of burns. J Am Geriat Soc 1980;28: 118–23.

[52] American College of Surgeons. Advanced trauma life support for doctors. 6th ed. Chicago (IL): Author; 1997.

[53] Rosin AJ, Exton-Smith AN. Hypothermia in the elderly—a clinical review. Curr Med Drugs 1964;48:3–16.

[54] Fox RH, Woodward PM, Exton Smith AN, et al. Body temperature in the elderly: a national study of physiological, social, and environmental conditions. BMJ 1973;1: 200–6.

[55] Goldman A, Exton Smith AN, Francis G, et al. A pilot study of low body temperatures in old people admitted to hospital. J R Coll Physicians Lond 1977;11:291–306.

[56] Weinberg AD. Hypothermia. Ann Emerg Med 1993;22:370–7.

[57] Official Website for the US Department of Health and Human Services. Administration on aging National Elder Abuse Incidence Study; 1998. Found at www.aoa.gov/eldfam/Elder_Rights/Elder_Abuse/ABuseReport_Full.pdf. Accessed Jan 5, 2005.

[58] Mann NC, Cahn RM, Mullins RJ, et al. Survival among injured geriatric patients during construction of a statewide trauma system. J Trauma 2001;50:111–6.

[59] Demetriades D, Sava J, Alo K, et al. Old age as a criterion for trauma team activation. J Trauma 2001;51(4):754–6.

[60] Bergeron E, Lavoie A, Belcaid A, et al. Should patients with isolated hip fractures be included in trauma registries? J Trauma 2005;58:793–7.

[61] Omert L, Zakhary S, Wilson R, et al. Falling down and falling out: management and outcome analysis. J Trauma 2004;56(1):58–63.

[62] Finelli FC, Jonsson J, Champion HR, et al. A case control study for major trauma in geriatric patients. J Trauma 1989;29(5):541–8.

[63] Oreskovich MR, Howard JD, Copass MK, et al. Geriatric trauma: injury patterns and outcome. J Trauma 1984;34(7):565–72.

[64] Davis JW, Kaups KL. Base deficit in the elderly: a marker of severe injury and death. J Trauma 1998;45(5):873–7.

[65] Demetriades D, Karaiskakis M, Velmahos G, et al. Effect of early intensive management of geriatric trauma patients. Br J Surg 2002;89:1319–22.

[66] Tisherman SA, Barie P, Bokhari F, et al. Clinical practice guideline: endpoints of resuscitation. J Trauma 2004;57(4):898–912.

[67] Brown CV, Shoemaker WC, Wo CC, et al. Is noninvasive hemodynamic monitoring appropriate for the elderly critically injured patient? J Trauma 2005;58:102–7.

[68] Wang HE, Callaway CW, Peitzman AB, et al. Admission hypothermia and outcome after major trauma. Crit Care Med 2005;33(6):1296–301.

[69] Mack LR, Chan SB, Silva JC, et al. The use of head computed tomography in elderly patients sustaining minor head trauma. J Emerg Med 2003;24:157–62.

[70] Reynolds FD, Dietz PA, Higgins D, et al. Time to deterioration of the elderly, anticoagulated, minor head injury patient who presents without evidence of neurologic abnormality. J Trauma 2003;54:492–6.

[71] Li J, Brown J, Levine M. Mild head injury, anticoagulants, and risk of intracranial injury. Lancet 2001;357:771–2.

[72] Rathlev N, Medzon R, Lowery D, et al. Intracranial pathology in the elderly with minor head injury. Acad Emerg Med 2003;10:478.

[73] Touger M, Gennis P, Nathanson N, et al. Validity of a decision rule to reduce cervical spine radiography in elderly patients with blunt trauma. Ann Emerg Med 2002;40(3):287–93.

[74] Lomoschitz FM, Blackmore CC, Mirza SK, et al. Cervical spine injuries in patients 65 years old and older: epidemiologic analysis regarding the effects of age and injury mechanism on distribution, type, and stability of injuries. AJR Am J Roentgenol 2002;178:573–7.

[75] Stiell IG, Wells GA, Vandemheen K, et al. The Canadian CT head rule for patients with minor head injury. Lancet 2001;357:1391–6.

[76] Regenbogen VS, Rogers LF, Atlas SW, et al. Cervical spinal cord injuries in patients with cervical spondylosis. AJR Am J Roentgenol 1986;146:277–84.

[77] Stawicki SP, Grossman MD, Hoey BA, et al. Rib fractures in the elderly: a marker of injury severity. J Am Geriatr Soc 2004;52:805–8.

[78] Bergeron E, Lavoie A, Clas D, et al. Elderly trauma patients with rib fractures are at greater risk of death and pneumonia. J Trauma 2003;54(3):478–85.

[79] Victorino GP, Chong TJ, Pal JD. Trauma in the elderly patient. Arch Surg 2003;138: 1093–8.

[80] Parker MJ, Pryor GA, Myles J. 11-year results in 2,846 patients of the Peterborough Hip Fracture Project: reduced morbidity, mortality and hospital stay. Acta Orthop Scand 2000;71(1):34–8.

[81] Dominguez S, Liu P, Roberts C, et al. Prevalence of traumatic hip and pelvic fractures in patients with suspected hip fracture and negative initial standard radiographs—a study of emergency department patients. Acad Emerg Med 2005;12(4):366–9.

[82] Papaioannou A, Watts NB, Kendler DL, et al. Diagnosis and management of vertebral fractures in elderly adults. Am J Med 2002;113(3):220–8.

[83] Alost T, Waldrop RD. Profile of geriatric pelvic fractures presenting to the emergency department. Am J Emerg Med 1997;15(6):576–8.

[84] Henry SM, Pollak AN, Jones AL, et al. Pelvic fracture in geriatric patients: a distinct clinical entity. J Trauma 2002;53(1):15–20.

[85] O'Brien DP, Luchette FA, Pereira SJ, et al. Pelvic fracture in the elderly is associated with increased mortality. Surgery 2002;132(4):710–4.

[86] Blake SP, Connors AM. Sacral insufficiency fracture. Br J Radiol 2004;77(922):891–6.

[87] Lourie H. Spontaneous osteoporotic fracture of the sacrum. An unrecognized syndrome of the elderly. JAMA 1982;248(6):715–7.

[88] Zietlow SP, Capizzi PJ, Bannon MP, et al. Multisystem geriatric trauma. J Trauma 1994; 37(6):985–8.

[89] Ferrera PC, Bartfield JM, D'Andrea CC. Outcomes of admitted geriatric trauma victims. Am J Emerg Med 2000;18(5):575–80.

[90] Gomberg BFC, Gruen GS, Smith WR, et al. Outcomes in acute orthopaedic trauma: a review of 130,506 patients by age. Injury Int J Care Injured 1999;30:431–7.

[91] Amacher AL, Bybee DE. Toleration of head injury by the elderly. Neurosurgery 1987;20: 954–8.

[92] Grossman M, Scaff DW, Miller D, et al. Functional outcomes in octogenarian trauma. J Trauma 2003;55(1):26–32.

[93] Richmond TS, Kauder D, Strumpf N, et al. Characteristics and outcomes of serious traumatic injury in older adults. J Am Geriatr Soc 2002;50:215–22.

[94] Carrillo EH, Richardson JD, Malias MA, et al. Long term outcome of blunt trauma care in the elderly. Surg Gynecol Obstet 1993;176:559–64.

[95] McConnell KJ, Newgard CD, Mullins RJ, et al. Mortality benefit of transfer to level I versus level II trauma centers for head-injured patients. Health Serv Res 2005;40(2):435–57.

[96] Sampalis JS, Denis R, Frechette P, et al. Direct transport to tertiary trauma centers versus transfer from lower level facilities: impact on mortality and morbidity among patients with major trauma. J Trauma 1997;43(2):288–95.

[97] Thomas SH, Orf J, Peterson C, et al. Frequency and costs of laboratory and radiograph repetition in trauma patients undergoing interfacility transfer. Am J Emerg Med 2000; 18(2):156–8.

[98] American Geriatrics Society, British Geriatrics Society, and American Academy of Orthopedic Surgeons Panel on Falls Prevention. Guideline for the prevention of falls in older persons. J Am Geriatr Soc 2001;49:664–72.

[99] Caplan GA, Williams AJ, Daly B, et al. A randomized, controlled trial of comprehensive geriatric assessment and multidisciplinary intervention after discharge of elderly from the emergency department—the DEED II study. J Am Geriatr Soc 2004;52(9):1417–23.

[100] Papaioannou A, Parkinson W, Cook R, et al. Prediction of falls using a risk assessment tool in the acute care setting. BMC Med 2004;2:1–7.

[101] Jacobs DG, Plaisier BR, Barie PS, et al. Practice management guidelines for geriatric trauma: the EAST Practice Management Guidelines Work Group. J Trauma 2003;54(2): 391–416.

ELSEVIER
SAUNDERS

Emerg Med Clin N Am
24 (2006) 433–448

EMERGENCY
MEDICINE
CLINICS OF
NORTH AMERICA

Infectious Emergencies in the Elderly

Adeyinka Adedipe, MD, Robert Lowenstein, MD*

*Department of Emergency Medicine, Boston Medical Center, 1 Boston Medical Center Place,
Dowling 1 South, Boston, MA 02188, USA*

As human life expectancy continues to increase, developed countries are reporting higher percentages of elderly in their respective populations [1]. Elderly, defined as people over the age of 65, comprised 6.2% of the world population in 1992, and is projected to reach 20% of the population by 2050 [2]. Caring for such patients presents many challenges in emergency medicine today. Not only is the elderly population more susceptible to infection, making common infectious diseases more prevalent in this age group, but the manifestations of infections are more severe, often leading to a poor outcome [1,3]. Mortality in the elderly population can be attributed to infections greater than 33% of the time [4]. Although the typical presentations of infections are commonly absent in the elderly it is imperative to recognize infection early and initiate treatment in a timely fashion. It is the purpose of this article to address contributing factors that predispose the elderly to infections, to review the clinical presentation of infections in the elderly, to illustrate preventative measures undertaken to limit infection-induced morbidity and mortality in the elderly population, and to discuss common infectious emergencies that include cellulitis, urinary tract infections, pneumonia, and meningitis.

Risk factors

There are numerous risk factors that predispose the elderly to infection, and consequently contribute to the morbidity and mortality in this population. The susceptibility to infection is multifactorial. Aging is associated with numerous chronic illnesses and comorbid conditions [5,6], polypharmacy and immunosuppressive medications, and changes in the immune system that include a reduction of T-lymphocyte function and cell-mediated immunity [5,7]. Functional impairment is common, and includes increased

---

* Corresponding author.
E-mail address: Robert.Lowenstein@bmc.org (R. Lowenstein).

0733-8627/06/$ - see front matter © 2006 Elsevier Inc. All rights reserved.
doi:10.1016/j.emc.2006.01.006   *emed.theclinics.com*

immobility, incontinence of the bladder, and limited activities of daily living (ADLs) [5,8]. There is an impairment of the normal physiologic reserves seen in the elderly, examples of which include decreased cough reflex leading to aspiration pneumonia, impaired arterial and venous circulation, and compromised wound healing, making cellulitis a common infection [2]. Living environments, such as assisted living facilities and nursing homes, allow for the development of infection and foster the transmission of infectious agents [5]. These facilities contribute to the rise and exposure of antibiotic-resistant bacteria (eg, methicillin-resistant *Staphylococcus aureus* and vancomycin-resistant enterococcus) [4]. Invasive devices, which include indwelling urinary catheters, intravenous catheters, feeding tubes, and tracheostomies, are more common in the elderly, and compromise host defenses enabling bacteria to enter the body and cause infection [5]. Malnutrition, common in the nursing home population, is associated with a limited immune response and impaired wound healing [5]. Polypharmacy is also frequently observed, and can contribute to infection.

Although there are numerous aforementioned predispositions toward infection in the elderly, challenges also exist in establishing a diagnosis in this patient population. The clinical presentation of infection in the elderly is often atypical, subtle, and elusive; thus, making an early diagnosis and initiating treatment a challenge [9]. Elderly may not only have fewer symptoms, but might present with nonspecific consequences of infection that on the surface appear unrelated. Examples of nonspecific symptoms include generalized malaise, falls, changes in mental status or cognitive impairment, and anorexia [10–12]. The classical manifestations of infection, fever, and leukocytosis, may be absent or blunted in 20% to 30% of serious elderly infections [9]. Only 59% of elderly patients mounted a fever in a large bacterial meningitis study [9]. In contrast to the young where fever is commonly attributed to a viral process, in the elderly it is associated with severe bactezrial infections [9,13]. As a result, in one study it was suggested that all such patients with a fever be considered for observation and admission [8]. It is important to note that criteria for fevers in the elderly are unique, and include elevations in body temperature from baseline of 1.1°C or greater [4]. Furthermore, hypothermia, a decrease in body temperature, is not an uncommon presentation of an underlying serious infection.

Cellulitis

Cellulitis is more common, more severe, and is associated with increased mortality in the elderly compared with the younger population. Cellulitis in the elderly can often be attributed to chronic venous insufficiency, peripheral vascular disease, malnutrition, and trauma [14]. It has been estimated that the prevalence of skin and soft tissue infection in the long-term care facility is 5% [2]. Outbreaks of bacteremia in nursing homes secondary to group A beta-hemolytic streptococci have been documented but are uncommon [2].

The microbial etiology is usually due to beta-hemolytic streptococci or *S aureus*. However, cellulitis complicated by diabetic ulcers or pressure ulcers may have different etiologies, and can include polymicrobial flora, *Enterobactenaceae*, and anaerobes [5,14]. Orbital cellulitis is another exception, and may be caused by *Streptococcus viridans* and Gram-negative bacteria. External otitis, cellulitis of the ear, is generally observed in the elderly, and is caused by Gram-negative bacteria, specifically Pseudomonas species [15].

It has been widely established that bacterial resistance is on the rise. Methicillin-resistant *Staphlococcus aureus* (MRSA) is an example of such resistant bacteria, and is more likely to occur in the elderly population, and is commonly seen in both hospitals and long-term care facilities [4,16,17]. Once colonized with MRSA the rate of MRSA infection increases up to 25%, as does the risk of mortality [17]. This can be attributed to the prevalence of resistance to traditional antibiotics. Additional risk factors for colonization include individuals with limited functional status, multiple hospitalizations, and the presence of any long-term catheters or feeding tubes [17]. Incidentally, the location of MRSA colonization generally includes the nasal mucosa and oropharynx.

Preventative measures employed in both hospitals and long-term care facilities include frequent hand washing, keeping colonized lesions covered, and isolating infected patients with contact precautions. Universal precautions must be employed when touching colonized patients, such as wearing clean gloves.

Treatment of cellulitis is dictated by the suspected organisms, the location of the cellulitis, underlying comorbidities, and the severity of the infection. These factors will determine whether the therapy should be administered orally or parenterally. MSRA and streptococci are treated with first-generation cephalosporins, antistaphylococcal penicillins, and clindamycin in penicillin allergic patients [16,18]. Polymicrobial infections frequently occur in decubiti and diabetic ulcerations. Broad-spectrum antibiotics are indicated for these infections, and must include coverage for Gram-positive and Gram-negative aerobes and anaerobes. MRSA colonization does not require antibiotic treatment; however, active infection with MRSA is treated with vancomycin, linezolid, or quinupristin-dalfopristin [16].

Herpes zoster

Herpes zoster (shingles) is another skin infection seen more frequently in the elderly population. It is a disease confined to the skin and nervous system, and is caused by the reactivation of the varicella-zoster virus (VZV). VZV is responsible for pediatric chicken pox, and remains dormant in the dorsal root ganglia. What reactivates VZV in the dorsal root ganglia remains unclear; however, it is usually a disease of the elderly and immunocompromised. As cellular immunity decreases with aging, the incidence of herpes zoster increases.

Pain and paresthesias over a particular dermatome usually precede the characteristic rash. This prodromal pain is lancinating, and is easily misdiagnosed as having cardiac, abdominal, and renal etiologies. Symptoms may last for several days before the hallmark lesions. These include an erythematous maculopapular rash over a dermatomal distribution followed by an eruption of grouped vesicles that form pustules and then crust over by day 10 of rash onset [4]. It is important to note that the pain can be severe and debilitating. Herpes zoster is a clinical diagnosis; however, laboratory confirmation can be obtained via a culture of the vesicular fluid or by observing giant cells on Tzanck preparation. A long-term sequela of herpes zoster is postherpetic neuralgia. The incidence of postherpetic neuralgia increases with age, with 50% to 75% of patients >70 experiencing chronic pain over the involved dermatome [14,15].

Treatment includes antiviral therapy which, if initiated within 72 hours of symptom onset, decreases viral replication, nerve damage, duration of eruption, and pain. Administration of therapy after 72 hours may reduce the incidence of post herpetic neuralgia, but will not impact on the duration of symptoms. The antiviral agents used include acyclovir, valacyclovir, and famciclovir.

Urinary tract infection

Urinary tract infections encompass a spectrum of disease, from asymptomatic bacturia and cystitis, to pyelonephritis and urosepsis. Urinary tract infections (UTIs) are among the most common infections affecting the elderly. A number of health factors contribute to genitourinary infections. Comorbid diseases, functional status, and living environments each play a role in a patient's susceptibility to infection, and each may complicate an otherwise simple urinary infection. Emergency physicians must be cognizant of each factor when making a diagnosis and initiating treatment. Quite frequently geriatric patients will have atypical presentations, and subsequently there is an increased risk of adverse events related to delayed treatment. Among healthy elderly patients, these infections are usually benign; however, in patients with significant comorbidities, UTIs can ultimately lead to more serious complications [19,20].

UTIs remain one of the leading causes of infection in elderly patients. Among otherwise healthy geriatric patients living in the community, rates of UTI range from 5% to 30%, with higher rates seen with advanced age. Among institutionalized patients, the prevalence rates increase remarkably; between 17% and 55% of women and 15% and 31% of men are bacteriuric [21]. There are multiple reasons for higher rates of infection when compared with younger patients. Anatomic variations during the aging process (such as changes in prostatic function in men and changes in vaginal flora associated with menopause in women) increase the risk of UTIs. Additionally, elderly patients are more likely than their younger counterparts to have obstructive uropathy or anatomic changes related to childbirth or reproductive surgery. Other factors to consider include higher rates of incontinence, more frequent urologic instrumentation, higher rates of catheterization, comorbid diseases, and medications that alter bladder function [22].

Among young, healthy patients, the vast majority of urinary infections are a result of *Escherichia coli*, *Proteus mirabilis*, *Klebsiella pneumoniae*, *Enterococcus*, *Pseudomonas*, and Staphylococcus species. Elderly patients have a lower incidence of *E coli* infection ($<50\%$ of isolates) and higher rates of polymicrobial infections (up to one in three geriatric patients with UTIs [22]. Patients with short-term urinary catheters are typically infected by a single organism, while long-erm catheters are associated with polymicrobial infections [21]. The prevalence of Gram-positive urinary tract infections in geriatric patients has been increasing [23].

Urinary frequency, incontinence, dysuria, fever, and flank pain are typical clinical presentations for patients with UTIs. Asymptomatic bacturia occurs in the majority of older patients. The elderly often present with atypical symptoms of UTI such as malaise, anorexia, weakness, and subtle mental status changes. Delirium and functional decline may be the first signs of bacteremia from a urologic source. Such "nonurinary" symptoms are more likely to occur in patients with existing comorbidities including dehydration [22].

Asymptomatic bacturia often complicates the diagnosis of urinary tract infections. Further complicating the diagnosis is the fact that some patients with acute symptoms of cystitis will have sterile urine [24]. Clinicians should therefore treat infections based on their degree of suspicion. Obtaining a midstream clean-catch urine specimen and submitting for dipstick analysis is the first step in diagnosis in the emergency department. Unfortunately, obtaining an uncontaminated specimen is frequently a problem in patients who are functionally impaired. The use of a condom catheter for male patients or a "straight" catheterization in female patients can aid in sample collection for such patients.

When analyzing urine specimens, the use of a urine dipstick to assess for leukocyte esterase and nitrates is invaluable as a screening tool. The absence of leukocytes has a negative predictive value of nearly 100% [25]. The presence of leukocytes, however, is not an adequate predictor of bacturia in elderly patients, and in fact, may be less reliable than in younger patients. Therefore, urine microscopy and culture should aid in making the ultimate diagnosis. Although urine cultures are rarely helpful for the emergency physician, obtaining urinary cultures for more complicated UTIs may help tailor the antibiotic regimen after an initial antibiotic has been initiated. Bacterial culture counts greater than 10^5 colony forming units/mL have traditionally been used as an indicator of infection; however, a few studies have shown that patients with symptoms of cystitis demonstrated counts below 10^4 [23]. Using a count of 10^3 in the symptomatic patient or a count of

10^4 in patients with indwelling catheters may be sufficient in establishing the diagnosis [23].

Treatment of urinary infections in elderly patients should be conservative when compared with younger, healthier individuals. Higher rates of failure and relapse are more often associated with advanced age [26]. Broad antibiotic coverage for a longer duration should be the cornerstone of any treatment plan. Seven to 10 days of treatment is preferred for women with symptoms for longer than 1 week, women with structural or functional changes, and for all men. Fourteen days of antibiotic treatment should be routine for elderly patients with uncomplicated pyelonephritis.

Fluoroquinolones are the preferred first-line treatment when the pathogen is not known, as they have a wider spectrum of coverage and greater penetration of the prostate gland compared with other antibiotics. Selection of the most appropriate fluoroquinolone is important in reducing the likelihood of adverse events associated with the antibiotic. Levoflaxacin and gatiflaxacin offer the broadest coverage; both Gram-positive and Gram-negative organisms are susceptible. Awareness of the potential for QTc prolongation (gatiflaxacin), potential for drug interactions (especially with coumadin), and other untoward effects is important when deciding to use a fluoroquinolone.

Trimethoprim-Sulfamethoxazole (TMP-SMX) may be given to elderly women, when the sensitivities are confirmed; however, there is a higher incidence of side effects and discontinuation when compared with fluoroquinolones [22]. In addition, greater rates of allergic reaction occur in TMP-SMX compared with other antibiotics.

Beta-lactam agents should be avoided in the geriatric patient as there is a higher incidence of beta-lactamase producing *E coli* in nursing home patients, rendering these antibiotics ineffective [25].

Treatment of patients with asymptomatic bacturia should be discouraged.

Pneumonia

Diseases of the respiratory tract have long been associated with morbidity and mortality among the elderly population. Rates of infection appear to rise with advanced age, and consequently, the rate of hospitalization is higher in the geriatric population. Understanding the epidemiology and microbiology in community-acquired pneumonia (CAP) and nursing home-acquired pneumonia will greatly facilitate diagnostic and management considerations in the elderly patient exposed to respiratory pathogens.

In the United States, pneumonia and influenza ranked sixth among the leading causes of death [27]. With advanced age, rates of morbidity and mortality for pneumonia increase dramatically. Nearly half of all cases of pneumonia involve patients ≥65 years of age [28], and among nursing home residents, pneumonia is the second most common cause of infection [29]. The nursing home population is particularly effected by pneumonia.

Although pneumonia accounts for 13% to 48% of infections among nursing home residents, mortality rates of those admitted to the hospital are as high as 44% [30]. It is also the second most common cause of bacteremia in a nursing home. Older patients appear more prone to pneumonia, and the disease course tends to be more protracted than in younger individuals. Recovery is prolonged in the elderly.

Several factors associated with the aging process of the respiratory tract and lung tissue predispose older people to respiratory infections. Changes in the mucociliary transport system associated with age and smoking have a negative effect with clearing of bacterial pathogens. In addition, changes in lung capacity, elasticity, and compliance are common with age [30]. Most cases of pneumonia in the elderly are, in fact, related to microaspiration of bacterial pathogens colonizing the oropharynx. Ineffective clearing of mucus and secretions from the respiratory tract makes patients more susceptible to aspiration pneumonia, a factor most frequently found in nursing home dwellers [30]. Other factors that may contribute to increased risk in the nursing home population include the presence of a gastric or nasogastric tube, difficulties swallowing, chronic obstructive lung disease, tracheostomy, and older age [29].

Microbiology

Streptococcus pneumoniae

The most common isolate from sputum culture is *Streptococcus pneumoniae* (recovered in 20–30% of CAP cases in the elderly). It is an important pathogen accounting for more than half of all cases of bacteremic CAP [31]. Pneumococcal pneumonia is also the most common pathogen found in nursing home residents. Meningitis, an uncommon extrapulmonary manifestation of *S pneumoniae* infection, is more likely to occur in the geriatric population (see below).

Haemophilus influenza

Patients infected with either the encapsulated H influenza type b or the unencapsulated strains typically have chronic lung disease, are male, and have a productive cough [32].

Legionella pneumophilia

Legionella pneumophila infections tend to occur sporadically; these infections usually appear in the summer and fall, and may be found in the water condensed from air conditioning systems.

Mycoplasma pneumoniae

M pneumoniae remains a common atypical pathogen causing pneumonia in patients under 60 years of age. Elderly patients have a somewhat lower proportion of cases of atypical infections compared with younger, healthier patients [32].

Staphylococcus aureus

More commonly associated with nosocomial infection, *S aureus* pneumonia causes a multilobe infiltration, and is frequently associated with bacteremia. A well-known manifestation of *S aureus* infection is the florid onset of pneumonia following recovery from influenza.

Gram-negative bacilli

Rare in younger patients, pneumonia due to enteric Gram-negative bacilli is more likely to affect nursing home residents compared with community dwellers. Nearly 12% of pneumonias in patients from nursing homes are related to Gram-negative bacilli [33].

Classically, cough, especially productive cough, and fever are the hallmarks of respiratory tract infections. Other clinical manifestations of pneumonia include pleurisy and rigors. In the elderly patient the clinical presentation is similar; however, the rates of patients presenting with these manifestations change. Although nearly 60% of patients with CAP presented with cough, only 34% of nursing home patients were noted to have a cough in the setting of pneumonia [31]. Confounding this picture is the fact that only 60% to 75% of nursing home patients are febrile on presentation [29]. Geriatric patients with pneumonia will tend to display more subtle signs and have more atypical presentations for pneumonia. An increased respiratory rate and the sensation of dyspnea are frequently noted in healthy geriatric patients. Mental status changes, lethargy, anorexia, abdominal pain, and failure to thrive occur predominantly in elderly patients with poor physical conditioning. Geriatric patients with "atypical" presentations make the diagnosis of pneumonia more challenging for the emergency physician, and thus a higher clinical suspicion must be maintained.

The initial emergency department workup of patients with respiratory infections includes pulse oximetry, radiography, complete blood count (CBC) with differential, blood cultures, serum electrolytes including Blood Urea Nitrogen (BUN) and rarely sputum culture with Gram stain and sensitivity.

Chest radiography remains the "gold standard" for diagnosis of pneumonia. A standard anteroposterior and lateral view are adequate for assessment of lung parenchymal involvement and the presence of pleural effusions.

Sputum culture can be used as an adjunct to isolate the pathogen and tailor antibiotic choices. Quite frequently, however, the sputum sample is inadequate for testing, and may be difficult to obtain. The optimal sputum sample has <10 epithelial cells and >25 white blood cells per low powered field. Some elderly patients may be unable to expectorate a sample from deep within the chest, thereby providing an oropharygeal colony sample instead. Even with a good respiratory sample, most studies have been unable to demonstrate a clear etiologic organism in 30% to 50% of cases [30].

Blood cultures do not need to be performed routinely on patients with pneumonia, as the yield is low, but should be performed on sicker patients. Only 6% to 10% of patients with pneumonia will be bacteremic [32]. Serum chemistries have little impact on patient outcome; however, the calculation of creatinine clearance may influence the provider's choice of antibiotic therapy. As there is a higher incidence of impaired renal function in this patient population, physicians should pay close attention to drug dosages.

Ensuring adequate oxygenation, adequate hydration, and possible cardiovascular support are key variables when initiating therapy for any patient with pneumonia. The principles of treatment of pneumonia in the elderly patient require the consideration of where the patient should be treated (at home, in the nursing care facility, or in the hospital), what antibiotic regimen to use, and the duration of treatment.

Numerous guidelines and prediction rules have been used to determine, based on clinical parameters, the mortality rate of patients with pneumonia. Site of care for elderly patients with pneumonia will depend on the severity of illness. Fine et al [34] developed a severity-of-illness score specific for pneumonia that uses 20 different variables (three demographic, five comorbid features, five physical examination findings, and seven laboratory data). Conte et al [35] developed a prognostic rule for geriatric patients with CAP. Higher scores are assigned to patients with advanced age (>85 years), impaired motor response, elevation in serum creatinine, comorbid conditions, and abnormalities in vital signs. A score of 0 was associated with low rates of mortality (4%), while higher scores were associated with mortality rates of over 40%.

With regard to antibiotic therapy, elderly patients who develop CAP should receive either a second-generation cephalosporin plus a macrolide, a nonpseudomonal cephalosporin plus a macrolide, or monotherapy with a fluoroquinolone. Patients from nursing care facilities require antibiotic therapy directed at the coverage of *S pneumoniae*, *H influenzae*, and *M catarrhalis*. Guidelines for the treatment of nursing home-acquired pneumonia have recommended the use of an oral quinolone, or amoxicillin–clavulanate plus a macrolide as second choice treatment [29]. Patient suspected of aspiration pneumonia require anaerobic coverage with clindamycin in addition to a cephalosporin.

The pneumococcal vaccine (Pneumovax) is currently recommended in the United States for patients over 65 years of age and those at higher risk due to underlying disease. Used in conjunction with the influenza vaccine, Pneumovax has the potential to prevent serious disease in the elderly population. Other measures advocated to decrease the rate of infection include attention to nutrition and smoking cessation in the community, along with staff hand washing, routine infection control, and respiratory isolation in long-term care facilities [27].

Influenza

Influenza infection ranks as one of the most common infectious diseases affecting the elderly population. Typically seen in the winter months in the United States, the influenza virus causes significant loss of workdays, morbidity, and mortality. For the elderly, respiratory viral infections pose a particular threat as older patients are more likely to have adverse outcomes. Baker and Mullooly [36] estimated that the risk of hospitalization during an influenza epidemic increased three to four times in patients 65 years or older. In addition, they found that 67% of total deaths were patients 65 years and older, with highest rates among elderly patients with comorbidities [37].

The influenza virus is a single-stranded RNA virus of which there are three major groups; influenza virus A, B, and C. The difference between these subtypes depends on the nucleoprotein of the virus. Influenza infection is transmitted via respiratory secretions. Once inside the respiratory tract of a susceptible host, the virus initiates cell damage, degeneration, and viral replication.

Infection from the influenza virus typically has an abrupt onset after an 18- to 72-hour incubation period. Symptoms of fever, chills, myalgias, cough, and rhinorrhea are most common. One important sequelae of influenza infection is pneumonia. Secondary bacterial infection occurs because of the influenza virus' ability to impair mucociliary function and the interruption of phagocytosis by immune cells. The most common strains causing secondary bacterial pneumonia are streptococci and staphylococci species [38].

Diagnosis of influenza A and B is performed via viral culture of the nasopharynx using Dacron swabs. Treatment of influenza virus rests primarily with symptomatic care; however, a few antiviral agents may decrease the duration of symptoms. Amantadine is an antiviral agent that prevents penetration of the virus by inhibiting viral uncoating. Oral oseltamivir has been shown to reduce both the duration and severity of symptoms of acute influenza [39]. The widespread use of amantadine is limited by central nervous system and gastrointestinal side effects. Oseltamivir is approved for use in patients who have been symptomatic with influenza for less than 48 hours [40].

A number of options are available as prophylaxis for elderly patients from the influenza virus. Oral (oseltamivir) and inhaled (zanamivir) neuraminidase inhibitors can be used to prevent influenza infection [41,42]. These agents can be used for prophylaxis in exposed patients who have not been immunized and for vaccinated immunosuppressed patients [40]. Routine immunization for influenza is recommended for patients 65 years and older. The vaccine is safe and effective in elderly people. Moreover, with vaccination, major reductions in economic costs and individual morbidity and mortality have been demonstrated [43].

c differences in the capsular polysaccharides. Recent strains have
ed multiple antibiotic resistance patterns, requiring treatment
mycin.

neningitidis

egative diplococcus is more commonly the cause of meningitis in
atients. Most cases of meningitis are a result of serotypes A, B,

lus influenza

enzae is a pleomorphic Gram-negative organism. Most cases of
due to this species are caused by encapsulated type b organisms,
capable of producing beta-lactamase.

nonocytogenes

a is an aerobic Gram-positive bacillus and is associated with de-
ost T-cell mediated response.

coccus aureus

-positive cocci that typically occur after intracranial injury or ma-
n, for example, head trauma, postneurosurgery, and in the presence
shunts.

gative bacilli

iella species, *Pseudomonas aeurginosa*, and less often *E coli* are the
nant Gram-negative bacilli as the causative agents of bacterial
tis.

ic presenting symptoms of meningitis include fever, headache, neck
, and photophobia. Other commonly encountered symptoms include
, malaise, altered sensorium, seizures, vomiting, and chills. Kernig's
idzinski's signs are present in approximately 50% of patients with
tis. Kernig's sign is noted when passive knee extension elicits ham-
r neck pain while the patient is supine with a flexed hip. Brudzinski's
noted when passive neck flexion elicits flexion of both hips or passive
of one hip is accompanied by a similar movement on the contralat-
e. Although the older patient may exhibit any of these signs and
ms, they are less often noted on presentation. Fever is a less fre-
encountered finding when compared with younger patients, and nu-
idity is not universally present [47]. In fact, nuchal rigidity is not as
e or as specific in the older patient. Older patients may exhibit a base-
iitation of neck mobility, making the physical finding of rigidity less
. Altered level of consciousness, respiratory symptoms, and seizures

Meningitis

Although the overall incidence of t
States has decreased, the proportion of
rently increasing [44]. Bacterial meningi
a more subtle fashion than in younger ind
ings are seen in the geriatric patient, a del;
significantly contributes to patient morbi
recognition of meningitis in the older pat
gency physicians must maintain a high lev
terial meningitis as the etiology of acute i

As the number of cases of meningitis in
clined due to the vaccine for *H influenza*
States has become a disease predominantly
cent studies have documented an increase i
ingitis in the elderly population. Higher mo
patients with meningitis, with case fatality
pneumococcal meningitis [45,46]. Older pati
impairment at presentation show morbidity
ing 50% [47].

The pathogenesis of meningitis has been
colonization of the nasopharyngeal mucos;
the subarachnoid space. Less often, bacterial
matogenous spread, most notably from patie
strumentation. Once bacteria have crossed
entered the cerebral spinal fluid (CSF), meni
inflammation occurs. With bacterial prolife
in CSF follows: the CSF glucose levels fall
The permeability of the blood–brain barrier ir
mation and elevation of intracranial pressure.
rise, the patient begins to have decreased aler
status. Left untreated, the patient's status rapi
mic brain injury, systemic hypotension, and de

The most likely organisms to cause bacterial
S pneumonia, *Neiserria meningitides*, *Listeria n*
and Gram-negative organisms. *S pneumonia* ac
all cases of meningitis among the elderly, with
most 25% of cases in patients over 60 years of ;
mophilus, common causes of meningitis in the yo
in the geriatric population.

Streptococcus pneumonia

A Gram-positive diplococcus on Gram's-stain
a fastidious bacterium. Many different serotypes

on antigen
demonstra
with vanc

Neisseria

Gram-
younger j
and C.

Haemoph

H influ
meningiti
which are

Listeria

Lister
creased

Staphylo

Gram
nipulatio
of CSF

Gram-ne

Klebs
predom
meningi
Class
stiffness
letharg
and Br
mening
string c
sign is
flexion
eral si
sympto
quently
chal ri
sensiti
line lir
reliabl

are more often found in elderly patients when compared with younger individuals [46]. As many patients will present with subtle clues, those with more pronounced symptoms are more likely to have a poor outcome. Among elderly patients admitted with the diagnosis of meningitis, risk factors for death were found to be age over 60 years, obtunded mental status on admission, and seizures within the first 24 hours [49].

Initial evaluation and diagnosis of patients suspected of having bacterial meningitis requires laboratory testing and CSF analysis. Appropriate testing includes CBC with differential, serum electrolytes to determine dehydration status, BUN and creatinine for medication dosing, and blood cultures. Blood cultures will be positive in 50% of cases of infection caused by N meningitidis, H influenzae, and S pneumoniae [44]. Radiologic evaluation by computed tomography is required for patients with evidence of head injury, focal neurologic deficits, or presence of papilledema. Although the absence of these findings may lead some practitioners to defer CT scanning, one must be cautious with geriatric patients. Elderly patients are more likely to have tumors, abscess formation, and other space-occupying lesions.

The diagnosis of bacterial meningitis is established by the analysis of CSF for cell count, protein and glucose level, and the presence of bacteria. Traditionally, tubes 1 and 4 are sent for cell count with differential, tube 2 is sent to chemistry lab for glucose and protein measurement, while tube 3 is sent to microbiology lab for Gram stain, culture, acid-fast bacillus stain, India ink, fungal cultures and cryptococcal antigen, if indicated. The general characteristics of CSF in bacterial versus aseptic meningitis are presented in Table 1. Some bacteria, such as Listeria, produce spinal fluid alterations that resemble the aseptic profile. Specifically, a more lymphocytic response may occasionally be seen on Gram's stain. Therefore, it is prudent to assume all cases of meningitis are bacterial until proven otherwise.

The objectives in the older patient with bacterial meningitis are prompt diagnosis and early institution of antibiotic therapy, which may improve patient outcome. Physicians waiting for CT and CSF results ultimately delay antibiotic administration. In fact, most delays in the initiation of antibiotics have been found to be physician generated [50]. If the possibility of bacterial

Table 1
Cerebral spinal fluid in bacterial and aseptic meningitis

CSF parameter	Bacterial meningitis	Aseptic meningitis
Opening pressure	>180 mm H_2O	Normal to slightly elevated
Glucose	<40 mg/dL	>45 mg/dL
Protein	>50 mg/dL	Normal or elevated
WBCs	>10 WBCs/mm^3 (PMNs)	50 to 2000/mm^3 (Lymphs)
Gram's stain	Positive in 70% to 90%	Negative
Lactic acid	>3.8 mmol/L	Normal

Abbreviations: CSF, cerebral spinal fluid; WBCs, white blood cells.
Data from Choi C. Bacterial meningitis. Clin Geriatr Med 1992;8:889–901.

meningitis is entertained after initial patient assessment, empiric antibiotic coverage should be initiated.

In deciding on an antibiotic regimen, elements to consider are organism susceptibility to the antibiotic, the ability of the drug to cross the blood–brain barrier, and appropriate dosing based on the patient's renal function. Empiric therapy should be directed against the most common etiologic agents, taking into account the patient's history and suspicion of underlying disease. In elderly patients, a combination of ampicillin plus a third-generation cephalosporin should be used for initial therapy, as these agents would be active against most species of *S pneumoniae*, *L monocytogenes*, aerobic Gram-negative bacilli, *H influenzae*, and *N meningitidis*. After the organism has been identified by Gram's stain and culture, the initial antibiotic therapy should be adjusted to the specific organism.

The use of dexamethasone in the management of bacterial meningitis remains controversial. In high-risk cases, adjunctive use of steroids may be beneficial [51]. Sanford recommends administering steroids to patients with positive Gram-stain, those who are in a coma, or those with increased CSF pressure. Dexamethasone, when given, should be administered 15 to 20 minutes before the first dose of antibiotics.

Other management considerations include intravenous fluid, antipyretics for fever, analgesics, supplemental oxygen, and ventilatory support when appropriate. For patients presenting with seizures, benzodiazepines should be administered.

All people who have had close contact with patients diagnosed with bacterial meningitis should be considered for prophylaxis. Rifampin 600 mg two times per day for four doses is adequate protection for *N meningitides*. Ciprofloxacin 500 mg orally as a single dose is an alternative if compliance is an issue.

Summary

As life expectancy continues to rise, the number of geriatric patients will increase, and the percentages of geriatric patients seen in the emergency department will reflect those numbers. Emergency physicians are responsible for making immediate diagnoses and initiating expeditious treatment. Infectious diseases in the elderly are more prevalent, challenging to diagnose, and are associated with greater morbidity and mortality than with the younger patient population [52].

References

[1] Gavazzi G, Krause KH. Ageing and infection. Lancet Infect Dis 2002;2(11):659–66.
[2] Crossley KB, Peterson PK. Infections in the elderly. In: Mandell: principles and practice of infectious diseases. 5th ed. London: Churchill Livingstone, Inc.; 2000. p. 3165–8.

[3] Yoshikawa TT. Epidemiology and unique aspects of aging and infectious diseases. Clin Infect Dis 2000;30:931–3.

[4] Mouton CP, Bazaldua OV, Pierce B, et al. Common infections in older adults. Am Fam Physician 2001;63:257–68.

[5] Nicolle LE, Strausbaugh LJ, Garibaldi RA. Infections and antibiotic resistance in nursing homes. Clin Microbiol Rev 1996;9:1–17.

[6] Jacobs LG. Infectious disease emergencies in the geriatric population. Clin Geriatr Med 1993;9:559–75.

[7] Yung RL. Changes in immune function with age. Rheum Dis Clin North Am 2000;26: 455–73.

[8] Marco CA, Shoenfeld CN, Hansen KN, et al. Fever in geriatric emergency patients: clinical features associated with serious illness. Ann Emerg Med 1995;26:18–24.

[9] Norman DC, Yoshikawa TT. Fever in the elderly. Infect Dis Clin North Am 1996;10:93–9.

[10] Chassagne P, Perol MB, Doucet J, et al. Is presentation of bacteremia in the elderly the same as in younger patients? Am J Med 1996;100:65–70.

[11] Jarrett PG, Rockwood K, Carver D, et al. Illness presentation in elderly patients. Arch Intern Med 1995;155:1060–4.

[12] Henschke PJ. Infections in the elderly. Med J Aust 1993;158:830–4.

[13] Miller D, Castle SC, Yoshikawa TT, et al. Effect of age on fever response to recombinant tumor necrosis factor alpha in a murine mode. J Gerontol 1996;46:176–9.

[14] Yoshikawa TT, Norman DC. Approach to fever and Infection in the nursing home. J Am Geriatr Soc 1996;44:74–82.

[15] Elgart ML. Skin infections and infestations in geriatric patients. Clin Geriatr Med 2002;18: 89–101.

[16] Weinburg JM, Vafaie J, Scheinfeld NS. Skin Infections in the elderly. Dermatol Clin 2004; 22:51–61.

[17] Stalam M, Kaye D. Antibiotic agents in the elderly. Infect Dis Clin North Am 2004;18: 533–49.

[18] Rajagopalan S, Yoshikawa TT. Antimicrobial therapy in the elderly. Med Clin North Am 2001;85:133–47.

[19] Mulholland SG. Urinary tract infection. Clin Geriatr Med 1990;6:43–53.

[20] Ginde AA, Rhee SH, Katz ED. Predictors in outcome in geriatric patients with urinary tract infections. J Emerg Med 2004;27:101–8.

[21] Yoshikawa TT, Nicolle LE, Norman DC. Management of complicated urinary tract infection in older patients. J Am Geriatr Soc 1996;44:1235–41.

[22] Shortliffe LDM, McCue JD. Urinary tract Infections at the age extremes: pediatrics and geriatrics. Am J Med 2002;113:55S–66S.

[23] Childs SJ, Egan RJ. Bacteriuria and urinary infections in the elderly. Urol Clin North Am 1996;23:43–54.

[24] Johnson JR, Stamm WE. Diagnosis and treatment of acute urinary tract infections. Infect Dis Clin North Am 1987;1:773–91.

[25] O'Donnell JA, Hofman MT. Urinary tract infections: how to manage nursing home patients with or without chronic catheterization. Geriatrics 2002;57:49–58.

[26] Nicolle LE, Bjornson J, Harding GKM, et al. Bacturia in elderly institutionalized men. N Engl J Med 1983;309:1420–5.

[27] Feldman C. Pneumonia in the elderly. Med Clin North Am 2001;85:1441–59.

[28] Chan ED, Welsh CH. Geriatric respiratory medicine. Chest 1998;114:1704–33.

[29] Mylotte JM. Nursing home-acquired pneumonia. Clin Infect Dis 2002;35:1205–11.

[30] Medina-Walpole AM, Katz PR. Nursing home-acquired pneumonia. J Am Geriatr Soc 1999;47:1005–15.

[31] Marrie TJ. Community-acquired pneumonia in the elderly. Clin Infect Dis 2000;31:1066–78.

[32] Marrie TJ. Pneumonia. Clin Geriatr Med 1992;8:721–31.

[33] Muder RR. Pneumonia in residents of long-term care facilities: epidemiology, etiology, management, and prevention. Am J Med 1998;105:319–30.

[34] Fine MJ, Auble TE, Yealy DM, et al. A prediction rule to identify low-risk patients with community-acquired pneumonia. N Engl J Med 1997;336:243–50.

[35] Conte HA, Chen YT, Mehal W, et al. A prognostic rule for elderly patients admitted with community-acquired pneumonia. Am J Med 1999;106:20–8.

[36] Barker WH, Mullooly JP. Pneumonia and influenza deaths during epidemics. Implications for prevention. Arch Intern Med 1982;142:85–9.

[37] Barker WH, Mullooly JP. Impact of epidemic type A influenza in a defined adult population. Am J Epidemiol 1980;112:798–811.

[38] Cesario TC, Yousefi S. Viral infections. Clin Geriatr Med 1992;8:735–43.

[39] Treanor JJ, Hayden FG, Vrooman PS, et al. Efficacy and safety of the oral neuraminidase inhibitor oseltamivir in treating acute influenza: a randomized controlled trial. US Oral Neuraminidase Study Group. JAMA 2000;283:1016–24.

[40] Olshaker J. Influenza. Emerg Med Clin North Am 2003;21:353–61.

[41] Hayden FG, Gubareva LV, Monto AS, et al. Inhaled zanamivir for the prevention of influenza in families. Zanamivir Family Study Group. N Engl J Med 2000;343:1282–9.

[42] Hayden FG, Atmar RL, Schilling M, et al. Use of the selective oral neuraminidase inhibitor oseltamivir to prevent influenza. N Engl J Med 1999;341:1336–43.

[43] Gross PA, Hermogenes AW, Sacks HS, et al. The efficacy of influenza vaccine in elderly persons. A meta-analysis and review of the literature. Ann Intern Med 1995;123:518–27.

[44] Choi C. Bacterial meningitis. Clin Geriatr Med 1992;8:889–901.

[45] Schuchat A, Robinson K, Wenger JD, et al. Bacterial meningitis in the United States in 1995. Active surveillance team. N Engl J Med 1997;337:970–6.

[46] Roos KL. Meningitis as it presents in the elderly: diagnosis and care. Geriatrics 1990;45:63–75.

[47] Miller LG, Choi C. Meningitis in older patients: how to diagnose and treat a deadly infection. Geriatrics 1997;52:43–4, 47–50, 55.

[48] Peeters A, Waer M, Michielsen P, et al. Listeria monocytogenes meningitis. Clin Neurol Neurosurg 1989;91:29–36.

[49] Durand ML, Calderwood SB, Weber DJ, et al. Acute bacterial meningitis in adults. A review of 493 episodes. N Engl J Med 1993;328:21–8.

[50] Talan DA, Guterman JJ, Overturf GD, et al. Analysis of emergency department management of suspected bacterial meningitis. Ann Emerg Med 1989;18:856–62.

[51] McIntyre PB, Berkey CS, King SM, et al. Dexamethasone as adjunctive therapy in bacterial meningitis. A meta-analysis of randomized clinical trials since 1988. JAMA 1997;278:925–31.

[52] Norman DC, Toledo SD. Infections in elderly persons. An altered clinical presentation. Clin Geriatr Med 1992;8:713–9.

ELSEVIER
SAUNDERS

Emerg Med Clin N Am
24 (2006) 449–465

EMERGENCY
MEDICINE
CLINICS OF
NORTH AMERICA

Pharmacologic Issues in Geriatric Emergency Medicine

Michelle P. Blanda, MD, FACEP

*Department of Emergency Medicine, Northeastern Ohio Universities College of Medicine,
Summa Health System, 41 Arch Street, Suite 518, Akron, OH 44304, USA*

The geriatric emergency care model emphasizes older emergency patients be considered a special population, analogous to pediatric patients [1]. This concept is especially relevant to pharmacologic issues in the elderly. The need for practitioners to create a balance between using medications with adverse effects while providing access to therapies that may have a beneficial effect on morbidity, mortality, function, and quality of life is challenging. Variables affecting this challenge in the elderly population include comorbidities, limited evidence for efficacy, increased risk of adverse drug reactions, polypharmacy, and altered pharmokinetics.

Elderly patients become involved in a vicious cycle described by Rochan as the "prescribing cascade" [2,3]. This cascade begins when an adverse drug reaction is misinterpreted as a new medical condition. A drug is prescribed to treat this new "medical condition" and another adverse drug effect occurs. Again, this is interpreted as a new condition and the patient is again subjected to unnecessary treatment and additional adverse effects of the drug. Because elderly patients have multiple medical problems they are prescribed multiple medications that lead to increased risk of adverse effects. Many of these adverse effects go unrecognized as such and lead to new drugs being added. This perpetuates the continued cycle of adverse effects.

This article describes the scope of the problem of drug prescribing in the elderly. It looks at the concept of adverse drug reactions and events, principles underlying clinical geriatric pharmacology, and reviews drugs that commonly cause adverse drug reactions. It includes recommendations about drugs to be avoided and substitutes and approaches to evaluate the evidence for risk and benefits when selecting drugs for an elderly person.

E-mail address: blandam@summa-health.org

0733-8627/06/$ - see front matter © 2006 Elsevier Inc. All rights reserved.
doi:10.1016/j.emc.2006.01.007   *emed.theclinics.com*

Scope of the problem

Drug prescribing in the elderly is an important topic to consider because of many factors. These include the growth of the aging population, the existence of chronic illness, and the use of multiple medications. In addition, because pharmacokinetics and pharmacodynamics may be altered by age and disease, this group is at high risk to be affected. All these points increase the susceptibility for adverse drug reactions in the elderly.

In the year 2003, there were 36 million people over the age of 65 years in the United States, representing 12% of the total population [4]. This group received approximately 40% of prescribed drugs, which is twice as much as their younger counterparts [5]. It is anticipated that significant growth will occur in this age group during the years 2011 to 2030 when baby boomers, the people born between 1946 and 1964, turn 65 years old [4]. Therefore, any issues that affect this growing population will continue not only to exist but to become more pronounced.

As stated, the incidence of chronic illness and pathology increases with age, leading to polypharmacy in this group. Although the term polypharmacy carries negative connotations, use of numerous medications is sometimes necessary [6]. Despite the view that there is widespread underuse of beneficial therapies in this population, drugs with known value in decreasing mortality in clinical trials are being offered more and more to the elderly. These include mainstays of therapy such as angiotensin converting enzyme inhibitors in heart failure, antiplatelet agents in stroke, and antiplatelet agents and beta-blockers in those with myocardial infarction [7].

The elderly have more adverse drug events than any other age group because their exposure to a greater number of medications provides more opportunities for medication errors and side effects. The Sloan Survey, which was a phone survey of a random sample of the nonistitutionalized US population, reported data on the range of drugs used by the general public. For patients aged at least 65 years, this survey found that 23% of women and 19% of men took at least five medications and 12% of both women and men took > 10 medications during the preceding week [5]. Others have reported similar numbers, with community-dwelling elders taking between two and six medications and one to three nonprescription medications on a routine basis [8].

The Sloan survey also reported on common vitamin and herbal use by this age group. The common vitamins used by both sexes in patients 65 years of age and older were multivitamins, vitamin E, and vitamin C. In addition, women used calcium and vitamin D. Common herbal supplements included *allium sativum*, glucosamine, and *serenoa repens* in men, and *ginkgo biloba* extract, glucosamine, and *allium sativum* in women [5] (Table 1). Awareness of the use of the full range of medications, both prescription and nonprescription, is essential for safety and to reduce risks associated with their consumption.

Table 1
Herbal medications and supplements used in the elderly

Herb/supplement	Reason for use
Allium sativum (garlic)	Immune enhancing Anticancer
Glucosamine/chondroitin	Osteoarthritis—pain relief and prevention
Serenoa repens	Treatment for benign prostatic hypertrophy
Ginkgo biloba extract	Prevention of dementia, Alzheimers disease
Calcium	Osteoporosis prevention
Vitamin D	Osteoporosis prevention
Vitamin E	Prevention of Alzeheimers, Parkinsons disease
Vitamin C	Anticancer, heart disease prevention

Adverse drug reactions

Adverse drug reactions are defined by the World Health Organization (WHO) as "any noxious, unintended, and undesired effect of a drug which occurs at doses used in humans for prophylaxis, diagnosis or therapy" [9]. This does not include therapeutic failures, poisonings (whether accidental or intentional), abuse of drugs, errors in administration, or noncompliance. Therefore, the term adverse drug reaction probably underestimates the true incidence of events related to drugs. Other terms are used instead of adverse drug reaction. "Adverse drug event" refers to any injury resulting from administration of a drug. A "drug-related problem" includes the above definitions but also includes failure to receive drugs for a medical problem and drug use without indication [10]. Most literature, however, tends not to use these broader definitions. The goal of research in adverse drug reactions is to alert physicians about the preventability of these reactions. However, one must keep in mind that literature on adverse drug reactions demonstrates that even when drugs are used properly there are still a large number of serious adverse drug reactions that occur [10].

Age-related changes affecting pharmacokinetics

Drug absorption, distribution, metabolism, excretion, and the physiologic response to drugs are altered in the elderly. The impairment of drug absorption due to resection of the gut, bacterial overgrowth, or achlorhydria is felt to have minimal clinical implications [11]. However, drug interactions can occur where one drug changes the absorption characteristics of another. The classic example of one drug binding another is the use of calcium and magnesium containing antacids. Absorption of drugs such as antibiotics, aspirin, and digoxin can be significantly impaired by concurrent administration of antacids. Drugs that change the gastrointestinal transit time may change a drug's pharmacologic action. Practitioners should be aware and monitor patients carefully when administering these drugs.

Drug distribution may be altered significantly due to decreased lean body mass, decreased total body water, and increased proportion of body fat in the aging body [12,13]. These changes in body composition lead to a decrease in the volume of distribution and an increase in the serum concentrations of drugs. Drugs that are water soluble such as coumadin, digoxin, and propanolol will have higher plasma concentrations at a given dose in the elderly. In drugs with low or narrow therapeutic windows (such as digoxin, aminoglycosides, lithium, or procainamide) this can lead to toxicity.

Serum protein, especially albumin, also decreases with age [13]. This leads to decreased binding sites for protein bound medications, higher serum concentrations, and the likelihood of more rapid clearance if normal excretion and clearance is occurring, or increased levels if not. Malnutrition is a cause of deceased serum albumin, and is common in older patients, especially those who are institutionalized. Competitive inhibition for protein binding sites by drugs can lead to displacement of one drug by another with increased levels of the drug being displaced. An example is aspirin and warfarin, where aspirin increases the unbound fraction of warfarin.

Metabolism and clearance of drugs are also changed in the elderly [12–16] (Table 2). Unfortunately, because elderly patients with comorbid conditions are excluded from many drug trials, the knowledge of drug metabolism is limited. There are age-related decreases in renal function that are not related to kidney disease. As the kidney ages there is a decrease in the glomerular filtration rate and tubular efficiency. A compensatory production of vasodilatory renal prostaglandins occurs to compensate for this decreased renal function. Drugs that impair this compensatory mechanism can cause a decrease in renally eliminated drugs. Nonsteroidal anti-inflammatory drugs are an example [17,18]. Because lean body mass decreases with age, the serum creatinine is a poor indicator of creatinine clearance, actually tending to overestimate clearance [19]. It is recommended that creatinine clearance be calculated with correction for age and weight using the Cockroft-Gault formula: (creatinine clearance = $[(140 - age) \times weight(kg)]/[72 \times creatinine (mg/dL) \times 0.85$ for females]). Results of decreased renal function include

Table 2
Common drugs that have decreased clearance in the elderly

Route of clearance	Drugs
Renal	Cardiovascular: atenolol, digoxin, furosemide, hydrochlorothiazide, procainamide, enalapril, lisinopril
	Antibiotics: ampicillin, ceftriaxone, gentamycin penicillin, ciprofloxacin, levofloxacin, ofloxacin
	Gastrointestinal: cimetidine, ranitidine, famotidine
	Neurologic: amantadine, lithium, pancuronium, phenobarbital
	Hypoglycemic drugs: chlorpropamide, glyburide
Hepatic	Cardiovascular: labetolol, lidocaine, prazosin, propanolol, quinidine, salicylates, warfarin
	Analgesics: acetaminophen, ibuprofen, meperidine, codeine
	Pulmonary: theophylline
	Neurologic: amitriptyline, barbiturates, phenytoin, benzodiazepines

prolonged half-life of renally cleared medications, increased serum levels, and prolonged clinical effects.

The other organ that contributes to metabolism of many drugs is the liver. Hepatic metabolism in the elderly is not only related to age, but to lifestyle, genotype, hepatic blood flow, hepatic disease, and interactions with other medications. It may be reduced up to 30% to 50% in the elderly [14–16]. Hepatic metabolism occurs through one of two biotransformation systems. Phase I reactions occur through the cytochrome P450 system, which either clears drugs or allows oxidation and activation of drugs. This occurs much more slowly in older adults. The change in Phase I reactions leads to change in the serum levels and clinical activity. Inhibitors of the P450 system cause an increase in the serum concentrations of drugs metabolized by the liver by impairing clearance of those drugs. Medications that induce the P450 system lead to decreased levels of medications metabolized by the liver. Phase II metabolism, which includes acetylation, sulfonation, conjugation, and glucuronidation, is minimally affected in the older population [14]. Cigarette smoking, alcohol use, and caffeine may also affect hepatic metabolism.

Other physiologic changes are occurring that affect the pharmacodynamics of many drugs. Age-related changes in cardiovascular function occur, and may explain the reduced compensatory capacity effect in the elderly to many drugs. Changes in cardiac morphology at a cellular level leads to decreased number of myocytes, stiffening of myocardial cells, reduced responsiveness to *B*-adrenergic stimulation, and clinically with decreased contractility of the heart with age. In parallel to these changes, large arteries dilate, have increased wall thickness, and increased smooth muscle tone with age [20–23]. This leads to increased systolic blood pressure and elevated left ventricular afterload, resulting in left ventricular wall thickening. This, in turn, causes decreased left ventricular compliance and impairment of diastolic function. Other changes in the older population include an increase in sympathetic outflow causing decreased sensitivity to *B*-adrenergic stimulation as well as autonomic and baroreceptor dysfunction leading to decreased response to posture and hypotension.

The central nervous system (CNS) is the other area where aging changes must be considered. Research now suggests that it is not a simple loss in the number of neurons that occurs with time, but subtler changes occurring at the level of synapses. Alterations in cellular Ca^{2+} capacity to deal with oxidative stress, reduced regeneration capacity (remyelination), and decrease in receptor sites as well as changes within these sites all have been identified as explanations for the diminution of CNS functioning and sensitivity to drugs in the elderly [20,24–26].

Consequences of adverse drug reactions

The consequences of medication-related problems are profound. Between 3% and 28% of hospital admissions can be attributed to drug-related problems or drug toxic effects [27–29]. If fatal adverse drug reactions were classified as a distinct entity, they would rank between the fourth and sixth leading cause of death in the United States. This would rank adverse drug reactions above pneumonia and diabetes as a cause of death. This is not unique to the United States, but has also been identified in other nations' health systems [30].

The cost of drug-related morbidity and mortality is estimated to be more than 136 billion dollars in the United States [11]. Admissions related to adverse drug reactions cost 847 million dollars in the United Kingdom, and account for 4% of hospital bed capacity [30]. Review of adverse drug reactions related to hospital admission found that 80% are directly responsible for the admission or known as "causal." The other 20% are "coincidental," and although not directly responsible for the admission, may have contributed to it. Almost three quarters are considered avoidable [30].

These adverse drug events are not limited to causing admissions. In hospitalized patients it is estimated that 2,216,000 patients experience an adverse drug reaction while being treated, and 106,000 of these are fatal [28]. For most hospitals this translates to about two out of every 100 admissions. These events increase the hospital cost by $4,700 dollars per admission, and if generalized to the whole US population, the cost is approximately 2 billion dollars [29].

Use of medications not documented or revealed to the physician while in the hospital is another problem. It has been described that, on average, about 1.5 additional drugs not mentioned on initial assessment of drug history, will be discovered on a second interview [31]. This has been verified by actual urine sampling of patients with analgesics, benzodiazepines, and ranitidine being reported as most commonly not disclosed [32]. This widespread phenomenon of physicians being unaware of medication used by the patient, has been described in emergency departments, surgical settings, and in office visits as well [33–35].

Drugs most commonly causing hospital admissions are listed in Box 1 [30,35,36]. Care must be exercised when reviewing this data because in the majority of studies it is difficult to say what the overall consumption of drugs is. Drugs implicated in causing adverse reactions may be more related to the frequency by which they are used. Also, no credit has been given to the benefits of the drugs. Aspirin is a classic example where there is convincing data of the long-term benefits of prophylactic use in high-risk patients [37].

Adverse drug events occur in the nursing home population as well. Rates for adverse drug reactions in nursing homes are 1.89 per 100 resident months and 0.65 per 100 resident months for potential adverse drug events [38]. For every dollar spent on drugs in nursing homes it is estimated that $1.33 in health care resources are consumed in the treatment of drug-related problems [39].

The most common drugs identified by practicioners as causing problems in nursing home residents are listed in Table 3 [38]. Warfarin is a drug that not only is identified as a problem in the hospital but in nursing homes

---

Box 1. Drugs implicated in Causing Hospital Admission (in order of frequency)

Diuretics
Warfarin
Nonsteroidal anti-inflammatory agents (includes aspirin)
Chemotherapy
Antidiabetic Agents
Cardiotonic Agents
Antiepileptic Drugs
Immunosuppressants
Antibiotics

Data from Postgrad Med J 1996;72:671–6 and Bandolier Extra 2002;1:1–15.

---

as well. Prescribers however, frequently do not make modifications in the warfarin dose even when drugs with well-established interactions with warfarin are prescribed [38]. Other drugs causing problems in the nursing home include psychoactive medications such as antipsychotics, antidepressants, and sedative/hypnotics. Percentages of nursing home patients using these drugs were 17%, 36%, and 24% respectively. Neuropsychiatric episodes such as oversedation, confusion, hallucinations, and delirium were the

Table 3
Top 10 dangerous drug interactions seen in nursing homes

Warfarin—NSAIDs	Increased bleeding
Warfarin—sulfonamides	Prolongation of warfarin's effects due to unknown mechanism. Need to decrease dose of warfarin by 50% during and 1 week after therapy with antibiotic
Warfarin—macrolide antibiotics	Prolongation of warfarin's effects due to inhibition of warfarin metabolism by macrolides
Warfarin—quinolone antibiotics	Prolongation of warfarin's effects due to unknown mechanism. May be due to decrease in vitamin K production and altered warfarin metabolism
ACE inhibitors—potassium	Hyperkalemia can occur due to decreased aldosterone production caused by ACE inhibitors
ACE inhibitors—spironolactone	Both drugs increase serum potassium and can cause hyperkalemia
Digoxin—amiodarone	Amiodarone decreases the clearance of digoxin leading to toxicity. Decrease the dose of digoxin by 50% and monitor levels
Theophylline—quinolone antibiotics	Some quinolones can affect the metabolism of theophylline and lead to its toxicity

Abbreviation: NSAIDs, nonsteroid anti-inflammatory drugs.
Data from Gurwitz JH, Fields TS, Avorn J, et al. Incidence and preventability of adverse drug events in nursing homes. Am J Med 2000;109:87–94.

most common types of adverse drug events in this population. Falls and bleeding were half as common, and ranked as second and third.

What goes wrong? Risk factors for adverse drug reactions

Problems of drug use in the elderly range from wrong or unnecessary drugs prescribed, use of medication without appropriate monitoring, dosage too high or too low, adverse drug reactions to nonadherence, and polypharmacy. Most of the time though, adverse drug reactions are an accentuation of the drug's known pharmacologic effect. Drugs with low therapeutic ratios (ratio between average therapeutic and toxic dose) such as cardiovascular drugs and analgesics are commonly implicated, as stated above. Also, drugs that are frequently used in the elderly are likely to be associated with adverse drug reactions. The actual effect of age alone and its relationship to adverse drug reactions has been questioned [40].

The direct relationship with the number of medications taken and adverse drug reactions is substantiated [27,41–44]. The concept of polypharmacy is challenging. It is known that several medical conditions can exist in the elder patient. These conditions may best be treated with multiple drugs resulting in "obligatory or rational pharmacy" [45]. Toxicity of drug combinations may be synergistic and be greater than the sum of the toxicity in either agent alone. This is reflected by Col's [27] work on adverse drug reactions related to hospital admission. It showed the odds ratio for an adverse drug reaction in those taking three to nine medications compared with with those taking less then three was 1.8. The odds ratio for those taking 10 or more medications compared with those taking three or less was 13.4.

Noncompliance is another issue leading to adverse drug reactions. Patients may underuse, overuse, and misuse medications. Elderly people who live alone, use two or more medications, have no assistance in taking their medications, and who use more then two pharmacies and more than two physicians are more likely to have noncompliance [27]. Medication regimens with a greater number of pills taken per day, greater number of kinds of medications, as well as a greater number of needed medications are cited as problematic. Noncompliance is felt to be almost equally split, with half being intentional and the other half unintentional. Forgetfulness, unpleasant side effects of medications perceived as unnecessary, confusion, cost, and dislike of taking medications are all cited by patients as causes for noncompliance.

Costs of medications are also related to adverse drug reactions. This may reflect use of newer, more costly medications that may have more side effects, more drug interactions, and are prescribed by practitioners with less awareness of potential reactions in this population.

Other risk factors for adverse drug reactions in older outpatients are in Box 2. Similar risk factors are found in the nursing home population. These

---

Box 2. Risk factors for adverse dug reactions in older outpatients

Polypharmacy (>5 medications)
Multiple (>2) chronic medical problems
Prior adverse drug reaction
Dementia
Renal Insufficiency (creatinine clearance <50 mL/min)
Advanced age (>85 years)
Multiple prescribers

---

include age 85 years and older, more then six active chronic medical diagnoses, low body weight or body mass index, nine or more medications, more than 12 doses of medication per day, and a previous adverse drug reaction [46,47].

Poisonings in the elderly

Data from poison control centers reveal that therapeutic errors are more common in the elderly (25% compared with 14.5% in younger patients). Elderly patients also contact poison centers more with acute or chronic conditions, especially women. This suggests that this population may not recognize the adverse drug reaction. Further prescribed drugs may be added, or self-medication may occur, complicating both the recognition and treatment of the adverse drug event [48]. Misuse of drugs also increased slightly with age, but then decreased in the oldest patients. Accidental exposures can be attributed to confusion, dementia, impaired vision, forgetfulness, or lack of knowledge or understanding of the product's intended use. Examples of unintentional exposures are listed in Box 3.

Inappropriate medications in the elderly

Consensus criteria have been used to identify safe medication use in the elderly [49–51]. This method uses expert consensus developed through

---

Box 3. Causes of unintentional exposures in the elderly

Taking extra dose of medication
Mistaking external preparations to be given orally
Taking nonmedicines in error
Mistaking eye for ear drops (or vice versa)
Mistaking another person or the pets prescription for one's own
Taking nonfood substances placed in food containers

---

literature review and questionnaire evaluation by nationally recognized experts in geriatric care, clinical pharmacology, and psychopharmacology using a modified Dephi technique for consensus building. Explicit criteria provide useful tools for assessing the quality of prescribing and potential risks from prescribing in the elderly. The initial criteria developed by Beers [50,51,52] were targeted to the frail nursing home patient. Updates have been done that are applicable to the general population of the elderly. The published list by Beers was adopted by the Health Care Financing Administration as a guideline for surveyors of long-term care institutions.

Medications with high severity rating for adverse reactions are in Table 4. Some discussion of the drugs and the reasoning behind the "inappropriate" label are discussed here. Many common themes are revealed in review of inappropriate drug lists. Anticholinergic drugs and drugs with anticholinergic effects are considered inappropriate. These drugs cause mild side effects (dry mouth, thirst, mydriasis), but can also cause toxicity with urinary retention, agitation, hallucinations, seizures, cardiac arrythmias, and heart block. Thermoregulation can be impaired, causing patients to be more at risk for heatstroke during hot weather. Delirium and cognitive impairment can also occur. Antiparkisonian drugs, tricyclic antidepressants (TCAs), phenothiazines, and antihistamines are all drugs that have anticholinergic effects.

TCAs are considered inappropriate not only due to their anticholinergic effects, but also due to their increased volume of distribution and slowed metabolism in the elderly. Cardiac toxicity occurs more frequently in patients with cardiac disease. This may result in heart block and fatal ventricular arrhythmias. Orthostatic hypotension is common. CNS effects such as confusion and seizures are more common in the elderly. Selective serotonin reuptake inhibitors are a better choice, although not beneficial for the treatment of neuropathic pain.

Antipsychotic medications are occasionally prescribed in the elderly patient with behavioral problems associated with dementia. Antipsychotics produce extrapyramidal and anticholinergic effects as well as tardive dyskinesia, which can occur after short-term and low-dose use. Newer generation antipsychotics (resperidone, olanzapine, and quetiapine) are available with efficacy that is similar to traditional antipsychotics but with a greater safety record. The Food and Drug Administration recently issued a black box warning stating that these newer antipsychotics may be associated with an increased risk of death in the elderly, making the choice of antipsychotic medications in elderly patients more difficult (see article on "Psychiatric Emergencies in the Elderly Population").

Barbiturates, except when used as anticonvulsants, are considered inappropriate for the elderly. This is due to their high lipid solubility and prolonged duration of action, which can lead to accumulation and toxicity. Tolerance to their sedating effects occurs and disruption of rapid eye movement sleep occurs, leading to unnatural sleep. Benzodiazepines are used in anxiety mood disorders. They are categorized according to half-life and the presence or absence of active metabolites. The older benzodiazepines (diazepam, chlordiazepoxide, and flurazepam) have an increased volume of distribution in the elderly. This is due to their lipid solubility and increase in adipose stores that increase with age. Also, because benzodiazepines are degraded by the liver, and hepatic function changes with age, their half life can increase up to four- to fivefold in an older patient compared with a young patient [6]. Low lipid soluble benzodiazepines (lorazepam and oxazepam) have less risk for accumulation and toxicity. Use of benzodiazepines should be limited in older patients, and when used, should be used in low doses and for short-term therapy.

Traditional antihistamines are not used in the older population due to their CNS effects and their anticholinergic properties. They are present in many over-the-counter medications for insomnia, respiratory symptoms, and allergic conditions. The sedative effects decrease motor reflexes and place older patients at risk for motor vehicle accidents, falls, and hip fractures. Second-generation antihistamines are a better choice if antihistamines are felt to be of benefit to the patient.

Nonsteroidal anti-inflammatory drugs (NSAIDs) are commonly used in the elderly for symptom management. NSAIDs are highly lipid soluble drugs with extensive protein binding. In the elderly there is widespread distribution of NSAIDs due to increased adipose stores. Unbound drug is also increased due to the reduction in plasma protein found in many older persons. NSAIDs are renally cleared and because there may be decreased renal function in older patients there is potential for excessive drug levels and toxicity.

Complications from NSAIDs are reported, with gastropathy being the most common [53]. These effects occur not only in the stomach, duodenum, and esophagus, but also in the small intestine and colon. Bleeding occurs, and is increased in patients taking anticoagulants and prednisone. NSAIDs may also inhibit the action of antihypertensive agents whose activity is via renal prostaglandins such as B-blockers and angiotensin converting agents. NSAIDs can also produce renal insufficiency, hyperkalemia, and fluid retention.

There is not adequate evidence to label NSAIDs as a class, as inappropriate for use in the elderly population. Beers specifically delineated indomethacin due to its CNS toxicity, and phenylbutazone because of its risk of bone marrow suppression as inappropriate. However, because NSAIDs benefit so many people, it is felt that cautious use with low doses and short-term therapy are appropriate.

Avoiding certain analgesics is recommended by the Beers guidelines. These included pentazocine, propoxyphene, and meperidine. Pentazocine is a mixed opiate agonist/antagonist with adequate efficacy but with increased risk of seizures and CNS effects compared with other analgesics. Propoxyphene is deemed inappropriate for elderly persons because of its doubtful efficacy and possibility of CNS toxicity due to the long half-life

Table 4
Inappropriate medications in the elderly

Medication (with example)	Reason for status
Amphetamines/anorexic agents	Potential for dependence, hypertension, angina, myocardial infarction
Analgesics	
Pentazocin	CNS adverse effects, also mixed agonist-antagonist
Meperidine	Not as effective as other narcotics
Indomethacin	CNS adverse effects
Ketorolac	Potential for GI bleed
NSAIDs	Potential for GI bleed, renal failure, high blood pressure, heart failure
Antianxiety agents/sedative/hypnotics	
Long-acting benzodiazepines	Highly addictive, cause more side effects than sedative/hypnotics. Better alternatives available
Short-acting benzodiazepines	Smaller doses are safer
Barbiturates	Highly addictive; better alternatives available
Meprobamate	Highly sedating anxiolytic; need to withdraw slowly
Antiarrythmic agents	
Disopyramide	Negative iontrope, can cause heart failure; strong anticholinergic
Amiodarone	Lack of efficacy in older patients, prolong QT interval/torsades
Anticoagulants	
Dipyridamole	May cause orthostatic hypotension
Ticlopidine	No better then aspirin, may be more toxic
Antidepressants	
Amitriptyline, chlordiazepoxide, Doxepin	Anticholinergic effects (arrythmia, dry mouth and eyes, urinary retention)
Daily fluoxetine	Excessive CNS stimulation, agitation
Antispasmodics/Muscle relaxants	
Dicyclomine, hyoscyamine, belladonna alkaloids carisprodop, cyclobenzaprine orphenadrine	Anticholinergic effects, questionable effectiveness
Blood glucose regulators	
Chlorpropamide	Prolonged half-life leads to prolonged hypoglycemia
First-and second-generation antipsychotics	
Thioridazine	
Mesoridazine	CNS adverse effects, extrapyramidal effects. Better alternatives available
First-generation antihistamines	Confusion and sedation
Diphenhydramine, hydroxine	
Guanethidine (Ismelin)	May cause orthostatic hypotension
Guanadrel (Hyloral)	May cause orthostatic hypotension
Long-term use of laxatives (biscodyl)	Exacerbate bowel dysfunction
Methyldopa (Aldomet)	Causes bradycardia and may exacerbate depression

Table 4 (*continued*)

Medication (with example)	Reason for status
Methyltestosterone	Potential for prostatic hypertrophy and cardiac problems
Mineral oil	Potential for aspiration
Nifedipine (short acting)	Potential for Orthostatic hypotension and CNS adverse effects
Nitrofurantoin	Potential for renal impairment
Thyroid (dessicated)	Cardiac effects
Trimethobenzamide (Tigan)	Extrapyramidal side effects

Drugs with low severity rating are not listed. These include: cimetidine, clonidine, cyclande-late, digoxin, doxazosin, ergot meyloids, estrogens, ethacrynic acid, ferrous sulfate, isoxurpine long acting dipyridamole, propoxyphene, and reserpine.

Abbreviations: CNS, central nervous system; GI, gastrointestinal; NSAIDs, nonsteroidal anti-inflammatory drugs.

Data from Beers MH. Explicit criteria for determining potentially inappropriate medication use by the elderly: an update. Arch Intern Med 1997;152:1531–6.

of its metabolite norpropoxyphene. It can also interact with warfarin and potentiate the anticoagulant effect. Meperidine is not recommended because of its poor analgesic activity when taken orally and toxicity related to the metabolite normeperidine that has a long half-life, especially in patients with impaired renal or hepatic function.

Dipyridamole had been classified as inappropriate; however, this was before there was evidence that it benefits some patients by preventing strokes. Its designation for being inappropriate for the elderly was due to hypotension seen early in therapy. However, the risk should not preclude its use if it is felt that there is potential benefit.

Preventability

Despite prescribing guidelines, inappropriate medications are still being used, and no improvement has occurred over time [54]. Improving drug benefits and limiting harm must be a goal of prescribers. The use of a large number of pharmaceuticals will always be an important component of the medical care of older patients. Resolving the tension of avoiding excessive medication use and providing access to therapies that are beneficial will only continue to be more difficult.

It is important to note that drug interactions account for one in six adverse drug reactions [54]. Therefore, regular review of prescriptions, the use of computerized prescribing, and pharmacist's review of prescribing behavior may limit adverse drug reactions [55,56]. Factors found in patients whose adverse drug reaction contributed to a possibly preventable hospital admission included lack of documentation of serum blood levels or laboratory tests in over two thirds of cases [57]. Other preventable factors included inappropriate dose for an individual, noncompliance, and drug interactions.

The majority of events, however, involved greater then one preventability factor.

Efforts must be made to expand the knowledge of benefits and risks in the elderly by including them in clinical trials. This is especially true for elderly patients with comorbid conditions. Without adequate research information on this population, clinicians are unable to decide whether drugs are beneficial for them and may withhold medication for fear of doing harm. The federal government has begun some programs to monitor drugs. The Food and Drug Administration's program MedWatch collects voluntary reports on suspected adverse drugs effects in the general population but it is not adequate to develop a large database for the elderly.

The use of interdisciplinary teams to care for complex elderly patients may improve the quality of care for these patients and avoid inappropriate prescribing [58]. This has been beneficial for disease management such as congestive heart failure [59]. However, for this approach to be successful, it needs to be comprehensive and not only consider medical and pharmacologic issues, but social and financial components as well.

Another piece that is crucial in avoiding inappropriate medications is a linked information system that allows physicians to easily review and prescribe medications. This would allow physicians and pharmacists to be alerted when inappropriate medications are used, and allow easy access to alternative suggestions. These information systems should also accommodate individual status of the patient, accounting for their age-related physiologic changes and concomitant diseases.

General concepts for prescribing that are useful are based in the ethical principles of beneficence, nonmaleficence, and autonomy. Practitioners need to ask, "How will this medication benefit this particular patient"? If evidence does not exist at all or is not based in the elder population, practitioners may trial the medication and make a clinical decision if there is an overall good that has been achieved [60]. Another question that may be asked, "How will this harm this particular patient"? The high rate of adverse drug reactions should be balanced against the efficacy or uncertain efficacy in older people before a decision to prescribe is finalized. Finally, prescribers need to include the concept of what the patient wants in the decision to prescribe. Older patients may be concerned about their independence and side effects of medication rather then whether their disease or risk factors are managed according to a published guideline.

Summary

The challenge for the practitioner is to balance incomplete evidence about efficacy of medications in frail older people against the problems related to adverse drug reactions, without denying patients potentially valuable pharmacotherapeutic interventions. Prescribers need to be diligent in reviewing medications periodically as well as when new medications are being considered. Review of updated explicit criteria is essential to understand and prescribe appropriately in this special population.

References

[1] Principles of care and application of the geriatric emergency care model. In: Sanders AB, editor. Geriatric Emergency Medicine Task Force: emergency care of the elder person. St. Louis (MO): Beverly Cracom Publications; 1996.

[2] Rochon PA, Gurwitz JH. Drug therapy. Lancet 1995;346:32–6.

[3] Rochon PA, Gurwitz JH. Optimising drug treatment for elderly people: the prescribing cascade. BMJ 1997;315:1096–9.

[4] Department of Health and Human Services, Administration on Aging (AoA). Statistics—a profile of older americans; 2003 (available at: http://www.aoa.gov/prof/Statistics/profile/2003/2_pf.asp).

[5] Kaufman DW, Kelly JP, Rosenberg L, et al. Recent patterns of medication use in the ambulatory adult population of the United States: the Slone Survey. JAMA 2002;287(3):337–44.

[6] Chutka DS, Takahashi PU, Hoel RW. Inappropriate medications for elderly patients. Mayo Clin Proc 2004;79:122–39.

[7] Delafuente JC. Understanding and preventing drug interactions in elderly patients. Crit Rev Oncol Hematol 2003;48:133–43.

[8] Stewart RB, Cooper JW. Polypharmacy in the aged. Practical solutions. Drugs Aging 1994; 4(6):449–61.

[9] World Health Organization (WHO). International drug monitoring: the role of the hospital. Geneva (Switzerland): World Health Organization; 1966. (Technical Report Series No. 425).

[10] Hepler CD, Strand LM. Opportunities and responsibilities in pharmaceutical care. Am J Hosp Pharm 1990;47:533–43.

[11] Johnson JA, Bootman JL. Drug-related morbidity and mortality: a cost of illness model. Arch Intern Med 1995;155:1949–56.

[12] Crome P. What's different about older people. Toxicology 2003;192:49–54.

[13] Grandison MK, Boudinot FD. Age-related changes in protein bindings of drugs: implications for therapy. Clin Pharmacokinet 2000;38(3):271–90.

[14] Zeeh J, Platt D. The aging liver. Gerontology 2002;48:121–7.

[15] Hammerlein A, Derendorf H, Lowenthal DT. Pharmakokinetic and pharmacodynamic changes in the elderly. Clin Pharmacokinet 1998;35:49–64.

[16] Schmucker DL, Woodhouse KW, Wang RK, et al. Effects of age and gender on in vitro properties of human liver microsomal monooxygenases. Clin Pharmacol Ther 1990;48: 365–74.

[17] Delafuente JC. Arthritis. In: Delafuente JC, Stewart RB, editors. Therapeutics in the elderly. 3rd ed. Cincinnati (OH): Harvey Whitney Books Co.; 2001. p. 499–513.

[18] Whelton A, Stout RL, Spilman PS, et al. Renal effects of ibuprofen, prioxicam, and sulindac in patients with asymptomatic renal failure. A prospective, randomized, crossover comparison. Ann Intern Med 1990;112:568–76.

[19] Swedko PJ, Clark HD, Paramsothy K, et al. Serum creatinine is an inadequate screening test for renal failure in elderly patients. Arch Intern Med 2003;163:356–60.

[20] Vuyk J. Pharmacodynamics in the elderly. Best Pract Res Clin Anaesthesiol 2003;17(2): 207–18.

[21] Gardin JM. Left ventricular diastolic function in the elderly. Am J Geriatr Cardiol 1994;3: 32–41.

[22] Gardin JM, Arnold AM, Bild DE, et al. Left ventricular diastolic filling in the elderly: the cardiovascular health study. Am J Cardiol 1998;82:345–51.

[23] Priebe HJ. The aged cardiovascular risk patient. Br J Anaesth 2000;85:763–78.

[24] Toescu EC, Verkhratsky A. Parameters of calcium homeostasis in normal neuronal ageing. J Anat 2000;197:563–9.

[25] Joseph JA, Denisova NA, Bielinski DS, et al. Oxidative stress protection and vulnerability in aging: putative nutritional implications for intervention. Mech Ageing Dev 2000;116: 141–53.

[26] Shields SA, Gilson JM, Blakemore WF, et al. Remyelination occurs as extensively but more slowly in old rats compared to young rats following gliotoxin-induced CNS demyelination. Glia 1999;28:77–83.

[27] Col N, Fanale JE, Kronholm P. The role of medication noncompliance and adverse drug reactions in hospitalizations of the elderly. Arch Intern Med 1990;150:841–5.

[28] Lazarou J, Pomeranz BH, Corey PN. Incidence of adverse drug reactions in hospitalized patients. JAMA 1998;279(15):1200–5.

[29] Bates DW, Spell N, Cullen DJ, et al. The costs of adverse drug events in hospitalized patients. Adverse Drug Events Prevention Study Group. JAMA 2997;277(4):307–11.

[30] Pirmohamed M, James S, Meakin S, et al. Adverse drug reactions as cause of admission to hospital: prospective analysis of 18,820 patients. BMJ 2004;329:15–9.

[31] Akwagyriam I, Goodyer LI, Harding L, et al. Drug history taking and the identification of drug related problems in an accident and emergency department. J Accid Emerg Med 1996; 13:166–8.

[32] Rieger K, Scholer A, Arnet I, et al. High prevalence of unknown co-medication in hospitalised patients. Eur J Clin Pharmacol 2004;60:363–8.

[33] Chung MK, Bartfield JM. Knowledge of prescription medications among elderly emergency department patients. Ann Emerg Med 2002;39(6):605–8.

[34] O'Connell MB, Johnson JF. Evaluation of medication knowledge in elderly patients. Ann Pharmacother 1992;26:919–21.

[35] Blenkiron P. The elderly and their medication: understanding and compliance in a family practice. Postgrad Med J 1996;72:671–6.

[36] Wiffen P, Gill M, Edwards J, et al. Adverse drug reactions in hospital patients. Bandolier Extra 2002;1–15 (http://www.jr2.ox.ac.uk/bandolier/Extraforbando/ADPRM.PDF).

[37] Gaspoz JM, Coxson PG, Goldman PA, et al. Cost effectiveness of aspirin, clopidogrel, or both for secondary prevention of coronary heart disease. N Engl J Med 2002;346:1800–6.

[38] Gurwitz JH, Fields TS, Avorn J, et al. Incidence and preventability of adverse drug events in nursing homes. Am J Med 2000;109:87–94.

[39] Bootman JL, Harrison DL, Cox E. The health care cost of drug-reltaed morbidity and mortality in nursing facilities. Arch Intern Med 1997;157:2089–96.

[40] Gurwitz JH, Avorn J. The ambiguous relation between aging and adverse drug reactions. Ann Intern Med 1991;114:956–66.

[41] Williamson J, Chopin JM. Adverse reactions to prescribed drugs in the elderly: a multicentre investigation. Age Ageing 1980;9:73–80.

[42] Davidsen F, Haghfelt T, Gram LF, et al. Adverse drug reactions and drug non-compliance as primary causes of admission to a cardiology department. Eur J Clin Pharmacol 1988;34: 83–6.

[43] Carbonin P, Pahor M, Bernabei R, et al. Is age an independent risk factor of adverse drug reactions in hospitalized medical patients? J Am Geriatr Soc 1991;39:1093–9.

[44] Hajjar ER, Hanlon JT, Artz MB, et al. Adverse drug reaction risk factors in older outpatients. Am J Geriatr Pharmacother 2003;1(2):82–9.

[45] Routledge PA, O'Mahony MS, Woodhouse KW. Adverse drug reactions in elderly patients. Br J Clin Pharmacol 2003;57(2):121–6.

[46] Williams CM. Using medications appropriately in older adults. Am Fam Physician 2002;66: 1917–24.

[47] Fouts M, Hanlon J, Pieper C, et al. Identification of elderly nursing facility residents at high risk for drug-related problems. Consult Pharm 1997;12:1103–11.

[48] Skarupski KA, Mrvos R, Krenzelok EP. A profile of calls to a poison information center regarding older adults. J Aging Health 2004;16(2):228–47.

[49] Beers MH, Ouslander JG, Rollingher I, et al. Explicit criteria for determining inappropriate medication use in nursing homes. Arch Intern Med 1991;151:1825–32.

[50] Beers MH. Explicit criteria for determining potentially inappropriate medication use by the elderly: an update. Arch Intern Med 1997;157:1531–6.

[51] Fick DM, Cooper JW, Wade WE, et al. Updating the Beers Criteria for potentially inappropriate medication use in older adults: results of a US consensus panel of experts. Arch Intern Med 2003;163:2716–24.

[52] Alliance for Aging Research and the American Society of Consultant Pharmacists. When medicine hurts instead of helps: preventing medication problems in older persons. Available at: http://ascp.com/medhelp/.

[53] Lanza FL, Umbenhauer ER, Melsom RS, et al. A double blind randomized placebo controlled gastroscopic study to compare the effects of indomethacin capsules and indomethacin suppositories on the gastric mucosa of human volunteers. J Rheumatol 1982;9:415–9.

[54] Goulding MR. Inappropriate medication prescribing for elderly ambulatory care patients. Arch Intern Med 2004;164:305–12.

[55] Anderson WK, Wahler R. Pharmacy management can reduce Medicare—and human costs. Aging Today January/February:2001.

[56] Hanlon JT, Lindblad CI, Gray SL. Can clinical pharmacy services have a positive impact on drug-related problems and health outcomes in community-based older adults? Am J Geriatr Pharmacother 2004;2(1):3–13.

[57] McDonnell PJ, Jacobs MR. Hospital admissions resulting from preventable adverse drug reactions. Ann Pharmacother 2002;36:1331–6.

[58] Schmader KE, Hanlon JT, Pieper CF, et al. Effects of geriatric evaluation and management on adverse drug reactions and suboptimal prescribing in the frail elderly. Am J Med 2004; 116:394–401.

[59] Rich MW, Beckham V, Wittenberg C, et al. A multidisciplinary intervention to prevent the readmission of elderly patients with congestive heart failure. N Eng J Med 1995;333:1190–5.

[60] Le Couteur DG, Hilmer SN, Glasgow N, et al. Prescribing in older people. Aust Fam Physician 2004;33(10):777–81.

ELSEVIER
SAUNDERS

Emerg Med Clin N Am
24 (2006) 467–490

EMERGENCY
MEDICINE
CLINICS OF
NORTH AMERICA

Psychiatric Emergencies in the Elderly Population

Joanna Piechniczek-Buczek, MD

*Division of Psychiatry, Boston University School of Medicine,
Robinson Building B-410, 88 East Newton Street, Boston, MA 02118, USA*

Treatment of psychiatric disorders among elderly has become a major public health concern. The number of Americans over the age of 65 with psychiatric conditions has reached 7 million in the year 2000, and is expected to double by the year 2030 [1]. Despite the growing requirement for mental health services for older persons, there is still substantial unmet need. Emergency psychiatric services are an important way by which elderly patients gain access to mental health services. New psychiatric symptoms in elderly patients often stem from an organic cause. It is essential for the emergency physician to look carefully for medical illnesses in this vulnerable patient population.

The goals of psychiatric evaluation in an emergency department (ED) are to conduct an adequate evaluation, identify a tentative diagnosis, provide emergency treatment, and arrange for an appropriate disposition. Frequent reasons for ED visits by persons 65 and older include psychotic and agitated behavior, suicidality, profound depression, substance abuse, and psychosocial problems such as elder abuse and neglect. Emergency physicians should take into consideration each of these diagnoses while assessing the geriatric patient presenting with behavioral disturbances. The disturbances may be caused by either early-onset psychiatric illness or late-onset illness; however, the majority of conditions presenting as psychiatric emergencies in the elderly stem from an underlying physical or organic cause.

This article identifies key psychiatric problems among the elderly presenting to the ED. It focuses on problems associated with elderly suicide, geriatric depression, and substance abuse. Also, psychotic presentations among older patients as well as the issue of elder mistreatment will be discussed. This article provides guidelines for diagnosis, assessment, and management of these common psychiatric emergencies in geriatric patients.

E-mail address: joanna.buczek@bmc.org

0733-8627/06/$ - see front matter © 2006 Elsevier Inc. All rights reserved.
doi:10.1016/j.emc.2006.01.008   *emed.theclinics.com*

Suicide

Older adults have the highest risk of death by suicide of all age groups in the United States. Suicidologists have cause to predict that a dramatic increase in suicide rates and total number of suicides will occur over the next several decades [2]. Clinicians face an urgent need for developing prevention and treatments strategies to combat this problem. Efforts should be made by clinicians, particularly in the ED and primary care settings, to identify risk factors, clues, and signs of imminent threats of late-life suicide [3].

Epidemiology

Suicide is the 11th leading cause of death in the United States [4], accounting for 31,655 deaths in the year 2002, with 11.0 completed suicides for every 100,000 people. Older adults are at higher risk for suicide than any other segment of the population, with the rate reaching 15.6 per 100,000 individuals in 2002. Among the oldest-old (defined as 85 and older) group the suicide rate was even higher at 18.0 per 100,000 individuals. White men aged 85 and over commit suicide at nearly six times the national age-adjusted rate [5]. On the other hand, attempted suicide is far less frequent in later life than in younger age groups [6]. The ratio of suicide attempts to completed suicide is estimated to be approximately 4:1 among the elderly compared with a ratio range of 8:1 to 20:1 in the general population [7]. Males 65 and older showed the greatest proportional increase in use of firearms as a method of suicide followed by jumping, hanging, and drowning, indicating that they resort to more violent means of suicide [4]. This population has more physical illness burden and less resilience, which may further contribute to increased lethality of suicide in this age group. Furthermore, older adults are more likely to be living alone; therefore, self-destructive acts are less likely to be discovered in time for them to be saved [8]. Suicide completers were more likely to have avoided intervention and to have taken precautions against discovery. They were less likely to communicate their intent to others, exhibiting greater intent to die than their younger counterparts [8,9]. Frierson et al [10] identified more planning of the act among older than younger attempters. Moreover, older men particularly were less likely to have had a history of previous attempts. The above characteristics indicate that elderly persons who are at high risk for suicide may be more difficult to identify as being at imminent risk [7].

Several retrospective studies have indicated that over 70% of older suicide victims have visited their physician within the month of the suicide. A third of this group was seen within the week before the suicide [11]. These findings imply that immediate and aggressive interventions are needed when suicide risk is identified in an older person. Because suicidal behavior in elderly is more planned and deliberate, and means are more lethal, all efforts then should be targeted at identification and treatment of conditions predisposing to the development of suicidal state [12].

Risk factors

Demographic, psychiatric, social, medical, and biologic determinants of suicide have been identified in numerous studies [13,14].

Demographic analysis of suicide data reveals three variables affecting elderly suicide rates: sex, race, and marital status. The analysis concludes that male gender, White race, and unmarried status significantly amplify risk of completed suicide [4].

Current or past *psychiatric* illness is perhaps the most powerful risk factor, as approximately 90% of people who commit suicide have diagnosable psychopathology [15]. Depression is the most common psychiatric diagnosis in elderly suicide victims, unlike the younger adult in whom substance abuse with comorbid mood disorder is encountered most frequently [16]. When compared with younger suicide victims, older victims were more likely to have had depression that was not comorbid with substance abuse nor complicated by psychosis nor associated with physical illness [17,18]. Older suicide victims are more likely to have suffered from a single episode of unipolar depression, the type of depression that tends to respond well to standard therapies [19].

Substance use disorders, particularly alcohol abuse and dependence, are the second most common psychiatric disorder associated with completed elder suicide. Estimates based on psychologic autopsy studies indicate that 3% to 44% of elderly suicide decedents had a substance use disorder [11,20,21]. The mechanism by which alcohol misuse in older adults is associated with suicide includes alcohol as an independent risk factor, alcohol abuse/dependence exacerbating cooccurring psychiatric or physical illness [22] or alcohol as the cause of loss of social supports [23].

Primary psychotic disorders, anxiety disorders, and personality disorders appear to play a smaller role in suicide among elderly than in younger cohorts [8]. Conner et al [24] conducted a comprehensive literature review on psychologic vulnerabilities to completed suicide, and identified five distinct psychologic constructs as potential correlates. They are impulsivity/aggression, depression, hopelessness, anxiety, and self-consciousness/social disengagement. These constructs distinguished suicides and controls, and were acknowledged as important factors interplaying with psychiatric, social, and medical liabilities in establishing an individual's risk profile.

Numerous studies have investigated association between *medical* illness and suicide risk, and despite their methodologic limitations, physical illness burden is considered to be a predisposing correlate of late life suicide [7,8,25]. In particular, Rich and colleagues [26] found illness to be the most frequent stressor in suicide victims over the age of 80 years. In Juurlink et al's [27] study of 1354 elderly patients who died of suicide several common medical illnesses were cited. Congestive heart failure, chronic lung disease, and seizures were independently associated with increased risk of suicide. Harris and Barraclough [28], in their review of 235 published reports, found that increased mortality from suicide is associated with HIV/AIDS, Huntington's disease, malignant neoplasm, multiple sclerosis, peptic ulcer disease, renal disease, spinal cord injuries, and systemic lupus erythematosus. Furthermore, visual impairment, neurologic disorder, and malignancy were independently associated with suicide in the elderly [29]. Untreated or undertreated pain, anticipatory anxiety regarding the progression of physical illness, fear of dependence, and fear of burdening the family are major contributing factors in the suicidal elderly with physical illness [30].

Multiple *social* stressors accompany late life, including retirement, loss of a loved one, social isolation, and increasing burden of disability. These stressors tend to cluster in the weeks or months preceding a suicide attempt [17,31–34]. Investigations suggest that living alone [21], having poor social support [25], and sustaining interpersonal loss through death [23] correlate highly with an increased incidence of suicide in an older age group with the risk being the highest during first 4 years of widowhood [12,35].

Several *biologic* correlates of suicide have been identified. Serotonergic, noradrenergic, and neuroendocrine systems are most frequently implicated in the neurobiology of suicide [36]. Abnormalities in the central serotonergic system have been linked to predisposition to impulsive and aggressive acts. Preliminary evidence suggests that persons with an impulsive/aggressive style are more likely to act on their suicidal thoughts than individuals without that predisposition [37]. A number of reviews have examined the evidence of the role of neurotransmitter systems in the biology of elderly suicide. However, an insufficient number of elderly persons were included to permit analysis or a conclusion.

Assessment

Clinical intervention strategies targeting individuals who are at high risk for suicide according to demographic, psychiatric, social, and medical factors may be more effective for preventing suicide than interventions that solely identify individuals with suicidal ideations or behavior. The fact that the majority of older adults are seen in a primary care setting within the month before their death, coupled with the finding that most late life suicide victims have had depressive episodes suggests that detecting and treating depression may be an effective way to prevent later life suicide [38–42].

Likelihood of suicide and nonfatal suicidal behaviors increases with additional risk factors. The role of the physician is to recognize patients at greater risk by determining psychosocial and medical domains associated with increased probability of suicide [27]. In addition to careful evaluation of medical conditions, assessment should include inquiries about previous suicide attempts, past episodes of depression, psychosis or mania, substance use disorders, impulse control, social supports, and recent stressful life events. [30]. There is some evidence that suicidal patients often do not spontaneously express their feelings or thoughts openly [43], but they are likely to admit to their suicidal thoughts when the topic is introduced by a physician [44]. All patients should be asked about their mood, sleep habits, appetite, interest, and feelings of hopelessness. Death wishes, thoughts of suicide, intent to harm self, and access to means should be elicited in indirect and direct inquires. For more comprehensive assessment of suicide ideation and behavior, standardized screening instruments may be administered. The Scale of Suicide Ideation is an example of such an instrument [45]. The geriatric population is at high risk for depression and suicide.

Management

The first step in managing a suicidal elder should focus on assessing the level and intensity of care based on a thorough risk assessment. Psychiatric hospitalization is an important treatment modality for patients in imminent danger. This measure prevents the patient from self-harm when adequate level of monitoring is provided [14]. In addition, hospitalization allows for induction of aggressive treatment, evaluation of coexisting psychiatric conditions, and subsequent transition to outpatient settings. If the individual who is assessed to be at acute risk for suicide refuses to be admitted, the physician then becomes responsible for initiating procedures for involuntary commitment in accordance to applicable civil laws.

If inpatient admission is not pursued, assuring adequate monitoring at home, facilitating prompt referral to outpatient psychiatric care, and reducing accessibility to means is considered to be a necessary intervention in management of suicidal patients [3,14].

Aggressive treatment of depression is essential following acute crisis as survivors of suicidal behavior in old age remain a high-risk group and require close monitoring. The NIH Consensus Conference of 1992 agreed that prevention of elderly suicide is best accomplished by increased recognition and adequate treatment of depression.

Depression

Although depression is the most common psychiatric disorder in the elderly, it remains poorly recognized and undertreated [46–49]. Even though late-life experiences are associated with a number of physical losses and difficult life events, and although sadness may be considered a normal response, depression is not a natural consequence of aging. When depressive disorder occurs, it is associated with marked disability, hastened functional decline, increased risk of hospitalization, diminished quality of life, increased medical service use, and mortality [50–52]. Depressed elders are four times more likely to die of any cause than are their nondepressed counterparts [53,54]. They present to EDs more frequently and have longer lengths of hospitalizations once admitted [55–58]. Use of ED resources by the growing geriatric population is increasing, whereas their mental health services use remains poor. This trend emphasizes the unique role emergency physicians play in recognizing and treating underlying depression in elderly patients.

Epidemiology

The prevalence of major depressive disorder in the elderly varies depending on criteria used for diagnosis and the population studied. Epidemiologic studies of community dwelling elders report up to a 5% prevalence of major depressive disorder and an 8% to 27% prevalence for minor depression [48,59,60] (often described as subsyndromal depression). Major depression is present in 5% to 12% of hospitalized patients and 12% to 16% of nursing home residents [61]. In an ED screening investigation conducted by Meldon, 27% of participating elders were found to be depressed [62]. In a study of the relation of comorbid depressive syndrome with the use of ED services, Himelhoch [63] found that patients with comorbid depressive syndrome are twice as likely to use medical emergency services compared with those without depression.

Risk factors and consequences

A number of biologic and psychosocial risk factors for depression have been identified in the elderly. Medical illness, functional disability, social isolation, accumulation of life stressors and losses, and genetic vulnerabilities frequently play a role as predisposing factors in late life mood disorders [64]. Medical illness is frequently cited as a predisposing and consequential correlate in depression implicating bidirectional relationship between these two conditions [65]. Depression is common in patients with coronary artery disease and other cardiac illnesses, affecting about one fifth of patients undergoing cardiac catheterization or recovering from recent myocardial infarction (MI) [66], and occurring in about one third of patients within the first 12 months after MI [67]. Conversely, post-MI mortality is higher in depressed than in nondepressed patients, implying that depression is contributory to the pathogenesis of heart disease [68]. Similar reciprocal correlation between depression and medical illness applies to a number of other conditions including cerebrovascular disease and dementia [69].

Functional disability is frequently cited as another factor linked to development of depression [70]. For community-dwelling older adults, the presence of disabilities (measured by activities of daily living limitation) increases risk of depression by 4.2 per 1 year [71]. Penninx et al's [72] investigation showed that depressive symptoms were predictive of up to 50% greater risk of decline in physical performance over 4 years of study duration providing evidence of bidirectional correlation between depression and functional disability. Other authors emphasized the role of social isolation, acute and chronic stress, and bereavement as risk factors for late life depression [73,74].

Assessment

Late-life mood disorders are significantly underdiagnosed, particularly in primary care settings where about one half of all elderly patients with mood disorders failed to be identified as depressed [1,75,76].

Because the ED services use by the geriatric population is growing, it has been postulated that assessment of social, functional, and psychologic factors need to be an integral part of emergency care in this population [55]. Recognition of depression remains poor as illustrated in an investigation conducted by Meldon et al [48], in which emergency physicians failed to clinically diagnose depression in patients identified as depressed on formal testing. Lack of awareness by emergency physicians may be a common problem, although several other factors contribute to the phenomena of underdiagnosis in the elderly. First, older patients frequently present with vague somatic complaints or overlapping symptoms of medical illness [77,78] that can mimic or mask underlying depressive symptoms [79]. Second, the symptoms frequently occur following a stressful life event and are therefore interpreted as "understandable," with no need for further intervention. Furthermore, co-occurrence of cognitive impairment and dementia might further complicate the diagnosis of late-life depression due to symptom overlap (eg, apathy, emotional withdrawal, regression, decreased concentration) and impaired recall of symptoms by cognitively impaired patients [80]. Third, elderly patients may attach stigma to depression, and therefore be less likely to accept the diagnosis and adhere to treatment [81].

The criteria outlined in the *Diagnostic Manual of Mental Disorders-IV-TR (DSM IV-TR)* should be used as a guideline for the diagnosis of major depression. According to these criteria patients must experience at least five of the following symptoms over the course of at least 2 weeks: depressed mood, diminished interest or pleasure in daily activities, significant changes in mood and appetite, sleep disturbances, psychomotor agitation or retardation, fatigue, feelings of guilt or worthlessness, impaired concentration, or suicidal ideation [82]. Many more patients, however, have depressive symptoms that do not fit full criteria for major depressive disorder. In fact, subsyndromal depression (minor depression, not described in the *DSM IV-TR*) is the most common form of depressive disorder in the elderly [83]. Minor depression has been equally associated with significant morbidity and disability [84], and therefore requires uniformly aggressive interventions as does major depression.

Standard screening tools may be helpful in diagnosing depressive disorders. The Self-rated Geriatric Depression Scale has been well validated and widely used in its various versions (30-, 15-, and 5-item versions) to assess depression and to monitor treatment response [85]. A brief three-question screening instrument has been validated for use in the ED setting to identify individuals with depression—Emergency Department-Depression Screening Instrument (ED-DSI) [86] (see Table 1).

Diagnostic workup should include detailed investigations of medical and neurologic problems, currently used medications and substances of abuse, thorough assessment of psychiatric history, and evaluation of cognitive status. Furthermore, investigation of functional abilities, supports in the community, living arrangements, and recent losses should take place [87]. Outside informants, such as family members, caretakers, and friends should be used to corroborate the history.

Management

As mentioned previously, untreated depression is associated with increased mortality from comorbid medical condition [54], suicide, increased risk of disability, and impaired psychosocial functioning. Failure to detect depression may cause overuse of physical and laboratory examinations, unnecessary referrals to medical specialists, frequent ED and office visits, costly medications, and other treatments [88]. Adequate recognition and referral is imperative to achieving treatment goals for the depressed patient. These include alleviating depressive symptoms, reducing risk of recurrence and relapse, improving quality of life, and decreasing morbidity and mortality [88].

Severe depressive disorder warrants hospitalization. Admission should be considered for patients who express suicidal ideations with intent, those who attempted suicide, patients who are having difficulties with compliance, those who are experiencing depression with psychotic symptoms, those who neglect themselves, and patients with significant medical illness that would complicate treatment for depression [89]. For less disturbed elders other forms of disposition should be used. These include referrals to their primary care provider, psychiatric consultants, or partial hospitalization programs. Indications for psychiatric referrals include: diagnostic difficulties, depression with coexisting other psychiatric symptoms (anxiety, psychosis, substance abuse), depression with comorbid medical and neurologic conditions, failed prior medication trials, or inability to tolerate

Table 1
Emergency department-depression screening instrument (ED-DSI)

1. Do you often feel sad or depressed?	Yes	No
2. Do you often feel helpless?	Yes	No
3. Do you often feel downhearted and blue?	Yes	No

A positive response to any of the three questions is considered a positive screen.

Adapted from Fabacher DA, et al. Validations of a brief screening tool to detect depression In elderly ED patients. Am J Emerg Med 2002;20:99–102.

antidepressants [90]. Pharmacologic interventions, psychotherapy, and electroconvulsive therapy are effective for treatment of geriatric depression [65]. Clinical recommendations frequently favor selective serotonin reuptake inhibitors (SSRIs) over tricyclic antidepressants due to a more benign side effects profile, although research studies failed to demonstrate SSRIs' superior effectiveness in alleviating depressive symptoms among geriatric patients [91,92].

Substance abuse

Substance abuse and dependence in the geriatric population has been identified as the fastest growing health problem in the country, yet these conditions are frequently overlooked by health care providers. Projected estimates indicate that the problem is likely to rise in coming years as the population of geriatric patients continues to expand [93,94]. The majority of patients with a substance abuse problem present in general medical settings making it imperative for clinicians to familiarize themselves with diagnostic criteria, risk factors, consequences, and treatment options to ensure adequate care [95].

Epidemiology

In population-based studies, prevalence estimates of alcohol abuse or dependence in older adults range from 0.6% to 3.7%. Using *DSM-IV* criteria, the National Longitudinal Alcohol Epidemiologic Survey reported a prevalence of alcohol abuse and dependence at 1.2% for men and 0.3% for women in the over 65 age group. In contrast, rates of heavy drinking among older adults are considerably higher, demonstrating that 15% to 20% of men and 8% to 10% of women drink at risk or at problem drinking level [96]. Prevalence estimates suggest that about 50% of persons over 65 years old report using alcohol at least occasionally, 40% drink alcohol regularly, and 10% to 22% consume it daily [97]. The prevalence of alcoholism is higher among elderly in health care settings than among the general elderly population. Approximately 4% to10% of patients seen by primary care physicians meet criteria for alcohol dependence (an additional 10–15% are heavy drinkers, but are not considered alcohol dependent). It is estimated that 14% of elderly ED patients [98,99] and 10% to 21% hospital inpatients [100] are abusing alcohol.

The rates of alcohol abuse and dependence in general appear to be lower in older individuals than in younger age groups [94], which may be due to a decline in alcohol problems with aging or underdetection of alcohol problems in the elderly. Cross-sectional studies that measured quantity of alcohol use have revealed that overall consumption of alcohol declines with age, rates of abstinence increase, and that significant gender differences in alcohol use exists with men drinking more than women [101]. Cross-section studies, however, fail to determine whether decreased alcohol consumption is due to cohort effect (older cohort consumed less alcohol throughout their lives compared with younger aged cohort) or a true age-related phenomenon (alcohol use decreases with advancing age [102].

Definitions and patterns

The *DSM IV-TR* defines alcohol abuse and alcohol dependence as distinct categories. Alcohol dependence is described as a pattern of drinking associated with at least three of the following occurring in the same 12-month period: tolerance, withdrawal symptoms, lack of control, preoccupation with acquisition or use, desire or unsuccessful efforts to quit, continued use despite adverse effects. These symptoms need to be associated with impairment in social, occupational, and recreational activities. Alcohol abuse is a maladaptive pattern of drinking associated with at least one of the following: failure to fulfill obligations, drinking in hazardous situations or causing legal problems, or continued use despite social or occupational problems. The World Health Organization recognizes harmful drinking ("evidence that use is causing adverse consequences") and hazardous use ("quality and pattern of use that places patients at risk of adverse consequences") as additional separate diagnoses.

About two thirds of elderly alcoholics are "early-onset drinkers," whose enduring problem with alcohol developed earlier in life [103]. On the other hand, "late-onset drinkers" begin problematic drinking later in life, often in response to traumatic life events, such as retirement, death of a spouse, medical illness, and increased disability [104]. Late-onset drinkers typically have fewer alcohol-related problems, less psychiatric comorbidities, are less likely to have family history significant for alcohol use disorders, and are more likely to compliant be with treatment [105].

Risk factors, vulnerabilities, consequences

Fink et al [106], in their review of determinants and consequences of alcohol abuse in the elderly, concluded that being a single, relatively well-educated male, living alone, and having personal history of prior alcohol use or abuse is associated with increased risk of alcohol abuse in later life.

Physiologic changes linked to the aging process make the older patient more vulnerable to the intoxicating effects of alcohol. Volume of distribution for water soluble substances (like alcohol) diminishes as the fat content increases, while lean body mass and total body water decrease, yielding higher peak concentrations for a given dose of alcohol [107]. Decreased activity of alcohol dehydrogenase in the stomach associated with aging may further amplify older adults' sensitivity to intoxicating effects of alcohol [108].

Adults over the age of 65 are more likely to be affected by at least one chronic illness [108,109], and be prescribed medications for underlying medical problems. Alcohol interacts with a number of commonly prescribed medications, and has direct effects on metabolic capacity of the liver, resulting in increased potential for considerable medication side effects and interactions in geriatric patients [110].

Elderly drinkers have increased rates of liver disease, cancers of head, neck, esophagus, as well as of the lung and breast [111]. Chronic alcohol consumption can cause myopathy, peripheral neuropathy, and cerebellar damage, which in combination with the direct impairing effect of alcohol on judgment and balance, critically contribute to gait abnormalities encountered in elderly alcoholics [112]. Osteoporosis combined with the detrimental effects of alcohol on gait and balance results in higher age-adjusted rates of hip fractures among elderly alcoholic patients [113]. Additionally, several syndromes that involve impairment in brain function can occur in elderly alcohol abusing individuals (delirium, Wernicke encephalopathy, Korsakoff's syndrome). These syndromes are frequently superimposed on the age-related medical conditions associated with cognitive deficits (dementia, mild cognitive impairment) [111]. Gastrointestinal disease and bleeding commonly bring older alcoholics to EDs [112].

Chronic alcohol use is further associated with significant psychiatric comorbidities, specifically affective disorders, anxiety, cognitive impairment, personality disorders, and schizophrenia [114]. Depressive disorders are of particular concern as they are implicated in increased morbidity and mortality in the elderly, including increased risk of suicide [113,115].

Assessment

The ED offers a unique opportunity for the detection of the elderly substance abuser. An adequate diagnosis is frequently missed due to ageist assumptions such as the belief that older adults' quality of life will remain poor even if they are successfully treated for their substance abuse. Failure to detect symptoms and lack of knowledge is commonly seen among health care providers [114]. Furthermore, many older drinkers attribute their alcohol problems to a breakdown in moral values, which in turn, creates a sense of shame and stigma ultimately preventing them from seeking help [113]. Difficulty applying criteria to a variety of nonspecific symptoms (falls, sleep problems, confusion, irritability) [103], stereotyping (physicians are less likely to detect alcohol problem in women, the educated and those of higher socioeconomic status) [116], and abbreviated office/ED visits [117], may further impede the clinician's ability to detect alcohol related problems in the elderly.

Screening is recommended in all older patients, particularly those undergoing major life transitions or presenting with nonspecific physical symptoms. Several brief, practical, and well-validated screening tools for alcoholism are available. The CAGE questionnaire [118] and MAST-G (Michigan Alcoholism Screening Test-geriatric Version) [119] are two commonly used tools that have been validated for use in older adults. These instruments do not distinguish, however, between current and past drinking behavior; therefore, supplemental data about the frequency and amounts of recent drinking should be acquired [112].

Management

It is an important task for the ED physician to detect substance abuse problems in the elderly and refer to the appropriate level of treatment. The American Society of Addiction Medicine offers patient placement guidelines allowing health care providers to determine the adequate level of intervention based on severity of substance abuse, significance of prior withdrawal, and comorbid medical and psychiatric problems [120]. In elderly substance abusers the comorbid medical problems, limited reserve, susceptibility to kindling, and adverse effects of drug treatment may increase the risk of complicated withdrawal [121]. History of prior complicated detoxifications, history of withdrawal seizures or delirium tremens, or unstable comorbid medical conditions should precipitate admission for inpatient detoxification [112,113]. After completing detoxification elderly patients should be referred to residential, day treatment, or outpatient programs where psychologic interventions such as psychoeducation, counseling, and motivational interviewing can be provided [122]. The use of medications promoting abstinence has not been studied extensively in elderly subjects. Disulfiram should be used with caution due to the risk of precipitating confusional state [123]. Naltrexone showed some efficacy (prevention of relapse) in subjects 50 to 74 years of age [122]. Project TREAT [96] and Project GOAL [96] investigated the impact of brief physician advice with at-risk, nondependent drinkers and demonstrated a positive effect on drinking patterns.

Geriatric psychoses

Psychotic manifestations are common in the elderly, and are defined as disturbances in thought processes and behavior leading to loss of contact with reality [124]. Psychoses in the elderly can be manifestations of a variety of neuropsychiatric conditions and pose a significant diagnostic challenge for a clinician. In the *DSM IV-TR*, psychotic disorders include schizophrenia, schizophreniform disorders, brief psychotic disorder, and psychotic disorder due to general medical condition. Psychotic symptoms can also accompany major depressive disorder, bipolar disorder, substance intoxication, and withdrawal, as well as dementia [82]. Psychotic manifestation in late life can be also broadly divided into early-onset psychosis with symptoms continuing through late life and late-onset psychosis. Onset of psychotic symptoms in late life may be the first sign of medical, neurologic, or a substance-induced condition; therefore, it warrants careful diagnostic evaluation [125].

Epidemiology

Geriatric data from the Epidemiologic Catchment Area study showed prevalence for schizophrenia and schizophreniform disorder ranging from 0.2% to 0.9% [126]. On the other hand, 16% to 23% of the elderly population had so-called "organic" psychoses, with dementia being the main contributing cause [127–129]. Dementia increases the vulnerability to psychosis and more than 50% of elderly patients with dementia have been noted to have paranoia and hallucinations [127,130,131].

Risk factors

Incidence of psychosis in general increases with age with a number of factors leading to an increase in vulnerability and expression [124,132]. Age-related deterioration of cortical areas such as the frontal and temporal lobes, as well as neurochemical changes common in aging, might be implicated in the increased incidence of psychosis. Other risk factors include hearing and visual impairment, social isolation, cognitive deficits, use of substances, and concomitant use of multiple medications [133]. Other researchers identify bedfast status [134] and premorbid personality with paranoid and schizoid traits [135,136] as likely correlates of late-onset psychotic symptoms.

Assessment

The emergency physician's role in dealing with the acutely psychotic patient is to control the patient's behavior, to delineate the etiology of the psychosis, and to provide appropriate initial treatment and disposition [137]. Late-life psychoses are a diverse group of disorders that pose a significant diagnostic challenge. They can be broadly divided into early- and late-onset psychoses. The late-onset psychoses should be further divided as with or without dementia [125]. The most common entities within the late-onset group are dementia, delirium, late-onset psychotic and mood disorders, as well as psychotic disorders due to general medical deterioration [82]. Evaluation of new onset psychotic symptoms in late life must include thorough medical, neurologic, and psychiatric evaluation to define causality of the symptoms. A routine workup typically includes laboratory tests, such as complete blood count, comprehensive metabolic panel, B12/folate levels, thyroid function tests, urinalysis, electrocardiogram, and brain imaging studies [133]. Careful evaluation of all medications and prior psychiatric and substance use history is of paramount importance. Psychiatric history should be obtained to determine whether the symptoms are a continuation of an early life psychiatric condition.

About 10% of cases of schizophrenia occur in patients who are older than 45 [124]. Very late-onset schizophrenia (age 60 and more) is extremely rare and not a commonly recognized entity [138]. Patients with late-onset schizophrenia, compared with early-onset counterparts, have more systematized delusions and hallucinations [139,140], fewer negative symptoms (affective flattening, social withdrawal) [141,142] and fewer thought disorders [143]. They are more likely to have sensory deficits, are less likely to have family history of schizophrenia [142,144], and are more likely to have comorbid depressive symptoms [145]. Further, several investigations have implicated a number of abnormalities seen on neuroimaging, such as increased ventricles-brain ratio, cortical atrophy [139], and increased deep white matter hyperintensities in late-onset psychosis [146]. Male to female ratios in late-onset schizophrenia showed a marked preponderance in females [147].

Agitation

A common manifestation of late-life psychosis (despite etiology) is agitation. Agitation is defined as an excessive motor or verbal activity, and is exemplified by hyperactivity, assaultiveness, verbal abuse, threatening gestures, physical destructiveness, vocal outbursts, and excessive verbalizations of distress [148]. Pacing, fidgeting, and resisting care are common behavioral disturbances occurring in the context of dementia [149]. Medical illness and environmental factors (overstimulation, understimulation, lack of familiar cues) may also contribute to agitation warranting prompt evaluation of a possible causative contribution [150].

Management of agitation and aggression in the elderly poses a significant challenge in the emergency service. Persons aged 65 and older are particularly susceptible to adverse drug reaction due to coexisting multimorbidity, high number of prescribed medications with enhanced potential for drug–drug interactions, and age-associated changes in pharmacokinetic and pharmacodynamic properties [151]. Therefore acute and long-term management of agitation in the elderly should combine medication and behavioral interventions. Behavioral management strategies should be instituted before medication interventions [64,152]. Adjusting the physical environment, redirecting distressed patients, talking calmly, and promoting appropriate social interactions and activities can decrease problem behaviors. Several investigations have implicated psychotic symptoms that occur during the course of dementia to be associated with faster cognitive deterioration, propensity toward aggression, and increased caregiver burden [153]. Psychosocial treatment of psychotic symptoms should therefore involve active family and caregiver participation. Education, support, and respite should be offered to all caregivers to prevent burnout that would interfere with caregiver's ability to care for the elder with psychosis.

Interventions should always focus on safety of the patient, caregivers, and ED personnel. The research data suggest that antipsychotic medications are effective for both psychotic symptoms and nonpsychotic agitated behavior [64,149]. Antipsychotic drugs are the most effective in patients with complex and bizarre delusions, hallucinations, and with agitated or violent patients. The choice of a particular antipsychotic medication should depend on the side effect profile of the medication. There is enough evidence from recent studies to support use of atypical antipsychotics over conventional ones [154]. Atypical antipsychotics have a lower risk of side effects such as extrapyramidal symptoms and tardive dyskinesia. In addition, conventional antipsychotics are associated with increased risk of sedation, orthostatic hypotension with associated increased risk of falls [155], hip fractures [156], and mortality [125]. New generation atypical antipsychotics seem to be safer and at least equally effective. Several trials investigated the efficacy of risperidone, olanzapine, quetiapine, and ziprasidone, and confirmed their benefit in management of agitation and psychosis in the context of dementia [152]. The side effect profile of atypical antipsychotics is also associated with significant risks, including sedation, weight gain, cardiac conduction changes, as well as glucose and lipid metabolism abnormalities [128]. The Food and Drug Administration recently issued a black box warning that older patients treated with atypical antipsychotics for dementia have an increased risk of death [157]. It is unclear at this time what are the best agents for sedating agitated elderly ED patients.

Elder mistreatment

Elder mistreatment, also described as elder abuse or neglect, is a widespread problem in today's society. The problem first gained broader attention about 20 years ago with first reports of "granny battering" in British literature [158]. It seems to be an escalating problem; however, the actual extent of elder mistreatment is not known due to limited detection, significant underreporting, and varying descriptions of the problem. The American Medical Association (AMA) defines elder abuse and neglect as "an act of omission which results in harm or threatened harm to the health or welfare of an elderly person [159]. Elder mistreatment may take many forms, including physical abuse, psychologic abuse, caregiver neglect, self-neglect, and financial exploitation [160].

Epidemiology

It has been estimated that over 2 million older adults are mistreated each year in the United States [161].

In one random sample community-based epidemiologic study of abuse in the elderly, over 2000 Boston area residents were asked about physical violence, psychologic abuse, and neglect. [162]; 3.2% of the participants experienced some form of maltreatment since turning 65. Elder abuse occurs in all segments of society and in all settings. The perpetrators are most frequently family members, and according to the 1996 US National Elder Abuse Incidence Study, about two thirds of the perpetrators were adult children or spouses of the victims [163]. Elders are also abused in the hospitals, nursing homes, and other institutions. In a survey conducted in the United States, 36% of the nursing home staff reported having witnessed at least one incident of physical abuse [163].

Risk factors

Several characteristics of elderly persons and their caretakers may be associated with increased risk of maltreatment. Victim's cognitive impairment, shared living arrangements with the abuser, and the need for the assistance in activities of daily living have strong empirical support as significant risk factors [164,165]. Other predisposing factors include social isolation, high degree of dependence on caretaker, advanced age, and minority status [161]. The profile of an abuser includes excessive dependence on the elderly for financial support and housing (reversed dependence), as well as presence of substance abuse and personality disorders [164].

Assessment

Identifying mistreatment is frequently difficult due to several factors. Victims may be reluctant or unable to provide adequate report due to fear of retaliation or cognitive impairment. Some others are afraid of placement in nursing facility, and therefore hesitate to acknowledge mistreatment at home [161]. AMA guidelines emphasize that all geriatric patients should be questioned about family violence even in the absence of symptoms suggestive of abuse or neglect.

In severe cases of physical abuse, physicians typically can easily recognize the problem. The diagnosis of elder abuse should be considered in all geriatric patients who present with multiple injuries in various stages of evolution or when the injuries are unexplained. Neglect should be suspected when an elderly person with adequate resources and designated caretaker presents with significant negligence in hygiene, nutrition or medical care, such as missed appointments or unfilled prescriptions [164].

Frequently however, physicians are likely to encounter more subtle forms of mistreatment. Careful history is crucial in identifying possible victims and clinicians should familiarize themselves with techniques most likely to yield accurate information. Generally the patient should be interviewed without the caregiver present. Interview should start with general questions about the patient's perceptions of safety in the home [164] and neighborhood. Subsequently the discussion should move on to inquiries about who is responsible for providing care and assistance, and then turn to more specific questions about maltreatment. Interviewing the person who is suspected of abuse or neglect poses a different set of challenges. A nonjudgmental approach, empathy, and validation of burden typically help to elicit more accurate information [166]. Careful documentation, including drawings of injuries and verbatim description of events is particularly important as the medical record can be entered as evidence in a criminal trial or guardianship hearing [161].

Management

Management should focus on assuring safety. Patients who are in potential danger should not be permitted to return to their living environment until the issue of abuse or neglect has been addressed [160]. In a less acute situation intervention should be specifically geared toward alleviating stressors that directly contributed to the situation. All health care providers and administrators are mandated by law to report suspected elder mistreatment. Reports of suspected elder mistreatment should be given to the state or county division of adult protective services. Elder abuse is covered in more detail in the article on elder abuse and neglect.

Summary

This article has reviewed the most common behavioral emergencies in the geriatric population. Psychiatric emergencies are seen frequently by emergency physicians who face the challenge of assessing and managing patients presenting with psychosis, severe depression, agitation, suicidal intent, and substance abuse in the ED. The evaluation is frequently complicated by the necessity to investigate numerous domains such as underlying medical conditions, prior psychiatric disorders and substance abuse, as well as psychosocial factors. It is crucial to rule out organic causes for what appears to be psychiatric disease in the elderly. The assessment might be further complicated by the patient's limited ability to recall pertinent aspects of the history due to either cognitive impairment or acute distress. ED personnel might have inadequate expertise in assessing emergencies in elderly persons, further impeding the ability to appropriately manage behavioral complications in geriatric patients. Availability of high-quality emergency care and tight collaboration with primary care providers, psychiatric consultants, and social services is crucial to optimal outcomes from acute psychiatric decompensations in the elderly.

Acknowledgments

The author thanks Fiona Abbott, Jeantel Degazon, Laurie Sickles and Clifford Knapp for their assistance in the preparation of this manuscript.

References

[1] Jeste DV, Alexopoulos GS, Bartels SJ, et al. Consensus statement on the upcoming crisis in geriatric mental health: research agenda for the next 2 decades. Arch Gen Psychiatry 1999; 56(9):848–53.

[2] Bharucha AJ, Satlin A. Late-life suicide: a review. Harv Rev Psychiatry 1997;5(2):55–65.
[3] Richardson R, Lowenstein S, Weissberg M. Coping with the suicidal elderly: a physician's guide. Geriatrics 1989;44(9):43–7, 51.
[4] Center for Disease Control and Prevention, National Center for Injury Prevention and Control. Web based Injury Statistics Query and Reposting System [online]. Accessed January 24, 2005.
[5] Kochanek KD, Murphy SL, Anderson RN, et al. Deaths: Final data for 2002. Hyattsville (MD): National Center for Health Statistics; 2004.
[6] Moscicki EK. Identification of suicide risk factors using epidemiologic studies. Psychiatr Clin North Am 1997;20(3):499–517.
[7] Pearson JL, Brown GK. Suicide prevention in late life: directions for science and practice. Clin Psychol Rev 2000;20(6):685–705.
[8] Conwell Y, Duberstein PR, Caine ED. Risk factors for suicide in later life. Biol Psychiatry 2002;52(3):193–204.
[9] Merrill J, Owens J. Age and attempted suicide. Acta Psychiatr Scand 1990;82(5):385–8.
[10] Frierson RL. Suicide attempts by the old and the very old. Arch Intern Med 1991;151(1): 141–4.
[11] Conwell Y, Olsen K, Caine ED, et al. Suicide in later life: psychological autopsy findings. Int Psychogeriatr 1991;3(1):59–66.
[12] Conwell Y, Duberstein PR. Suicide in elders. Ann N Y Acad Sci 2001;932:132–47 [discussion: 147–150].
[13] Blumenthal SJ, Kupfer DJ. Generalizable treatment strategies for suicidal behavior. Ann N Y Acad Sci 1986;487:327–40.
[14] Nemeroff CB, Compton MT, Berger J. The depressed suicidal patient. Assessment and treatment. Ann N Y Acad Sci 2001;932:1–23.
[15] Szanto K, Mulsant BH, Houck PR, et al. Treatment outcome in suicidal vs. non-suicidal elderly patients. Am J Geriatr Psychiatry 2001;9(3):261–8.
[16] Waern M, Runeson BS, Allebeck P, et al. Mental disorder in elderly suicides: a case–control study. Am J Psychiatry 2002;159(3):450–5.
[17] Conwell Y, Brent D. Suicide and aging. I: patterns of psychiatric diagnosis. Int Psychogeriatr 1995;7(2):149–64.
[18] Conwell Y. Suicide in elderly patients. In: Schneider LS, Reynolds CF, Lebowitz BD, Friedhoff AJ, editors. Diagnosis and treatment of depression in late-life. Washington (DC): American Psychiatric Association; 1994. p. 397–418.
[19] Conwell Y, Duberstein PR, Cox C, et al. Relationships of age and axis I diagnoses in victims of completed suicide: a psychological autopsy study. Am J Psychiatry 1996;153(8):1001–8.
[20] Carney SS, Rich CL, Burke PA, et al. Suicide over 60: the San Diego study. J Am Geriatr Soc 1994;42(2):174–80.
[21] Barraclough BM. Suicide in the elderly. Br J Psychiatry 1971;6(suppl):87–97.
[22] Blow FC, Brockmann LM, Barry KL. Role of alcohol in late-life suicide. Alcohol Clin Exp Res 2004;28(5 Suppl):48S–56S.
[23] Murphy GE, Wetzel RD, Robins E, et al. Multiple risk factors predict suicide in alcoholism. Arch Gen Psychiatry 1992;49(6):459–63.
[24] Conner KR, Duberstein PR, Conwell Y, et al. Psychological vulnerability to completed suicide: a review of empirical studies. Suicide Life Threat Behav 2001;31(4):367–85.
[25] Alexopoulos GS, Bruce ML, Hull J, et al. Clinical determinants of suicidal ideation and behavior in geriatric depression. Arch Gen Psychiatry 1999;56(11):1048–53.
[26] Rich CL, Warstadt GM, Nemiroff RA, et al. Suicide, stressors, and the life cycle. Am J Psychiatry 1991;148(4):524–7.
[27] Juurlink DN, Herrmann N, Szalai JP, et al. Medical illness and the risk of suicide in the elderly. Arch Intern Med 2004;164(11):1179–84.
[28] Harris EC, Barraclough BM. Suicide as an outcome for medical disorders. Medicine (Baltimore) 1994;73(6):281–96.

[29] Waern M, Rubenowitz E, Runeson B, et al. Burden of illness and suicide in elderly people: case–control study. BMJ 2002;324(7350):1355.

[30] Szanto K, Gildengers A, Mulsant BH, et al. Identification of suicidal ideation and prevention of suicidal behaviour in the elderly. Drugs Aging 2002;19(1):11–24.

[31] Berglund M, Ojehagen A. The influence of alcohol drinking and alcohol use disorders on psychiatric disorders and suicidal behavior. Alcohol Clin Exp Res 1998;22(7 Suppl): 333S–45S.

[32] Draper BM. Prevention of suicide in old age. Med J Aust 1995;162(10):533–4.

[33] Petronis KR, Samuels JF, Moscicki EK, et al. An epidemiologic investigation of potential risk factors for suicide attempts. Soc Psychiatry Psychiatr Epidemiol 1990;25(4):193–9.

[34] Shulman K. Suicide and parasuicide in old age: a review. Age Ageing 1978;7(4):201–9.

[35] Duberstein PR, Conwell Y, Cox C. Suicide in widowed persons. A psychological autopsy comparison of recently and remotely bereaved older subjects. Am J Geriatr Psychiatry 1998;6(4):328–34.

[36] Rifai AH, Reynolds CF, Mann JJ. Biology of elderly suicide. Suicide Life Threat Behav 1992;22(1):48–61.

[37] Mann JJ, Waternaux C, Haas GL, et al. Toward a clinical model of suicidal behavior in psychiatric patients. Am J Psychiatry 1999;156(2):181–9.

[38] Pearson JL. Recent research on suicide in the elderly. Curr Psychiatry Rep 2002;4(1):59–63.

[39] Isacsson G, Bergman U, Rich CL. Epidemiological data suggest antidepressants reduce suicide risk among depressives. J Affect Disord 1996;41(1):1–8.

[40] Rutz W, von Knorring L, Walinder J. Long-term effects of an educational program for general practitioners given by the Swedish Committee for the Prevention and Treatment of Depression. Acta Psychiatr Scand 1992;85(1):83–8.

[41] Rihmer Z, Rutz W, Pihlgren H. Depression and suicide on Gotland. An intensive study of all suicides before and after a depression-training programme for general practitioners. J Affect Disord 1995;35(4):147–52.

[42] Stoppe G, Sandholzer H, Huppertz C, et al. Family physicians and the risk of suicide in the depressed elderly. J Affect Disord 1999;54(1–2):193–8.

[43] Moscicki EK, Caine ED. Opportunities of life: preventing suicide in elderly patients. Arch Intern Med 2004;164(11):1171–2.

[44] Waern M, Beskow J, Runeson B, et al. Suicidal feelings in the last year of life in elderly people who commit suicide. Lancet 1999;354(9182):917–8.

[45] Beck AT, Schuyler D, Herman I. Development of suicidal intent scales. In: Beck AT, Resnick HCP, Lettieri D, editors. The prediction of suicide. Bowie (MD): Charles Press; 1974. p. 45–56.

[46] Weissman MM, Leaf PJ, Tischler GL, et al. Affective disorders in five United States communities. Psychol Med 1988;18(1):141–53.

[47] Weissman MM, Myers JK. Affective disorders in a US urban community: the use of research diagnostic criteria in an epidemiological survey. Arch Gen Psychiatry 1978;35(11): 1304–11.

[48] Meldon SW, Emerman CL, Schubert DS. Recognition of depression in geriatric ED patients by emergency physicians. Ann Emerg Med 1997;30(4):442–7.

[49] Borson S, Barnes RA, Kukull WA, et al. Symptomatic depression in elderly medical outpatients. I. Prevalence, demography, and health service utilization. J Am Geriatr Soc 1986;34(5):341–7.

[50] Ganguli M, Dodge HH, Mulsant BH. Rates and predictors of mortality in an aging, rural, community-based cohort: the role of depression. Arch Gen Psychiatry 2002;59(11): 1046–52.

[51] Unutzer J, Patrick DL, Diehr P, et al. Quality adjusted life years in older adults with depressive symptoms and chronic medical disorders. Int Psychogeriatr 2000;12(1):15–33.

[52] Huang BY, Cornoni-Huntley J, Hays JC, et al. Impact of depressive symptoms on hospitalization risk in community-dwelling older persons. J Am Geriatr Soc 2000;48(10):1279–84.

[53] Bruce ML, Leaf PJ. Psychiatric disorders and 15-month mortality in a community sample of older adults. Am J Public Health 1989;79(6):727–30.

[54] Schulz R, Drayer RA, Rollman BL. Depression as a risk factor for non-suicide mortality in the elderly. Biol Psychiatry 2002;52(3):205–25.

[55] Sanders AB. Care of the elderly in emergency departments: conclusions and recommendations. Ann Emerg Med 1992;21(7):830–4.

[56] Johnson J, Weissman MM, Klerman GL. Service utilization and social morbidity associated with depressive symptoms in the community. JAMA 1992;267(11):1478–83.

[57] Callahan CM, Kesterson JG, Tierney WM. Association of symptoms of depression with diagnostic test charges among older adults. Ann Intern Med 1997;126(6):426–32.

[58] Unutzer J, Patrick DL, Simon G, et al. Depressive symptoms and the cost of health services in HMO patients aged 65 years and older. A 4-year prospective study. JAMA 1997;277(20): 1618–23.

[59] NIH consensus conference. Diagnosis and treatment of depression in late life. JAMA 1992; 268(8):1018–24.

[60] Blazer D. Depression in the elderly. N Engl J Med 1989;320(3):164–6.

[61] Koenig HG. Depressive disorders in older medical inpatients. Am Fam Physician 1991; 44(4):1243–50.

[62] Meldon SW, Emerman CL, Moffa DA, et al. Utility of clinical characteristics in identifying depression in geriatric ED patients. Am J Emerg Med 1999;17(6):522–5.

[63] Himelhoch S, Weller WE, Wu AW, et al. Chronic medical illness, depression, and use of acute medical services among Medicare beneficiaries. Med Care 2004;42(6):512–21.

[64] Alexopoulos GS, Borson S, Cuthbert BN, et al. Assessment of late life depression. Biol Psychiatry 2002;52(3):164–74.

[65] Charney DS, Reynolds CF 3rd, Lewis L, et al. Depression and Bipolar Support Alliance consensus statement on the unmet needs in diagnosis and treatment of mood disorders in late life. Arch Gen Psychiatry 2003;60(7):664–72.

[66] Carney RM, Freedland KE, Eisen SA, et al. Major depression and medication adherence in elderly patients with coronary artery disease. Health Psychol 1995;14(1):88–90.

[67] Lesperance F, Frasure-Smith N, Talajic M. Major depression before and after myocardial infarction: its nature and consequences. Psychosom Med 1996;58(2):99–110.

[68] van Melle JP, de Jonge P, Spijkerman TA, et al. Prognostic association of depression following myocardial infarction with mortality and cardiovascular events: a meta-analysis. Psychosom Med 2004;66(6):814–22.

[69] Krishnan KR. Biological risk factors in late life depressin. Biol Psychiatry 2001;52:185–92.

[70] Rovner BW, Ganguli M. Depression and disability associated with impaired vision: the MoVies Project. J Am Geriatr Soc 1998;46(5):617–9.

[71] Prince MJ, Harwood RH, Thomas A, et al. A prospective population-based cohort study of the effects of disablement and social milieu on the onset and maintenance of late-life depression. The Gospel Oak Project VII. Psychol Med 1998;28(2):337–50.

[72] Penninx BW, Guralnik JM, Ferrucci L, et al. Depressive symptoms and physical decline in community-dwelling older persons. JAMA 1998;279(21):1720–6.

[73] Rosenzweig A, Prigerson H, Miller MD, et al. Bereavement and late-life depression: grief and its complications in the elderly. Annu Rev Med 1997;48:421–8.

[74] Bruce ML. Psychosocial risk factors for depressive disorders in late life. Biol Psychiatry 2002;52(3):175–84.

[75] Harman JS, Schulberg HC, Mulsant BH, et al. The effect of patient and visit characteristics on diagnosis of depression in primary care. J Fam Pract 2001;50(12):1068.

[76] Shah S, Harris M. A survey of general practitioner's confidence in their management of elderly patients. Aust Fam Physician 1997;26(Suppl 1):S12–7.

[77] Gallo JJ, Rabins PV, Anthony JC. Sadness in older persons: 13-year follow-up of a community sample in Baltimore, Maryland. Psychol Med 1999;29(2):341–50.

[78] Gallo JJ, Rabins PV, Lyketsos CG, et al. Depression without sadness: functional outcomes of nondysphoric depression in later life. J Am Geriatr Soc 1997;45(5):570–8.

[79] Schwenk TL. Diagnosis of late life depression: the view from primary care. Biol Psychiatry 2002;52(3):157–63.

[80] Mulsant BH, Ganguli M. Epidemiology and diagnosis of depression in late life. J Clin Psychiatry 1999;60(Suppl 20):9–15.

[81] Thompson TL 2nd, Mitchell WD, House RM. Geriatric psychiatry patients' care by primary care physicians. Psychosomatics 1989;30(1):65–72.

[82] Diagnostic and Statistical Manual of Mental Disorders. 4th ed. Washington (DC): American Psychiatric Association; 2000.

[83] Fischer LR, Wei F, Solberg LI, et al. Treatment of elderly and other adult patients for depression in primary care. J Am Geriatr Soc 2003;51(11):1554–62.

[84] Steffens DC, Skoog I, Norton MC, et al. Prevalence of depression and its treatment in an elderly population: the Cache County study. Arch Gen Psychiatry 2000;57(6):601–7.

[85] Hoyl MT, Alessi CA, Harker JO, et al. Development and testing of a five-item version of the Geriatric Depression Scale. J Am Geriatr Soc 1999;47(7):873–8.

[86] Fabacher DA, Raccio-Robak N, McErlean MA, et al. Validation of a brief screening tool to detect depression in elderly ED patients. Am J Emerg Med 2002;20(2):99–102.

[87] Evans JF, Ciraulo DA, Zysik MF, et al. Antidepressant treatment of geriatric depression. In: Ciraulo DA, Shader RI, et al, editors. Pharmacotherapy of depression. Totowa (NJ): Humana Press; 2004. p. 119–63.

[88] DasGupta K. Treatment of depression in elderly patients: recent advances. Arch Fam Med 1998;7(3):274–80.

[89] Macdonald AJ. ABC of mental health. Mental health in old age. BMJ 1997;315(7105): 413–7.

[90] Lapid MI, Rummans TA. Evaluation and management of geriatric depression in primary care. Mayo Clin Proc 2003;78(11):1423–9.

[91] Bartels SJ, Dums AR, Oxman TE, et al. Evidence-based practices in geriatric mental health care. Psychiatr Serv 2002;53(11):1419–31.

[92] Salzman C, Wong E, Wright BC. Drug and ECT treatment of depression in the elderly, 1996–2001: a literature review. Biol Psychiatry 2002;52(3):265–84.

[93] Patterson TL, Jeste DV. The potential impact of the baby-boom generation on substance abuse among elderly persons. Psychiatr Serv 1999;50(9):1184–8.

[94] Liberto JG, Oslin DW, Ruskin PE. Alcoholism in older persons: a review of the literature. Hosp Community Psychiatry 1992;43(10):975–84.

[95] D'Onofrio G, Bernstein E, Bernstein J, et al. Patients with alcohol problems in the emergency department, part 1: improving detection. SAEM Substance Abuse Task Force. Society for Academic Emergency Medicine. Acad Emerg Med 1998;5(12):1200–9.

[96] Fleming MF, Barry KL, Manwell LB, et al. Brief physician advice for problem alcohol drinkers. A randomized controlled trial in community-based primary care practices. JAMA 1997;277(13):1039–45.

[97] Adams WL, Barry KL, Fleming MF. Screening for problem drinking in older primary care patients. JAMA 1996;276(24):1964–7.

[98] Adams WL, Magruder-Habib K, Trued S, et al. Alcohol abuse in elderly emergency department patients. J Am Geriatr Soc 1992;40(12):1236–40.

[99] Friedmann PD, Jin L, Karrison T, et al. The effect of alcohol abuse on the health status of older adults seen in the emergency department. Am J Drug Alcohol Abuse 1999;25(3): 529–42.

[100] Curtis JR, Geller G, Stokes EJ, et al. Characteristics, diagnosis, and treatment of alcoholism in elderly patients. J Am Geriatr Soc 1989;37(4):310–6.

[101] McKim WA, Quinlan LT. Changes in alcohol consumption with age. Can J Public Health 1991;82(4):231–4.

[102] Reid MC, Anderson PA. Geriatric substance use disorders. Med Clin North Am 1997; 81(4):999–1016.

[103] Finlayson RE, Hurt RD, Davis LJ Jr, et al. Alcoholism in elderly persons: a study of the psychiatric and psychosocial features of 216 inpatients. Mayo Clin Proc 1988;63(8):761–8.

[104] Hurt RD, Finlayson RE, Morse RM, et al. Alcoholism in elderly persons: medical aspects and prognosis of 216 inpatients. Mayo Clin Proc 1988;63(8):753–60.

[105] Liberto JG, Oslin DW. Early versus late onset of alcoholism in the elderly. Int J Addict 1995;30(13–14):1799–818.

[106] Fink A, Hays RD, Moore AA, et al. Alcohol-related problems in older persons. Determinants, consequences, and screening. Arch Intern Med 1996;156(11):1150–6.

[107] Morse RM. Substance abuse among the elderly. Bull Menninger Clin 1988;52(3):259–68.

[108] Blow FC. Substance abuse among older adults. Vol 26. Rockville (MD): US Department of Health and Human Services; 1998.

[109] Bucholz KK, Sheline Y, Helzer JE. The epidemiology of alcohol use, problems, and dependence in elders: a review. In: Beresford TP, Gomberg E, editors. Alcohol and aging. New York: Oxford University Press; 1995. p. 19–41.

[110] Scott RB, Mitchell MC. Aging, alcohol, and the liver. J Am Geriatr Soc 1988;36(3):255–65.

[111] Smith JW. Medical manifestations of alcoholism in the elderly. Int J Addict 1995;30(13–14): 1749–98.

[112] Rigler SK. Alcoholism in the elderly. Am Fam Physician 2000;61(6):1710–6, 1883–1714, 1887–1718 passim.

[113] Alcoholism in the elderly, Council on Scientific Affairs, American Medical Association. JAMA 1996;275(10):797–801.

[114] Blow FC, Cook CA, Booth BM, et al. Age-related psychiatric comorbidities and level of functioning in alcoholic veterans seeking outpatient treatment. Hosp Community Psychiatry 1992;43(10):990–5.

[115] Waern M. Alcohol dependence and misuse in elderly suicides. Alcohol Alcohol 2003;38(3): 249–54.

[116] Moore RD, Bone LR, Geller G, et al. Prevalence, detection, and treatment of alcoholism in hospitalized patients. JAMA 1989;261(3):403–7.

[117] Keeler EB, Solomon DH, Beck JC, et al. Effect of patient age on duration of medical encounters with physicians. Med Care 1982;20(11):1101–8.

[118] Ewing JA. Detecting alcoholism. The CAGE questionnaire. JAMA 1984;252(14):1905–7.

[119] Blow FC, Brower KJ, Schulenberg JE, et al. The Michigan Alcoholism Screening Test — Geriatric Version (MAST-G): a new elderly-specific screening instrument. Alcohol Clin Exp Res 1992;16:372.

[120] Patient Placement Criteria for the Treatment of Substance-Related Disorders. 2nd ed. Washington (DC): American Society of Addiction Medicine; 1996.

[121] Kraemer KL, Conigliaro J, Saitz R. Managing alcohol withdrawal in the elderly. Drugs Aging 1999;14(6):409–25.

[122] O'Connell H, Chin AV, Cunningham C, et al. Alcohol use disorders in elderly people—redefining an age old problem in old age. BMJ 2003;327(7416):664–7.

[123] Dunne FJ. Misuse of alcohol or drugs by elderly people. BMJ 1994;308(6929):608–9.

[124] Lacro JP, Jeste DV. Geriatric psychosis. Psychiatr Q 1997;68(3):247–60.

[125] Soares JC, Gershon S. Therapeutic targets in late-life psychoses: review of concepts and critical issues. Schizophr Res 1997;27(2–3):227–39.

[126] Myers JK, Weissman MM, Tischler GL, et al. Six-month prevalence of psychiatric disorders in three communities 1980 to 1982. Arch Gen Psychiatry 1984;41(10):959–67.

[127] Targum SD, Abbott JL. Psychoses in the elderly: a spectrum of disorders. J Clin Psychiatry 1999;60(Suppl 8):4–10.

[128] Khouzam HR, Battista MA, Emes R, et al. Psychoses in late life: evaluation and management of disorders seen in primary care. Geriatrics 2005;60(3):26–33.

[129] Koenig HG, George LK, Schneider R. Mental health care for older adults in the year 2020: a dangerous and avoided topic. Gerontologist 1994;34(5):674–9.

[130] Wragg RE, Jeste DV. Overview of depression and psychosis in Alzheimer's disease. Am J Psychiatry 1989;146(5):577–87.

[131] Rabins PV, Mace NL, Lucas MJ. The impact of dementia on the family. JAMA 1982; 248(3):333–5.

[132] Thorpe L. The treatment of psychotic disorders in late life. Can J Psychiatry 1997; 42(Suppl 1):19S–27S.

[133] Zayas EM, Grossberg GT. The treatment of psychosis in late life. J Clin Psychiatry 1998; 59(Suppl 1):5–10 [discussion: 11–2].

[134] Ohi G, Kai I, Ichikawa S, et al. Psychotic manifestations in the bed-fast elderly—a preliminary communication. J Hum Ergol (Tokyo) 1989;18(2):237–40.

[135] Jeste DV, Harris MJ, Krull A, et al. Clinical and neuropsychological characteristics of patients with late-onset schizophrenia. Am J Psychiatry 1995;152(5):722–30.

[136] Eastwood MR, Corbin SL, Reed M, et al. Acquired hearing loss and psychiatric illness: an estimate of prevalence and co-morbidity in a geriatric setting. Br J Psychiatry 1985;147: 552–6.

[137] Frame DS, Kercher EE. Acute psychosis. Functional versus organic. Emerg Med Clin North Am 1991;9(1):123–36.

[138] Barak Y, Aizenberg D, Mirecki I, et al. Very late-onset schizophrenia-like psychosis: clinical and imaging characteristics in comparison with elderly patients with schizophrenia. J Nerv Ment Dis 2002;190(11):733–6.

[139] Hassett A. A descriptive study of first presentation psychosis in old age. Aust N Z J Psychiatry 1999;33(6):814–24.

[140] Howard R, Rabins PV, Seeman MV, et al. Late-onset schizophrenia and very-late-onset schizophrenia-like psychosis: an international consensus. The International Late-Onset Schizophrenia Group. Am J Psychiatry 2000;157(2):172–8.

[141] Pearlson GD, Kreger L, Rabins PV, et al. A chart review study of late-onset and early-onset schizophrenia. Am J Psychiatry 1989;146(12):1568–74.

[142] Wynn Owen PA, Castle DJ. Late-onset schizophrenia: epidemiology, diagnosis, management and outcomes. Drugs Aging 1999;15(2):81–9.

[143] Castle DJ, Wessely S, Howard R, et al. Schizophrenia with onset at the extremes of adult life. Int J Geriatr Psychiatry 1997;12(7):712–7.

[144] Brodaty H, Sachdev P, Rose N, et al. Schizophrenia with onset after age 50 years. I: phenomenology and risk factors. Br J Psychiatry 1999;175:410–5.

[145] Howard RJ, Graham C, Sham P, et al. A controlled family study of late-onset non-affective psychosis (late paraphrenia). Br J Psychiatry 1997;170:511–4.

[146] Howard R, Cox T, Almeida O, et al. White matter signal hyperintensities in the brains of patients with late paraphrenia and the normal, community-living elderly. Biol Psychiatry 1995;38(2):86–91.

[147] Castle DJ, Abel K, Takei N, et al. Gender differences in schizophrenia: hormonal effect or subtypes? Schizophr Bull 1995;21(1):1–12.

[148] Bellnier TJ. Continuum of care: stabilizing the acutely agitated patient. Am J Health Syst Pharm 2002;59(17, Suppl 5):S12–8.

[149] Tueth MJ. Dementia: diagnosis and emergency behavioral complications. J Emerg Med 1995;13(4):519–25.

[150] Carlson DL, Fleming KC, Smith GE, et al. Management of dementia-related behavioral disturbances: a nonpharmacologic approach. Mayo Clin Proc 1995;70(11):1108–15.

[151] Turnheim K. When drug therapy gets old: pharmacokinetics and pharmacodynamics in the elderly. Exp Gerontol 2003;38(8):843–53.

[152] Alexopoulos GS, Jeste DV, Chung H, et al. Treatment of dementia and its behavioral disturbances. Minneapolis (MN): McGraw-Hill; 2005.

[153] Sweet RA. Taking a new look at psychosis in Alzheimer's disease. Psychiatr Times 2002; 19(11) [online].

[154] Tariot PN, Profenno LA, Ismail MS. Efficacy of atypical antipsychotics in elderly patients with dementia. J Clin Psychiatry 2004;65(Suppl 11):11–5.

[155] Tinetti ME, Speechley M, Ginter SF. Risk factors for falls among elderly persons living in the community. N Engl J Med 1988;319(26):1701–7.

[156] Ray WA, Griffin MR, Schaffner W, et al. Psychotropic drug use and the risk of hip fracture. N Engl J Med 1987;316(7):363–9.

[157] Drug Specific Information. Center for Drug Evaluation and Research, http://www.fda.gov/cder/index.html.

[158] Burston GR. Letter: granny-battering. BMJ 1975;3(5983):592.

[159] Diagnostic and treatment guidelines on elder abuse and neglect. Chicago (IL): American Medical Association; 1994. p. 4–24.

[160] Kruger RM, Moon CH. Can you spot the signs of elder mistreatment? Postgrad Med 1999; 106(2):169–73 [177–168, 183].

[161] Swagerty DL Jr, Takahashi PY, Evans JM. Elder mistreatment. Am Fam Physician 1999; 59(10):2804–8.

[162] Pillemer K, Finkelhor D. The prevalence of elder abuse: a random sample survey. Gerontologist 1988;28(1):51–7.

[163] Nelson D. Violence against elderly people: a neglected problem. Lancet 2002;360(9339): 1094.

[164] Lachs MS, Pillemer K. Abuse and neglect of elderly persons. N Engl J Med 1995;332(7): 437–43.

[165] Lachs MS, Williams C, O'Brien S, et al. Older adults. An 11-year longitudinal study of adult protective service use. Arch Intern Med 1996;156(4):449–53.

[166] Quinn MJ, Tomita SK. Elder abuse and neglect: causes, diagnosis, and intervention strategies. New York: Springer; 1986.

ELSEVIER
SAUNDERS

Emerg Med Clin N Am
24 (2006) 491–505

EMERGENCY
MEDICINE
CLINICS OF
NORTH AMERICA

Elder Abuse

Adam J. Geroff, MD*, Jonathan S. Olshaker, MD, FACEP

*Department of Emergency Medicine, Boston Medical Center,
1 Boston Medical Center Place, Boston, MA 02188-2393, USA*

The ugly specter of elder abuse casts as dark a pall over our society as other forms of domestic violence. Although recent years have brought increased awareness of this problem, elder abuse and maltreatment still lags woefully behind child abuse and intimate partner violence in with regard to research, education, and funding. Despite specific laws designed to protect the rights of America's senior citizens and to punish abusers, the prevalence of elder mistreatment is alarmingly high and the consequences are significant. Even when adjusting for confounding variables, studies have discovered higher mortality rates among abused elders [1]. The results of these studies should be quite disturbing to the medical community and the general public.

Medical personnel have an opportunity to play an important role in the detection of elder abuse. The emergency physician in particular may find him or herself with a unique opportunity to recognize a perhaps previously unrecognized situation. As always, the emergency physician is on the front line of disease and its treatment, whether that disease process is as glaring as an ST-segment elevation myocardial infarction or a hip fracture resulting from an accidental fall (or perhaps a deliberate push), or as subtle as an elderly person suffering from a less dramatic form of abuse or neglect. The emergency department may serve as a gateway for the detection of an abusive or neglectful circumstance, and can be the place where the first steps toward intervention are taken.

This discourse shall serve to educate and update physicians and emergency medical clinicians in the broad range of issues that encompass elder abuse, neglect, and mistreatment. These elements include a review of history, a definition of terms, and a presentation of the clinical features of abuse and neglect. The relevant characteristics of victims and their abusers and risk factors for maltreatment will be clarified. Legal implications will be

* Corresponding author.
E-mail address: ageroff@smail.umaryland.edu

0733-8627/06/$ - see front matter © 2006 Elsevier Inc. All rights reserved.
doi:10.1016/j.emc.2006.01.009   *emed.theclinics.com*

discussed, such as reporting requirements in the context of ethical obligations to patients. It is the authors' hope that readers of this article will use this manual as an instrument by which to better understand this scourge and ultimately to enable the practicing provider to recognize it and intervene appropriately.

History

The abuse, neglect, or mistreatment of the elderly has unfortunately accompanied human existence since the ancient era, and has spanned the globe. Classical Greek literature and mythology chronicle accounts of children killing their parents, called parricide, to consolidate power [2]. An extreme form of self-abuse and neglect is known in the medical lexicon as Diogenes Syndrome, whose namesake was a fourth century BCE philosopher who shunned common comforts and lived much of his life in a tub [3]. The Greek culture also found euthanasia acceptable for the ill and incurable older population. Shakespeare wrote in *King Lear* about the king's maltreatment by his sons [4]. Tales of vampirism from Europe often have centered on an elderly man accused of aberrant behavior, whose pallid appearance may have been the result of an anemia of chronic disease. Some tribal cultures in Africa will isolate and abandon elder members by accusing them of witchcraft and blaming them in times of scarce resources [5]. Some cultures have promoted the ritual suicide of tribal elders during famine or drought so that precious food and water could be allocated to the more productive younger people [2]. Colonial American history reminds us that victims of witch hunts who were stoned or burned were often postmenopausal women [6]. Like other forms of family violence, elder abuse had historically been deemed a private affair and exempt from outside inquiry.

Despite its historic prevalence, elder abuse was not formally recognized by the medical community until 1975. Two British journal published reports on "Granny battering" 1 month apart to finally shed some light on this longstanding problem [7,8]. Since then, reports have surfaced worldwide, and increasingly more research is being done on the topic [5,9–18].

In the United States, Congressional hearings first occurred in the late 1970s and early 1980s and heralded the gradual expansion of resources devoted to elder abuse. A 1987 amendment to the Older Americans Act defined certain terms. The Elder Abuse Task Force was created in 1990 by the Department of Health and Human Services, which enlarged the scope of the federal government's contribution to solving the problem. Following this, the United States Administration on Aging created the National Resource Center on Elder Abuse, which has evolved into today's agency called the National Center on Elder Abuse (NCEA). The Joint Commission on Accreditation of Health Care Organizations then began to specifically include elder abuse as a form of domestic violence to raise awareness in its directive for the recognition and treatment of all forms of domestic violence [9,19,20]. Elder abuse is joining the ranks of the other forms of domestic violence as they slowly are making their way out from the veil of secrecy, embarrassment, and shame, which had formerly hidden these maladies from scrutiny.

As a tangible benefit from this political awareness, President Clinton's first legislative signing was the Family Medical Leave Act in 1993. Among other changes, this act provided families with an easier means to care for their elder relatives. The Clinton administration also expanded Medicare benefits for senior citizens and saw the NCEA receive a one million dollar grant to expand its services and further its research. Hopefully, future administrations will be as progressive.

Despite heightened awareness of elder abuse and improvements in elder care, medical providers should anticipate treating more cases of elder abuse, neglect, and mistreatment in the coming years simply because the population is aging. The aged bring a myriad of special challenges to their health care in the emergency department, one of which is elder abuse. Overall advances in medical care are keeping Americans alive for more years than ever before. Many will enter institutions with varying levels of supervision and care before their deaths, which will introduce them to the possibility of an institutional abuser.

The population statistics and projected life expectancies are indeed astounding. The average American child born in 1990 will live to be more than 75 years old. Compare this to the average lifespan of 47 years for a child who had been born in 1900 [21]. Reaching the milestone of age 65 in the year 1990 meant to that fortunate senior citizen that he or she could expect to live an additional 17 years, thereby exceeding the average lifespan by over 7 years [21]. The most rapidly growing segment of the elderly population is referred to as the "old-old," that is, age over 75. The Census Bureau has subdivided this group to identify the "oldest-old" of age over 85. This number of this group's living members increased by 38% from 1980 to 1990. Additionally, the number or American centenarians doubled in this decade [2,21]. Senior citizens comprise an ever-increasing proportion of all Americans. In 1980, there were over 25 million Americans at age 65 or older [21]. By the year 2000, this number increased to 35 million. Predictions estimate that by the year 2020, more than 52 million Americans will be 65 or over [22]. The elder boom is not just an American phenomenon. Currently, 20% of the population of the United Kingdom is over age 60, and by the year 2050 this proportion will increase to 40% [23].

The marked increase in the elderly population will necessarily increase total interactions with the health care system, particularly the emergency department. Studies have shown that elders use emergency departments with relatively greater frequency than the general population [24–28]. These statistics should come as no surprise to practicing emergency physicians, who readily recognize the stressors that this special population places on ED resources [29]. The elderly are more frequently admitted to the hospital, more likely to require an intensive care unit, and more likely to require a comprehensive level of emergency department service [24]. Therefore, one may actually conclude that the elderly are more in need of emergency medical resources than younger patients. Indeed, the elderly may actually access emergency services on a more justified and efficient bases than the young. The emergency medical community must recognize this calling and prepare itself to see and treat elders with all of their medical problems and nonmedical issues. These may more increasingly include abuse and neglect.

Terms, definitions, and types of abuse

There exists considerable variability among authors with regard to what constitutes elder abuse. Different disciplines, representing the medical, legal, and social work arenas all seem to place their particular perspectives on terminology. Even providers within each arm cannot agree. No generally accepted meanings for the terms abuse, mistreatment, or maltreatment exist [18,30,31]. Some authorities include neglect in these terms while others do not. [20,32,33]. The somewhat gentler expression "inadequate care" has been used as an umbrella phrase by some authors [34].

Although there exist many variations among individual authors, it is worthwhile to review the published definitions by three key groups in the past 20 years likely to have the greatest impact. In 1985, the US Congress passed the Elder Abuse Prevention, Identification and Treatment Act, which clarified terminology (Table 1) [35]. Another reasonable collection of terms was defined in 1992 by the American Medical Association in this organization's guidelines (Table 2) [36]. These sets were seemingly used by a later project, the National Elder Abuse Incidence Study (NEAIS) to produce an updated, comprehensive list of definitions (Table 3) [37]. The NEAIS was sanctioned by the NCEA in 1996 to study the problem of domestic elder abuse. The US Department of Health and Human Services Administration on Aging authorized a group of national experts to research and conduct surveys on potential definitions to use before creating and selecting their final terms for publication. This list should become the standard to which all those who provide care to the elderly should be held.

Table 1
Congressional definitions

Abuse	Willful infliction of injury, unreasonable confinement, intimidation, or cruel punishment with resulting physical harm, pain, or mental anguish; or the willful deprivation by a caretaker of goods or services that are necessary to avoid physical harm, mental anguish or mental illness
Physical harm	Bodily pain, injury, impairment, or disease
Exploitation	Illegal or improper act of a caretaker using the resources of an elder for monetary or personal benefit, profit or gain
Neglect	Failure of a caretaker to provide the goods or services that are necessary to avoid physical harm, mental anguish or mental illness

Table 2
AMA definitions

Physical abuse	Acts of violence that may result in pain, injury, impairment, or disease
Physical neglect	Failure of the caregiver to provide the goods or services that are necessary for optimal functioning of, or avoidance of the older adult
Psychologic abuse	Conduct that causes mental anguish in an older person
Psychologic neglect	Failure to provide a dependent elderly individual with social stimulation
Financial or material abuse	Misuse of the elderly person's income or resources for the financial or personal gain of a caretaker or advisor
Financial or material neglect	Failure to use available funds and resources necessary to sustain or restore the health and well being of the older adult
Violation of personal rights	Caretaker or providers ignoring the older person's rights and capability to make decisions for himself or herself.

The term neglect can be even more confusing than abuse. Some panelists regard neglect as a lesser form of elder maltreatment and suggest that neglect should comprise those situations whereby intent to cause harm is absent [38]. However, an act of neglect may be just as willful and just as harmful as a more overt act of abuse. Indeed, such an action, or inaction, may be even more sinister and disturbing, because cases of neglect necessarily involve a person with whom the victim has an established relationship, either personal or professional. Many authorities do not even mention or describe self-neglect in their works. Self-neglect is perhaps the most deeply psychologically challenging concept of all, and calls significant ethical considerations into question.

All this lingo can cause bewilderment in the medical community. Emergency providers should familiarize themselves with these terms so that they

Table 3
NEAIS definitions

Physical abuse	The use of physical force that may result in bodily injury, physical pain or impairment
Sexual abuse	Nonconsensual sexual contact of any kind with an elderly person
Emotional or psychologic abuse	The infliction of anguish, emotional pain, or distress
Neglect	The refusal or failure to fulfill any part of a person's obligations or duties to an elder
Abandonment	The desertion of an elderly person by an individual who has assumed responsibility for providing care or by a person with physical custody of an elder
Financial or material exploitation	The illegal or improper use of an elder's funds, property, or assets
Self-neglect	The behaviors of an elderly person that threaten his or her own health or safety

can recognize cases of elder maltreatment and alert the necessary law enforcement or government agency. This is the ultimate benefit that can be conferred to the elder that has been victimized by abusive or neglectful circumstances.

The most easily recognizable form is physical abuse. This involves the deliberate infliction of force upon a victim with resulting pain, injury, suffering, or impairment. Examples include slapping, pinching, striking with objects, kicking, biting, shaking, shoving, burning, rough handling, and force feeding [39,40]. The abuser's own hand is the most common instrument of damage used to cause harm. Other more subtle behaviors that would constitute physical abuse include unindicated or inappropriate use of physical or chemical restraints or the administration of or overmedication with a drug such as a sedative or a tranquilizer. Sexual abuse is sometimes included as a form of physical abuse. Obvious examples include rape, fondling, or unwanted touching. Other less direct violations may be just as unbecoming: coerced nudity, indecent exposure, and lewd talk. Although the subject of the sexual assault of an elderly person is loathsome, emergency physicians must not dismiss this as a possibility. There is not much data on the topic, but one study reported that only 1% of elder abuse victims suffered a sexual assault [41]. Most of these victims sustained the mistreatment while living in an institutional setting, not at home. Furthermore, prohibiting or restricting consensual sexual activity involving a competent elder may be considered abusive. Senior citizens have as much right to continue to explore human sexuality as any other adults do, as long as they have the capacity to make such decisions.

Physical neglect in general involves bodily harm brought about by the failure of a provider to supply the means for an elder's well-being. Examples include inadequate hydration, nourishment, physical activity, or therapy. Failing to provide or maintain in working order basic appliances that assist daily living like glasses, hearing aids, dentures and canes or walkers constitute neglectful conduct. Inadequate home safety measures to prevent injury such as handrails or siderails also qualify. Neglect may be active or passive, depending upon the presence or absence of intent [42]. From a legal perspective, intent is often difficult to prove. From a purely medical perspective, intent is probably immaterial to the medical evaluation and decision making. The practicing clinician in the emergency department should not attempt to evaluate this issue too deeply, if at all. He or she must identify and treat any injury discovered and consider the possibility of abuse or neglect. The next step should be to ensure safe disposition of the patient. Regardless of whether or not a significantly adverse occurrence to an elder was the result of an intentional act of omission or commission, that it occurred at all should heighten the suspicion of the clinician that the elder should not return immediately to the environment from which he or she came, unless additional help or supervision can be arranged.

The matter of self-neglect may present a particular quandary in the emergency department. This situation involves value judgments on the part of the physician and provokes ethical dilemmas. For example, a patient may present to the emergency department with foot ulcers or skin lesions or dental infections resulting from poor hygiene and inadequate basic care, but may choose to shun the level of personal care that most other people would choose for themselves. As long as patients have decisional capacity, they cannot be forced into another social situation against their will. The clinician should naturally educate these patients as to the importance of such basic care with regard to its therapeutic and preventative benefits, but should recognize that it is outside the scope of medical practice to impose his or her personal values upon the patient. If, however, such a patient demonstrates signs of reduced decisional capacity, it may be justified and ethical and obligatory for an emergency physician to ensure that the patient is indeed removed from the living situation contributing to the problem, perhaps against the patient's will. Signs of concern would include hypoxia, perhaps high fever, disorientation, active psychosis, and other significant abnormal findings on a mental status examination.

Psychologic or emotional abuse wreaks mental anguish by means of threat, humiliation, fear, or other cruel conduct. It may be inflicted via verbal or nonverbal communication cues. Examples include harassment, scolding, and stalking. Threatening an elderly person with physical punishment or deprivation of basic needs is a particularly heinous form of this type of abuse. Psychologic neglect deprives an elder of healthy mental well-being. Examples include prolonged periods of solitude and failure to provide adequate companionship. A caregiver might be providing an elder with adequate essential needs such as food, water, and shelter, but neglect to provide this person with adequate social stimulation. This can lead to feelings of isolation and low-self esteem. Many of the elderly suffer from clinical depression already [43]; psychologic abuse and neglect can advance such mental health problems.

The financial exploitation of an elder includes direct criminal behaviors such as theft of money or property and coercion to sign any unwanted agreement. Many professional scam artists target the elderly as a particularly vulnerable segment of the population upon whom to prey. More commonly, however, an elder who falls victim to material abuse is exploited by a family member or caregiver. These victims may possess considerable assets, or may live on the fixed income of a government subsidy. Even small monthly sums can entice an exploiter to take advantage of an elderly person [44].

Elder abuse may also be classified by its setting. Domestic abuse or maltreatment occurs in the home of the victim [31,37]. The abuser has an established personal relationship with the elder, such as spouse, child, relative, friend, or in-home caregiver. Conversely, institutional mistreatment transpires outside a private residence, such as in a nursing home, hospital, assisted living center, or group home. The perpetrators have a professional or contractual duty to provide care and can be nurses, aides, or techs. Additionally, a complex form of institutional financial abuse occurs when

executives and administrators of such facilities take advantage of elderly patients' monetary resources or file false claims with an insurance company or
Medicare. These white-collar criminals defraud companies out of thousands
of dollars and deprive elderly victims of needed services.

Epidemiology and demographics

The actual incidence and prevalence of elder abuse in this country and
worldwide is unknown. Studies performed over the past 20 years are quite
varied in their methods and analysis. Most have reported a prevalence
rate of 3% to 5% of all elders as having been at some time a victim
[18,45]. A common source of criticism for all of these early accounts is
that they have been based on cases that have been reported to authorities.
Thousands of incidents of abuse and maltreatment go unreported each
year. One recently published population based study undertaken by the
NCEA attempted to extrapolate data on reported cases to estimate the incidence of elder abuse and neglect nationwide. This study (NEAIS) was
well designed, although it was limited to domestic elder mistreatment
only. These researchers concluded that, in the study year, approximately
551,000 cases of elder abuse and neglect occurred in over 450,000 victims
[37]. Although the statistical range on this estimate was wide, the absolute
number is still shocking. This total is even more humbling when one con-
siders that it, by design, does not include any cases of institutional abuse.
Other studies have estimated the total number of abused seniors annually
to be even higher, ranging from 1 million to 2.5 million [46]. The NEAIS investigators determined that the most common form of maltreatment was neglect, as delineated in Table 4 [37].

Neglect was also the most common harm type discovered in another
study of a smaller cohort of elders [47]. The NEAIS also undertook the ef-
fort to independently substantiate the reports of mistreatment that it received. Physical abuse was the most readily substantiated; while neglect
was the hardest to validate [37]. The NEAIS performed many meticulous
statistical analyses on its raw data. Rather than focus on the minutia of
the numbers, it is most helpful to the practicing clinician to recognize the

Table 4
Percentage of cases that involved a particular harm type

Neglect	48.7%
Psychologic	35.4%
Financial	30.2%
Physical	25.6%
Abandonment	3.6%
Miscellaneous/other	1.4%
Sexual	0.3%

enormous scale of the problem and the order of magnitude of the numbers discussed. The emergency physician would be remiss to trivialize the incidence of this crisis.

Who is most likely to become a casualty of abuse? Risk factors and victim characteristics have been evaluated by various investigators. Exact conclusions are difficult to draw, but the data suggest that the typical victim is as old as or older than 75 to 80 years, suffers from some form of mental illness, and to some extent is unable to provide complete independent self-care. The NEAIS found a median age of 78 years, and determined that the elderly in the over-80 age group were two to three times more likely to be abused or neglected than all elders [37]. This data corroborated earlier investigators' conclusions that the most elderly were the most at risk for abuse and neglect, in part due to the greater likelihood of overall poor health and dependency [2,13,18,25]. Interestingly, other research has failed to demonstrate a link between infirmity and probability of mistreatment [14,47,48]. Similarly, the data with regard to any gender predilection is also incongruous. Some studies report a significant majority among females [14,47,48], while another describes the exact opposite [18]. The NEAIS proved what many authorities had long held as dogma: that the reduced mental health of an elder placed that elder at significant risk of mistreatment. Depression and dementia were the two illnesses that were overwhelmingly encountered by the NEAIS researchers among victims, occurring in 45% to 50% of victims, respectively [37], with some persons displaying signs of both disorders. These percentages vastly exceed the prevalence of these illnesses among the general elder community [49,50].

Who is most likely to be responsible for these deeds? By far, the most common perpetrator of domestic abuse or neglect is a close relative, most likely an adult child or spouse [2,18,37,48,51]. As incredible as this may seem, these conclusions have been consistently drawn by nearly all investigators who have been able to independently reproduce similar data. This conclusion represents perhaps the only "sure thing" that is known about elder abuse and mistreatment. Reports from Adult Protective Services agencies documented that an adult child committed the abuse in over 47% of cases, and that a spouse was at fault in over 19% of cases [37]. NEAIS data collectors found that children and spouses were involved in about 30% of cases each [37]. It will not surprise most clinicians to discover that a history of substance abuse in the caregiver, most likely alcoholism, is perhaps the single most important characteristic predictive of abusive behavior [51,52]. The incidence of addiction in an abuser can be as high as 35% [53] (Box 1).

The discovery of elder abuse and neglect may be as simple as walking into a room and seeing an obviously nonaccidentally injured patient or as daunting as examining a nonverbal, demented person who has arrived at 2 AM by an ambulance from home without the benefit of speaking with a reliable historian. The emergency provider must maintain vigilance and a high index of

Box 1. Risk factors for elder abuse

Age greater than 75 years
History of depression or other mental illness
Dementia
Inability to completely self care
Substance abuse in the caregiver
Depression

suspicion at all times to uncover a mistreatment situation. This holds true for all elderly patients, whether they present from a private home or from an institution.

The history-taking process is challenging. Many authors have proposed screening tools and instruments. Many of these are elaborate and time-consuming and most applicable for a social work provider and not for the busy emergency physician. The American Medical Association (AMA) has created a set of screening questions that are concise and to the point. These are indeed practical for use in an emergency department (Box 2):

The technique employed by the clinician is of utmost importance. The interview should be conducted privately so that the elderly patient is the first person making contact with the clinician. This can instill in a victim a sense of confidence and confidentiality with the stranger wearing the stethoscope. The consultation should take the form of a dialog where possible, rather than a rapid-fire question and answer session. The savvy examiner will incorporate the screening questions to make them seem like a routine part of the appraisal, to place a potential victim at ease. He or she should express empathy and concern in a nonjudgmental manner. Any description given of mistreatment or neglect should be documented meticulously, using the victim's own words. Likewise, physical findings of abuse should be carefully

Box 2. AMA screening questions

1. Has anyone ever touched you without your consent?
2. Has anyone ever made you do things you didn't want to do?
3. Has anyone taken anything that was yours without asking?
4. Has anyone ever hurt you?
5. Has anyone ever scolded or threatened you?
6. Have you ever signed any documents you didn't understand?
7. Are you afraid of anyone at home?
8. Are you alone a lot?
9. Has anyone ever failed to help you take care of yourself when you needed help?

charted. Using sketches with notation of lesion type, size, color, and exact location in relation to a fixed anatomic site is helpful. Photographs are even better, although maintenance of chain of custody for anything other than instant photography may preclude their use by the emergency physician.

The physical examination of the elderly must always be performed using the most meticulous scrutiny, regardless of whether or not abuse is suspected. The importance of a head-to-toe physical examination cannot be stressed enough. Careful attention must be paid particularly to the head and neck, the skin, and the neurologic and musculoskeletal systems, because often the most obvious signs of abuse or neglect will manifest here. Table 5 lists pertinent findings that one might discover on exam. Ancillary testing is likewise important to the evaluation. The provider should already have a low threshold to order diagnostic tests in the elderly. At a minimum, a complete blood count, a basic chemistry profile, a urinalysis, and a chest radiograph should be ordered. These may reveal findings suggestive of malnutrition, dehydration, and rib fractures. Additional tests must be obtained, naturally, as the clinical scenario warrants. As a guideline, any body part that is tender, swollen, grossly deformed or bruised should be imaged with a radiograph to look for either an acute of remote fracture. The clinician should have a low index of suspicion in ordering a cranial CT scan to detect an intracranial hemorrhage, such as a traumatic subdural hematoma, which can occur in even minor to moderate trauma, such as shaking or a ground-level fall [54]. An alteration in consciousness should also prompt the clinician to obtain an analysis for toxins such as alcohol and drugs of abuse, even in a patient whose age or social situation does not conform to the stereotypic person in whom one might expect to find a positive result. Of course, the presence of a significant abnormality does not conclusively rule in abuse or neglect. There is no one pathognomonic finding. Any pathology must be considered within the context of each individual situation and each patient's pertinent history. Older people in particular can be prone

Table 5
Physical findings of abuse or neglect

Bruises—especially of varying ages and not over bony prominences
Wounds—decubitus ulcers, untreated lacerations or abrasions
Patterned injuries—hand slap or fingertip marks, ligature imprints on the wrists or ankles, bite marks
Burns—cigarette burns or a scald burn with an immersion line
Genital lesions—urethral or vaginal discharge or bleeding, signs of trauma
Anorectal findings—mucosal tears or fecal impaction
Fractures—particularly spiral in orientation or without an accompanying mechanism, or fractures in various stages of healing
Poor hygiene—excrement soilage, infestation
Poor nutrition—dehydration, cachexia

to problems such as bruises and fractures purely due to physical consequences of aging or concurrent medical conditions.

The emergency provider should realize that it is not his or her role to perform the most comprehensive of evaluations for elder abuse. This clinician's primary responsibilities are threefold: to recognize or suspect elder abuse and neglect when present, to treat any medical problems associated with such maltreatment, and to ensure a safe disposition for the patient. There exist other services and providers within the hospital and the community to provide additional evaluations, assessments, and more long-term recommendations. The first contact for an elder to these adjunct providers may indeed be made via a referral from the emergency department. Therefore, the initial, de novo assessment made by the emergency physician may be the most crucial.

Legal and ethical considerations

Physicians must become familiar with their state's laws with regard to elder abuse, especially with regard to reporting. Such laws have considerable variability from jurisdiction to jurisdiction. Most states have mandatory reporting laws for physicians. Some states' laws extend such a provision to other non-physician health providers, but ultimately this responsibility will fall on the physician. Not surprisingly, one study found significantly higher investigation rates in states that required mandatory reporting and tracking of the numbers of reports [55]. Unfortunately, physicians have still performed poorly in this regard. Numerous studies have documented physicians' overall dismal reporting rate [46,56,57]. Much of this can be attributed to a lack of education and training. Only a minority of residency training programs in emergency medicine include any formal education in elder abuse. Furthermore, there are still many practicing emergency physicians who are not residency trained in emergency medicine. Presumably, these physicians would have had even less of an opportunity to be formally educated in this discipline. Perhaps this accounts for several surveys' documentation of physicians' major underestimation of the incidence of elder mistreatment [47,58]. Fortunately, other individuals and professionals have traditionally performed better in this regard, so overall reporting has increased steadily [31,37].

The decision to report a case of suspected or admitted elder abuse or neglect is not quite as simple for the physician as it might seem. Certainly, a clinician's first response to such a situation would be to involve the appropriate law enforcement or adult protective services agent. Indeed, this would be a requirement by statute in most states. However, the psychosocial issues involved in elder abuse and mistreatment are quite complex, and can transcend the black and white requirement of the letter of the law. An elder may not want his or her case reported. Such reasoning may be based on antiquated thinking that such a situation is a private family matter, or illogically founded in simple embarrassment. However, a victim may harbor well-founded fears if his or her case is reported. Many fear repercussion by the abuser or separation from family. Victims may be afraid that such a revelation will uproot them from their homes. Others are dependent on that very person to maintain activities of daily living. Some may even feel the need to protect a perpetrator from an investigation, especially if he or she is a family member. Most disturbingly, some abused and neglected elders have succumbed to a pattern of victimization for such a long time that they may come to accept such treatment.

In these cases, the law may place the physician in direct conflict with a patient's wishes. Furthermore, the American College of Emergency Physicians has published a clinical policy that supports a competent elder's right to decide for him or herself to have a case reported [59]. This directive supports the autonomy of the patient and the maintenance of confidentiality in its opposition to mandatory reporting. This can place the emergency physician in a difficult dilemma. Hopefully, compassionate discussion with a patient, consensual involvement of concerned family or friends, discussion with the patients primary care physician, and consultation with a nonphysician provider such as a social worker in the emergency department will help convince a maltreated elder that it is best to be in compliance with any mandatory reporting statutes. One strategy to employ in a clinician's efforts is to divert a victim's trepidation away from the immediate concerns surrounding the filing of a report and to focus on the future benefits. One should explain to a victim that he or she most likely would come to willingly accept, and benefit from, assistance that would come in the future because of the reporting done today. This scenario was supported by a California study implemented the year after that state enacted a mandatory reporting statute [60].

Summary

Elder abuse and neglect is a prevalent, underrecognized problem among today's senior citizens. Fortunately, awareness is increasing, and services are being provided to elders on a more ready basis. Still, the emergency care provider must act as a patient advocate and assume responsibility for the detection, treatment, and safe disposition of unfortunate victims.

References

[1] Lachs MS, Williams MA, O'Brien S, et al. The mortality of elder mistreatment. JAMA 1998; 280:428–32.
[2] Quinn MJ, Tomita SK. Elder abuse and neglect. 2nd ed. New York: Springer Publishers; 1997. p. 9–10.
[3] Levine JM. Elder neglect and abuse. A primer for primary care physicians. Geriatrics 2003; 58:37–44.
[4] Shakespeare, W. King Lear. RA Foakes, editor. London: The Arden Shakespeare; 2004.
[5] Lachs MS, Pillemer K. Elder abuse. Lancet 2004;364:1263–72.
[6] Stearns PN. Old age conflict: the perspective of the past. In: Wolf R, Pillemer K, editors. Elder abuse: conflict in the family. Dover: Auburn House; 1986. p. 3–29.

[7] Burston GR. Granny-battering. BMJ 1975;3:592.

[8] Baker AA. Granny battering. Mod Geriatr 1975;5:20–4.

[9] Wolf RS. Elder abuse: ten years later. J Am Geriatr Soc 1988;36:758–62.

[10] Kurrle SE, Sadler PM, Cameron ID. Elder abuse: an Australian case series. Med J Aust 1991; 155:150–3.

[11] Kurrle S. Abuse of the elderly: a hidden problem. Aust Family Phys 1992;21:1742–8.

[12] Ogg J, Bennett G. Elder abuse in Britain. BMJ 1992;305:998–9.

[13] Homer AC, Gilleard C. Abuse of elderly people by their careers. BMJ 1990;301:1359–62.

[14] Comijs HC, Pot AM, Smit JH, et al. Elder abuse in the community: prevalence and consequences. J Am Geriatr Soc 1998;46:885–8.

[15] Pillemer K, Moore DW. Abuse of patients in nursing homes: findings from a survey of staff. Gerontologist 1989;29:314–20.

[16] Coyne AC, Reichman WE, Berbig LJ. The relationship between dementia and elder abuse. Am J Psychiatry 1993;150:643–6.

[17] Reis M, Nahmiash D. Validation of the Indicators of Abuse (IOA) screen. Gerontologist 1998;38:471–80.

[18] Pillemer K, Finkelhor D. The prevalence of elder abuse: a random sample survey. Gerontologist 1988;29:51–7.

[19] Aravanis SC, Adelman RD, Breckman R, et al. Diagnostic and treatment guidelines on elder abuse and neglect. Arch Fam Med 1993;2:371–81.

[20] Rosenblatt DE. Elder mistreatment. Crit Care Nurs Clin North Am 1997;9:183–92.

[21] US Bureau of the Census. Sixty-five plus in America. Curr Popul Rep (Special Studies) Series 1992;1023–178.

[22] Schneider EL, Guralnik JM. The aging of America: impact on health care costs. JAMA 1990; 263:2335–40.

[23] Greenbaum AR, Donne J, Wilson D, et al. Intentional burn injury: an evidence-based, clinical and forensic review. Burns 2004;30:628–42.

[24] Strange GR, Chen EH, Sanders AB. Use of emergency departments by elderly patients: projections from a multicenter data base. Ann Emerg Med 1992;21:819–24.

[25] Lowenstein SR, Crescenzi CA, Kern DC, et al. Care of the elderly in the emergency department. Ann Emerg Med 1986;15:529–35.

[26] Baum SA, Rubenstein LZ. Old people in the emergency room: age-related differences in emergency department use and care. J Am Geriatr Soc 1987;35:398–404.

[27] Gerson LW, Skvarch L. Emergency medical service utilization by the elderly. Ann Emerg Med 1982;11:610–2.

[28] Spaite DW, Cris EA, Valenzuela TD, et al. Geriatric injury: an analysis of prehospital demographics, mechanisms, and patterns. Ann Emerg Med 1990;19:1418–21.

[29] McNamara RM, Rousseau E, Sanders AB. Geriatric emergency medicine: a survey of practicing emergency physicians. Ann Emerg Med 1992;21:796–801.

[30] Geroff AJ, Olshaker JS. Elder abuse. In: Olshaker JS, Jackson MC, Smock WS, editors. Forensic emergency medicine. Philadelphia (PA): Lippincott Williams & Wilkins; 2001. p. 173–202.

[31] Tatara T. NARCEA's suggested state guidelines for gathering and reporting domestic elder abuse statistics for compiling national data. Washington (DC): NARCEA; 1990.

[32] Lachs MS, Berkman L, Fulmer T, et al. A prospective community-based pilot study of risk factors for the investigation of elder mistreatment. J Am Geriatr Soc 1994;42: 169–73.

[33] Hudson MF. Elder mistreatment: its relevance to older women. J Am Med Womens Assoc 1997;52:142–6.

[34] Fulmer TT, O'Malley TA. Inadequate care of the elderly: a health perspective on abuse and neglect. New York: Springer Publishers; 1987.

[35] Jones J, Dougherty J, Schelble D, et al. Emergency department protocol for the diagnosis and evaluation of geriatric abuse. Ann Emerg Med 1988;17:1006–15.

[36] Aravanis SC, Adelman RD, Breckman R, et al. Diagnostic and treatment guidelines on elder abuse. Chicago (IL): American Medical Association; 1992.

[37] US Department of Health and Human Services Administration on Aging and the Administration for Children and Families. The National Elder Abuse Incidence Study. Washington (DC): NCEA; 1998.

[38] Johnson T. Critical issues in the definition of elder mistreatment. In: Pillemer K, Wolf R, editors. Elder abuse: conflict in the family. Dover: Auburn House; 1986. p. 167–96.

[39] McCreadie C. Introduction: the issues, practice and policy. In: Eastman M, editor. Old age abuse: a new perspective. London: Chapman & Hall; 1994. p. 3–22.

[40] O'Malley TA, O'Malley HC, Everitt DE, et al. Categories of family mediated abuse and neglect of elderly persons. J Am Geriatr Soc 1984;32:362–9.

[41] Tatara T. Elder abuse in the United States: an issue paper. Washington (DC): NARCEA; 1990.

[42] Fulmer TT, Gould ES. Assessing neglect. In: Baumhover LA, Beall SC, editors. Abuse, neglect, and exploitation of older persons: strategies for assessment and intervention. Baltimore (MD): Health Professions Press; 1996. p. 89–103.

[43] Blazer DG. The epidemiology of psychiatric disorders in late life. In: Busse EU, Blazer DG, editors. Geriatric psychiatry. Washington (DC): American Psychiatric Press; 1989. p. 235–62.

[44] Sengstock MC, Steiner SC. Assessing nonphysical abuse. In: Baumhover LA, Beall SC, editors. Abuse, neglect, and exploitation of older persons: strategies for assessment and intervention. Baltimore (MD): Health Professions Press; 1996. p. 105–22.

[45] Davidson JL. Elder abuse. In: Block MR, Sinnott JD, editors. The battered elder syndrome: an exploratory study. College Park (MD): University of Maryland; 1979. p. 49–66.

[46] Kleinschmidt KC. Elder abuse: a review. Ann Emerg Med 1997;30:463–72.

[47] Lachs MS, Williams C, O'Brien S, et al. Risk factors for reported elder abuse and neglect: a nine-year observational cohort study. Gerontologist 1997;37:469–74.

[48] Paveza GJ, Cohen D, Eisdorfer C, et al. Severe family violence and Alzheimer's disease: prevalence and risk factors. Gerontologist 1992;32:493–7.

[49] German PS, Shapiro S, Skinner EA, et al. Detection and management of mental health problems of older patients by primary care providers. JAMA 1987;257:489–93.

[50] Jolley S, Jolley D. Psychiatry. In: Pathy MSJ, editor. Principles and practice of geriatric medicine. 3rd ed. London: John Wiley & Sons; 1998. p. 1031–53.

[51] Kosberg JI, Nahmiash D. Characteristics of victims and perpetrators and milieus of abuse and neglect. In: Baumhover LA, Beall SC, editors. Abuse, neglect, and exploitation of older persons: strategies for assessment and intervention. Baltimore (MD): Health Professions Press; 1996. p. 31–49.

[52] Lachs MS, Pillemer K. Abuse and neglect of elderly persons. N Engl J Med 1995;332:437–43.

[53] Steiner RP, Vansickle K, Lippmann SB. Domestic violence: do you know when and how to intervene? Domestic Violence 1996;100:103–16.

[54] Levy DB, Hanlon DP, Townsend RN. Geriatric trauma. Geriatr Emerg Care 1993;9:601–20.

[55] Jogerst GJ, Daly JM, Brinig MF, et al. Domestic elder abuse and the law. Am J Public Health 2003;93:2131–6.

[56] Bird PE, Harrington DT, Barillo DJ, et al. Elder abuse: a call to action. J Burn Care Rehabil 1998;19:522–7.

[57] Rosenblatt DE, Cho K, Durance PW. Reporting mistreatment of older adults: the role of physicians. J Am Geriatr Soc 1996;44:65–70.

[58] Clark-Daniels CL, Daniels RS, Baumhover LA. Abuse and neglect of the elderly: are emergency department personnel aware of mandatory reporting laws? Ann Emerg Med 1990;19:970–7.

[59] American College of Emergency Physicians. Policy statement: management of elder abuse and neglect. Ann Emerg Med 1998;31:149–50.

[60] Garfield AS. Elder abuse and the states' adult protective services response: time for a change in California. Hastings Law J 1991;42:809–932.

ELSEVIER
SAUNDERS

Emerg Med Clin N Am
24 (2006) 507–512

EMERGENCY
MEDICINE
CLINICS OF
NORTH AMERICA

Index

Note: Page numbers of article titles are in **boldface** type.

emed.theclinics.com

Changing Your Address?

Make sure your subscription changes too! When you notify us of your new address, you can help make our job easier by including an exact copy of your Clinics label number with your old address (see illustration below.) This number identifies you to our computer system and will speed the processing of your address change. Please be sure this label number accompanies your old address and your corrected address—you can send an old Clinics label with your number on it or just copy it exactly and send it to the address listed below.

We appreciate your help in our attempt to give you continuous coverage. Thank you.

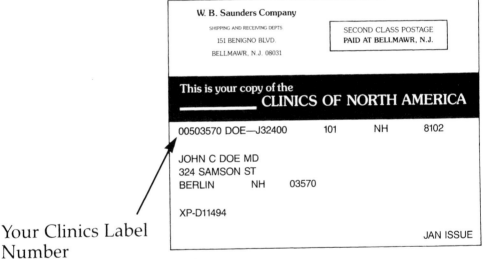

Your Clinics Label Number

Copy it exactly or send your label
along with your address to:
Elsevier Periodicals Customer Service
6277 Sea Harbor Drive
Orlando, FL 32887-4800
Call Toll Free 1-800-654-2452

Please allow four to six weeks for delivery of new subscriptions and for processing address changes.